D1682708

# Radiology Imaging Words and Phrases

*Diagnostic Imaging*
*Interventional Radiology*
*Therapeutic Radiology*
*Nuclear Medicine*
*Neuroradiology*
*Ultrasonography*
*Computed Tomography*
*Magnetic Resonance Imaging*

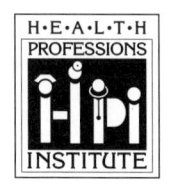

Health Professions Institute • Modesto, California • 1997

## Radiology Imaging Words and Phrases

*Diagnostic Imaging, Interventional Radiology, Therapeutic Radiology, Nuclear Medicine, Neuroradiology, Ultrasonography, Computed Tomography, Magnetic Resonance Imaging*

**©1997, Health Professions Institute**
**All rights reserved.**

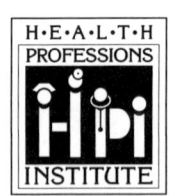

Sally Crenshaw Pitman
Editor & Publisher
Health Professions Institute
P. O. Box 801
Modesto, CA 95353-0801
Phone 209-551-2112
Fax 209-551-0404
E-mail: hpi@ainet.com
Web site: http://www.hpisum.com


*Printed by*
Parks Printing & Lithography
Modesto, California

ISBN 0-934385-68-8

Last digit is the print number: 9 8 7 6 5 4

*To*

*Bud Parks*

# Preface

*Radiology Imaging Words and Phrases* is more than an update of *Radiology Words and Phrases,* second edition, published in 1990. It has been greatly expanded to include over 50,000 entries from diagnostic imaging, interventional radiology, therapeutic radiology, nuclear medicine, neuroradiology, ultrasonography, computed tomography (CT), magnetic resonance imaging (MRI), and hundreds of imaging agents.

Terminology in the field of radiology imaging crosses all body systems and medical specialties, thus challenging us to cover all the bases with a minimum amount of redundancy. With so many new developments in medicine, surgery, and technology in the past six years, it was easy to find new terms and new products.

We tried to limit this quick-reference book to the basic words and phrases widely used in radiology reports, and to new terminology that might appear in imaging reports in the future. Technology advances in radiology have spawned monoclonal antibody-labeled isotopes, giving rise to the radiopathology laboratory. Advances in neuroradiology, microradiology, and holography have made possible the imaging of very small anatomical structures that heretofore could not be imaged using standard radiology techniques. Radiation therapy in combination with monoclonal antibody imaging has made the science of oncology more precise. Thus, the reader will note the addition of relevant pathology terms in this edition.

This book is by no means an exhaustive list of words and phrases in the radiology imaging specialties. We've culled words and phrases from hundreds of transcripts of radiology imaging dictation, references and textbooks, scholarly journals in all specialties, and have taken liberal advantage of the educational material available on the Internet.

Physicians and other healthcare professionals who dictate patient health records often refer to radiology imaging diagnostic and therapeutic studies. We hope that this book will be useful for medical transcriptionists in all specialties, not just those who work exclusively in radiology imaging departments.

Research and editing for this book were done primarily by Linda Campbell and Kathy Cameron, with proofreading assistance provided by Vera Pyle and John H. Dirckx, M.D. My warmest gratitude to all.

Sally Crenshaw Pitman<br>
Editor & Publisher

# How to Use This Book

The words and phrases in this book are alphabetized letter by letter of all words in the entry, ignoring punctuation marks and words or letters in parentheses. The possessive form ('s) is omitted from eponyms for ease in alphabetizing. Numbers are alphabetized as if written out, with the exception of subscripts and superscripts which are ignored.

Eponyms may be located alphabetically as well as under the nouns they modify. For example, *Cholebrin imaging agent* is found alphabetically under the C's as well as under the main entry *imaging agent*. *Technetium* is found in the T's as well as under *imaging agent*, which includes a list of nearly a thousand imaging agents. Under alternate terms such as *contrast medium, isotope, radioisotope,* and *radionuclide,* there is a *see imaging agent* reference.

Names of various radiology imaging studies have been combined under the broad category *imaging,* while names of various kinds of technology used in radiology imaging are listed under the broad term *system.*

Many anatomical terms are found in the book, but no attempt was made to be comprehensive. Rather, we refer readers to our recent *Laboratory/Pathology Words and Phrases* (1996), which includes tables of arteries, bones, muscles, nerves, and veins, with both English and Latin forms in tabular form for quick reference.

Main entries with a lengthy list of subentries include the following:

| | |
|---|---|
| artery | node |
| bone | scanner |
| catheter | shunt |
| deformity | sign |
| fracture | stenosis |
| imaging | system |
| imaging agent | technique |
| lesion | ultrasound |
| ligament | vein |
| muscle | view |

# A, a

AA (ascending aorta)
AAA (abdominal aortic aneurysm)
Abbott artery
ABC (aneurysmal bone cyst)
abdomen
    acute
    acute surgical
    boat-shaped
    distended
    nondistended
    postlymphangiography
    postsurgical
    scaphoid
    surgical
abdominal abscess
abdominal aneurysm
abdominal aorta
abdominal aorta thrombosis
abdominal aortic aneurysm (AAA)
abdominal aortic coarctation
abdominal aortography
abdominal carcinosis
abdominal circumference (AC)
abdominal contents
abdominal distention
abdominal iron deposition
abdominal mass
abdominal paracentesis, ultrasonic guidance for
abdominal pregnancy
abdominal situs inversus
abdominal vascular accident
abdominis rectus muscle
abdominopelvic mass
abducens (or abducent) nucleus
abducens nerve (sixth cranial nerve)
abduction fracture
abduction stress test
abductor muscle of little finger
abductor muscle of little toe
abductor digiti quinti (ADQ) muscle
abductor hallucis muscle
abductor pollicis brevis (APB) muscle
abductor pollicis longus (APL) muscle
abductovalgus, hallux
aberrant
aberrations, intersegmental
ABGd imaging agent
ABI (ankle/brachial index)
ablation
    percutaneous radiofrequency
    radiofrequency (RF)

**ablation • abscess**

ablation *(cont.)*
  saline-enhanced RF tissue
  stereotactic or stereotaxic
  surgical
  thermal
  total
  ultrasound-guided percutaneous interstitial laser
ablative laser therapy
abnormality
  accumulation
  acral
  arch of aorta
  augmentation
  bony
  bulbar
  cranial nerve
  cytoarchitectonic
  definitive
  fetal
  figure-of-eight
  focal
  frontal plane growth
  functional
  gestational sac
  gray matter
  obstructive
  perfusion
  restrictive
  screening-detected
  soft tissue
  torsional
  tracer
  ultrastructural
  white matter
  vasculature
  vessel wall
aboral direction
Abrikosov tumor
abrupt vessel closure
abruptio placentae (abruption of placenta)

abscess (pl. abscesses)
  abdominal
  actinomycotic brain
  acute
  amebic liver
  anaerobic lung
  appendiceal
  arthrifluent
  *Aspergillus* cerebral
  bone
  brain
  Brodie
  Brodie metaphyseal
  cerebral
  collar-button
  cuff
  daughter
  deep interloop
  deep pelvic
  encapsulated brain
  enteroperitoneal
  epidural
  extradural
  frontal
  gallbladder wall
  growth plate
  hepatic
  horseshoe (in the hand)
  interloop
  intermesenteric
  intersphincteric
  intra-abdominal
  intradural
  intrahepatic
  intramesenteric
  intraosseous
  intraperitoneal
  ischiorectal
  liver
  lung
  metaphyseal
  midpalmar

abscess *(cont.)*
  Paget
  pancreatic
  paracolic
  pararectal
  pararenal
  perianal
  periappendiceal
  pericecal
  pericolic
  pericolonic
  perinephric
  perirectal
  phoenix
  postoperative
  Pott
  psoas
  pyogenic liver
  rectal
  retroperitoneal
  retroperitoneal-iliopsoas
  serous
  spinal epidural (SEA)
  splenic
  subaponeurotic
  subdiaphragmatic
  subdural
  subgaleal
  subhepatic
  subperiosteal
  subphrenic
  subungual
  suture
  thecal
  thenar space
  tubo-ovarian
absence of uptake
absence seizure
absent aortic knob
absolute artery dimensions
absolute emission probability
absolute-peak efficiency calibration
absolute scotomata
absorbed dose per unit
absorbed dose range
absorber
absorptiometry
  double photon (DPA)
  dual x-ray
  single photon (SPA)
  single-energy x-ray (SXA)
  x-ray
absorption
  actinide
  bony
  impaired
  linear
  lysosomal (of cartilage in rheumatoid arthritis)
absorption cavity
absorption coefficient
absorption of radionuclide
abstraction
abut, abutted
abutment
abutting
AC (abdominal circumference)
AC (acromioclavicular) joint separation
AC (anterior commissure)
AC-PC (anterior commissure-posterior commissure)
  AC-PC line
  AC-PC plane
ACA (anterior cerebral artery)
ACA (anterior choroidal artery)
ACAD (atherosclerotic carotid artery disease)
acalculous cholecystitis
acanthopelvis
ACAT (automated computed axial tomography)
ACB (asymptomatic carotid bruit)
accelerated acute rejection
accelerated fractionation

accelerated hyperfractionated
  radiotherapy
accelerated peristalsis
acceleration time
accelerator
  alpha particle
  Bevatron
  dual-energy
  electron linear
  linear
  medical linear
  particle
  Philips linear
  Siemens Mevatron 74 linear
accelerator mass spectrometry (AMS)
accentuation of markings
access, vascular
accessory atlantoaxial ligament
accessory bones
accessory lobe
accessory organ
accident
  cardiovascular
  cerebrovascular (CVA)
  vascular
accidental correction
Accu-Flo CSF reservoir
Accu-Flo ventricular catheter
accumulation, abnormal tracer
accumulation of air in interlobar
  spaces
accumulation of gas
ACE fixed-wire balloon catheter
ACE inhibition scintigraphy
ace of spades sign on angiogram
acetabular bone
acetabular cup
acetabular depth to femoral head
  diameter (AD/FHD)
acetabular fossa
acetabular labrum
acetabular notch

acetabular osteolysis
acetabular roof
acetabuli, os
acetabulum (pl. acetabula)
  deep-shelled
  dysplastic
acetazolamide (Diamox) challenge test
acetazolamide-enhanced SPECT
acetylcholine receptor antibody
  (AChRab)
ACF (anterior cervical fusion)
ACG (apexcardiogram, apexcardiography)
ACh (acetylcholine) receptor
achalasia
  classic
  cricopharyngeal
  pelvirectal
  sphincteral
  ureteral
  vigorous
Achiever balloon dilatation catheter
Achilles bulge sign
Achilles bursa
Achilles+ ultrasound bone densitometer
Achilles tendon (tendo Achillis)
achillodynia
achlorhydria, gastric
achlorhydric
acholic stool
achondroplasia
achondroplastic dwarfism
AChR (acetylcholine receptor)
  antibody
AChRab (acetylcholine receptor
  antibody)
acid
  DTPA (diethylenetriamine
    pentaacetic)
  low-dose folinic
acidophilic pituitary tumor

Ackerman criteria for osteomyelitis
Ackrad balloon-bearing catheter
ACL (anterior cruciate ligament)
ACM (automated cardiac flow measurement) ultrasound technology
ACMI ulcer measuring device
ACoA (anterior communicating artery)
Acoma scanner
acoprosis
acoprous
acoustic backscatter characteristics of blood
acoustic impedance
acoustic interface
acoustic nerve
acoustic nerve tumor
acoustic neurinoma
acoustic neuroma
acoustic quantification, left ventricular ejection fraction
acoustical shadowing (in ultrasonography)
acoustic window
acquired disease
acquired toxoplasmosis
acquired tracheobronchomalacia
acquired unilateral hyperlucent lung
acquired ventricular septal defect (AVSD)
acquisition
   data
   ECT
   image
   multisection multirepetition
   multislice
   sequential image
   spirometric
   volume
acquisition technique
acquisition time
ACR teleradiology standard
acral abnormality

Acrel ganglion
acro-osteosclerosis
acropectorovertebral dysplasia
acrocephalosyndactyly
acromegaly
acromial angle
acromial bone
acromioclavicular (AC) joint
acromiocoracoid ligament
acromiohumeral interval (AHI)
acropachy
acrosyndactyly
ACS (Advanced Cardiovascular Systems)
ACS Endura coronary dilation catheter
ACS JL4 (Judkins left 4) French catheter
ACS Mini catheter
ACS Multilink coronary stent
ACS RX coronary dilatation catheter
ACS SULP II balloon
ACTH (adrenocorticotrophic hormone) antibody
ACTH independent hyperplasia
ACTH-producing pituitary adenoma
ACTH-producing pituitary tumor
actinomycosis, retroperitoneal
actinomycotic brain abscess
active biplanar MR imaging guidance
active emptying fraction (left atrium)
Acuson computed sonography
Acuson linear array transducer
Acuson 128EP imager
Acuson 128XP ultrasound system
Acuson transvaginal sonography
acutance, image edge profile
acute abdominal series
acute avulsion fracture
acute cholecystitis

acute coronary insufficiency
acute myocardial infarction (AMI)
acute phase gene expression
acute renal failure (ARF)
AD (Alzheimer disease)
AD (aortic diameter)
adactyly (adactylia)
adamantinoma
Adamkiewicz (also Adamkiewitz)
   Adamkiewicz artery
ADC (analog-to-digital) conversion
   quantization error
Addison point
adduct
adduction fracture
adduction to neutral
adductor canal
adductor hiatus
adductor magnus
adductor sweep of thumb
adductor tubercle
adductus
   metatarsus (MTA)
   true metatarsus (TMA)
adenocarcinoma
   annular
   colloid
   exophytic
   giant cell
   infiltrating
   metastatic
   papillary
   scirrhous
   ulcerating
adenohypophysial
adenohypophysis
adenoma
   acidophilic
   acinous
   ACTH-producing pituitary
   basophilic
   bile duct (BDA)

adenoma *(cont.)*
   bronchial
   chromophobic
   colonic
   cutaneous
   eosinophilic
   gallbladder
   glycoprotein-secreting
   gonadotropin-secreting
   hepatic
   hepatocellular (HCA)
   intraspinal
   liver cell
   moderately differentiated
   mucinous
   null cell
   papillary
   parotid pleomorphic
   pituitary
   poorly differentiated
   prolactin-secreting
   sebaceum
   sessile
   suprasellar
   toxic
   tubular
   tubulovillous
   undifferentiated
   villoglandular
   villous
   well-differentiated
adenomatoid malformation
adenomatosis
adenomatous hyperplasia
adenomatous polyposis coli
adenomyomatosis
adenomyosis
   diffuse
   uterine
adenopapillomatosis, gastric
adenopathy
Adenoscan contrast medium

adenosine echocardiography
adenovirus, enteric
AD/FHD (acetabular depth to femoral head diameter)
adherent thrombus
adhesed
adhesion
adhesive
ADI (atlanto-dens interval)
adiabatic demagnetization
adiabatic fast passage
adiabatic off-resonance spin-locking
adiabatic RF (radiofrequency) pulses
adiabatic slice-selective RF pulses
adiadochokinesia
adipose ligament
adipose tissue
adiposogenital dystrophy
aditus pelvis
adjacent voxels
adjuvant radiation therapy
adjuvant therapy
adnexa (*not* adnexae)
adnexal masses
adolescent hallux valgus
adolescent idiopathic scoliosis (AIS)
ADQ (abductor digiti quinti) muscle
ADR ultrasound
adrenal cortical adenoma
adrenal gland
adrenal hyperandrogenism
adrenal hyperplasia
adrenal imaging MIBG (meta-iodobenzylguanidine)
adrenal medulla
adrenal medullary hyperplasia
adrenal scintiscanning
adrenal tuberculosis
adrenogenital syndrome
ADR Ultramark 4 ultrasound
adult respiratory distress syndrome (ARDS)

advanced cortical disease
Advanced NMR Systems scanner
adventitia
adventitious bursa
adynamic ileus
AE (above-elbow) amputation
AE1, AE3 antibody
AEG (acute erosive gastritis)
AER (apical ectodermal ridge)
aerate, aerated
aeration
aerophagia
aerosol ventilation study
aerosolized Tc-DTPA evaluation
aerosolized Tc-PYP
AF (arcuate fasciculus)
A-FAIR (arrhythmia-insensitive flow-sensitive alternating inversion recovery) imaging
afferent digital nerve
afferent loop
afferent view
affix, affixed
AFP (alpha-fetoprotein) test
afterloader
  $^{192}$I high-dose-rate remote
  remote
afterloading, high-dose-rate
AG (angular gyrus)
aganglionic segment of colon
AGC (anatomically graduated component)
age
  bone
  chronologic
  gestational
  menstrual
AGE (acute gastroenteritis)
AGE (angle of greatest extension)
agenesis
  corpus callosum
  lung

agenesis *(cont.)*
  renal
  sacral
agenetic fracture
agent (see *imaging agent*)
AGF (angle of greatest flexion)
Agfa CR system
Agfa Medical scanner
Agfa PACS system
aglutition
agonist muscle groups
agyria
AHI (acromiohumeral interval)
AHO (acute hematogenous osteomyelitis)
AICA (anterior inferior cerebellar artery)
AICA (anterior inferior cerebral artery)
AICA ("i'-ka") (anterior inferior communicating artery)
Aicardi syndrome
AICS (artery of inferior cavernous sinus)
AIDS dementia complex (ADC)
AI 5200 diagnostic ultrasound system
air
  bowel loop
  colonic
  free
  intracranial
  intramural colonic
  intraorbital
  intraperitoneal
  pleural cavity
  subcutaneous
air-block syndrome
air bolus
air bronchogram
air cavity
air cisternography
air column, corrugated
air-conditioner lung
air contrast barium enema
air cyst
air cystogram
air density
air embolism
air enema
air enema fluoroscopic imaging
air exchange
air-filled lungs
air-fluid level
air gap
air hunger
air inflation
air insufflation
air interface on x-ray
air leak
airless lung
airlessness, alveolar
air luminogram
air myelogram
air plethysmography
air pocket
air sac
air space
  apical
  terminal
air-space consolidation
air-space disease
air-space opacity
air-tissue interface
air trapping, localized
airway fluoroscopy
airway narrowing
airway obstruction
airway opening
airway pressure
airways disease, reversible
airways tuberculosis
airway trees
AIS (adolescent idiopathic scoliosis)
Aitken classification of epiphyseal fracture

AJC (ankle joint complex)
Ajmalin liver injury
AK (above-knee) amputation (AKA)
Akerlund deformity
akinetic posterior wall
akinetic segmental wall motion
ala (pl. alae)
    nasal
    sacral
ala cerebelli
ala magna
Alagille syndrome
Alanson amputation
alar bone
alar ligament
Albers-Schönberg (Schoenberg) disease
Albers-Schönberg marble bones
Albright-McCune-Sternberg syndrome
Albunex ultrasound imaging agent
Alcock canal
alcohol embolization
alcoholic cirrhosis of liver
alcoholic liver disease (ALD)
ALD (alcoholic liver disease)
aldosteronoma
Alexander disease
algorithm
    annealing
    bioeffects
    clustering
    cone-beam reconstruction
    contour-following
    correlation (CR)
    decryption
    defuzzification
    DIP
    document-recognition
    dual lookup table
    dynamic range control (DRC)
    edge-enhanced error diffusion
    edge-enhancing
    encryption

algorithm *(cont.)*
    Feldkamp
    fringe thinning
    histogram equalization
    image restoration
    interpolation
    iterative
    JPEG (joint photographic experts group)
    K-means clustering
    least-squares (LS)
    lossy
    mapping
    maximum-likelihood
    memory-intensive
    mensuration
    MIP (maximum intensity projection)
    neural evaluation
    pixel-oriented
    quantizer-design
    Ramesh and Pramod
    reconstruction
    SSD (shaded-surface display)
    3D elastic subtraction
    wavelet scalar quantization (WSQ)
    word segmentation
    z-interpolation
alias artifact
aliasing (wrap-around ghosting) artifact
aliasing phenomenon in Doppler studies
aliasing, temporal
alien hand sign
alignment
    anatomic
    angular
    field
    fracture fragment
    integrity and
    rotational
    torsional

**alignment • amenorrhea**

alignment *(cont.)*
   transverse-plane
   vertebral body
alignment and registration of 3D
   images
alimentary canal
alimentary system
alimentary tract
alkaline reflux gastritis
ALL (anterior longitudinal ligament)
Allis sign
Allman classification of acromioclavicular injury
allocortex
allodynia
alloesthesia
allogenic marrow transplantation
allogenous bone graft
alloy
   cobalt-chromium
   stainless steel
   Ti-Nidium
   Ti6A14V
   Wood
All-Tronics scanner
Aloka color Doppler imaging
Aloka echocardiograph machine
Aloka linear scanner
Aloka sector scanner
Aloka SSD ultrasound system
AL-1 catheter
Alouette amputation
Alpers disease
alphafetoprotein level
alpha index
alpha motor neuron
alpha particle bombardment
alpha particle emitter
ALS (amyotrophic lateral sclerosis),
   carcinomatous
alta, patella
alteration in blood-brain barrier

alterations
   bilateral
   hemodynamic
alternator, film
altitudinal anopsia
altitudinal hemianopsia
alveolar bone fracture
alveolar clouding
alveolar consolidative process
alveolar edema
alveolar infiltrate
alveolar opacities
alveolar rhabdomyosarcoma
alveolar sarcoid
alveolus (pl. alveoli)
Alzate catheter
Alzheimer disease (AD)
Alzheimer neurofibrillary degeneration
Alzheimer-type, senile dementia
   (SDAT)
AMA-Fab scintigraphy
amaurosis
   central
   cerebral
   uremic
amaurosis fugax
ambient air
ambient cistern
ambifixation
ambilevosity
ambilevous
amblyaphia
ambulant
ambulatory equilibrium angiocardiography
AME (American Medical Electronics)
AME (Austin Medical Equipment)
amebiasis (see *amoebiasis*)
amebic abscess
ameboma
amelia
amenorrhea

amentia
American Shared-CuraCare scanner
americium (Am) radioactive source
ameroid occluder
AMI 121 contrast medium
AMI 227 contrast medium
amine
  basophilic
  macrolytic
aminopolycarboxylic acid imaging agent
Amipaque contrast medium
AML (amyotrophic lateral sclerosis)
Ammon horn (mesial temporal) sclerosis
amniocentesis, ultrasonic guidance for
amniography
amniotic fluid
amniotic sac
A-mode echocardiography
A-mode encephalography
A-mode ultrasound
amorphous collection of contrast
Amoss sign
amphetamine precursor
Amplatz catheter
amplifier, linear
amplitude image
amplitude limits
ampulla of Vater
ampulla, rectal
ampullary carcinoma
ampulloma
amputation
  above-elbow (AE)
  above-knee (AK, AKA)
  Alanson
  Alouette
  Beclard
  below-knee (BK, BKA)
  Berger interscapular
  Bier

amputation *(cont.)*
  Boyd ankle
  Bunge
  Burgess below-knee
  button toe
  Callander
  Carden
  chop
  Chopart
  Chopart hindfoot
  circular supracondylar
  closed flap
  complete
  congenital
  digital
  femoral head
  fingertip
  fish-mouth
  forearm
  forefoot digital
  forequarter
  Gritti-Stokes distal thigh
  guillotine
  Hey
  hindquarter
  incomplete
  index ray
  interinnominoabdominal
  interphalangeal
  interscapular
  interscapulothoracic
  Jaboulay
  Kirk distal thigh
  Le Fort
  Lisfranc
  midthigh
  nonreplantable
  one-stage
  Pirogoff
  ray
  replantable

amputation (cont.)
  supramalleolar open
  Syme
  Syme ankle disarticulation
  Teale
  toe
  transcarpal
  transcondylar
  translumbar
  transmetatarsal (TMA)
  traumatic
  two-stage
  Vladimiroff-Mikulicz
amputation neuroma
amputation stump
AMS (accelerator mass spectrometry)
AMT-25-enhanced MR images
amygdala of cerebellum
amygdalofugal pathway
amygdaloid area
amygdaloid nuclear complex
amyloid disease
amyloidoma
amyostatic syndrome
amyotonia congenita
amyotrophic lateral sclerosis (ALS)
anal atresia
anal bulging
anal column
anal crypt
anal dilatation
anal endosonography
anal fissure
anal protrusion
anal stricture
anal verge
analog (see *analogue*)
analog-to-digital (ADC) conversion
  quantization error
analog-to-digital converter
analogous

analogue (analog)
  adenosine
  dysprosium
  L-arginine
  tamoxifen
analysis
  activation
  biomechanical
  cephalometric
  Cerenkov scintillation
  clinicopathological
  diagnostic efficacy
  digital frequency
  discriminant
  duplex ultrasound
  eigenvector
  electro-oculographic
  fission track (of urine)
  flow cytometry DNA
  folding-potential
  footprint
  fractal
  gamma spectrometric
  kinetic parameter
  late effect
  liquid scintillation
  multi-elemental neuron activation
  neutron activation
  nuclide
  phase
  pole figure texture
  power spectral (PSA)
  prospective
  pulse height spectral
  range-gated Doppler spectral flow
  residual stress
  risk
  Sassouni
  signal
  sonographic feature
  stepwise regression
  teboroxime resting washout (TRW)

analysis *(cont.)*
   thin film
   total body neutron activation
     (TBNAA)
   volumetric
anaplastic astrocytoma
anaplastic glioma
anastomosis (pl. anastomoses)
   (anatomical or surgical)
   aorta-to-vein
   aortic
   aorticopulmonary or aorto-
     pulmonary
   arterio-arterial
   arteriolovenularis
   arteriovenous
   ascending aorta to pulmonary
     artery
   beveled
   bidirectional cavopulmonary
   Billroth II
   cavopulmonary
   cobra-head
   coiling of
   colocolic
   diamond
   diamond-shaped
   dilatation of
   distal
   embryonic
   end-to-end
   end-to-side portacaval
   extradural
   extrapericardial
   glomeriform arteriovenous
   heterocladic
   homocladic
   ileorectal
   intercavernous
   intercoronary
   internal mammary artery to
     coronary artery

anastomosis *(cont.)*
   intradural
   intrapericardial
   laser-assisted microvascular
     (LAMA)
   left pulmonary artery to
     descending aorta
   LIMA (left internal mammary
     artery)
   mesocaval
   microvascular
   outflow
   portacaval
   portosystemic
   precapillary
   proximal
   pyeloileocutaneous
   right atrium to pulmonary artery
   right internal mammary artery
   right pulmonary artery to
     ascending aorta
   right subclavian to pulmonary
     artery
   Roux-en-Y
   side-to-end
   side-to-side
   simple arteriovenous
   splenorenal
   superior vena cava to distal right
     pulmonary artery
   superior vena cava to pulmonary
     artery
   systemic to pulmonary artery
   tendon
   terminoterminal
   tracheal
   transureteroureteral
   ureteroileocutaneous
   ureteroureteral
   vascular
anastomotic defect
anastomotic disruption

anastomotic leakage
anastomotic pseudoaneurysm
anastomotic site
anastomotic stoma
anastomotic stricture
anatomic alignment
anatomic distribution
anatomic landmarks
anatomic moment erratum
anatomic neck
anatomic position
anatomic snuffbox
anatomic variability
anatomic variant
anatomical dead space
anatomical snuffbox
anatomically dominant
anatomy
   anomalous
   distorted
   left-dominant coronary
   medullary venous
   right-dominant coronary
   Saltzman
   sectional
   segmental
anconeal fossa (also anconal fossa)
anconeus
anconoid
ancyroid cavity (also ankyroid)
Anderson-Hutchins tibial fracture
android pelvis
anechoic area
anechoic center
anechoic fluid collection
anencephaly
anesthesia
anesthetic
aneurysm
   abdominal
   abdominal aortic (AAA)
   acquired

aneurysm *(cont.)*
   ampullary
   aortic
   aortic arch
   aortic sinus
   aortic sinusal
   aortoiliac
   arterial
   arteriosclerotic
   arteriovenous
   arteriovenous pulmonary
   ascending
   ascending aortic
   aspergillotic
   atherosclerotic
   atrial septal
   axillary
   bacterial
   basilar artery
   berry
   berry intracranial
   bland aortic
   brachiocephalic arterial
   brain
   bulge of
   bulging
   calcified wall of
   cardiac
   carotid artery
   cavernous carotid
   cavernous sinus
   cavity of
   cerebral
   circle of Willis
   circumscript
   cirsoid
   clinoid
   clip ligation of
   clipping of
   coating of
   coiling of
   compound

**aneurysm** *(cont.)*
   congenital
   congenital aortic sinus
   congenital arteriosclerotic
   congenital cerebral
   contained leak of aortic
   coronary artery
   coronary vessel
   cranial
   cylindroid
   de novo
   debulking of
   descending thoracic
   dilatation of
   dissecting
   dissecting abdominal
   dissecting aortic
   dissecting intracranial
   distal aortic arch
   dome of
   ductal
   ectatic
   embolic
   extracerebral
   extracranial
   false
   feeding artery of
   fundus of
   fusiform
   giant
   great cerebral vein of Galen
   hematoma of
   hemorrhage of
   hernial
   hunterian ligation of
   imperforate
   infected
   infrarenal abdominal aortic
   innominate
   internal carotid artery
   intracerebral
   intracranial

**aneurysm** *(cont.)*
   intramural coronary artery
   isthmus
   juxtarenal
   juxtarenal aortic
   late false
   lateral
   left ventricular
   luetic aortic
   M1 segment
   miliary
   mixed
   mural
   mycotic
   mycotic intracranial
   mycotic suprarenal
   neck of
   neoplastic
   nodular
   orbital
   pararenal aortic
   pelvic
   phthisis of
   PICA (posterior inferior cerebellar artery)
   popliteal
   posterior communicating artery
   postinfarction ventricular
   precursor sign to rupture of
   prerupture of
   pulmonary arteriovenous
   pulmonary artery compression ascending aorta
   pulmonary artery mycotic
   racemose
   rebleeding of
   renal
   renal artery
   rerupture of
   ruptured
   ruptured atherosclerotic
   ruptured intracranial

aneurysm (cont.)
   sacciform
   saccular
   sacculated
   sac of
   serpentine
   Shekelton
   sinus of Valsalva
   spindle-shaped
   spontaneous infantile ductal
   spurious
   subclavian
   suprarenal
   suprasellar
   syphilitic
   thoracic
   thoracic aorta
   thoracoabdominal
   thoracoabdominal aortic
   thrombosed
   thrombotic
   trapping of
   traumatic
   traumatic intracranial (TICA)
   true
   tubular
   unruptured
   uterine cirsoid
   Valsalva sinus
   varicose
   varix of
   vein of
   venous
   ventricular
   ventricular septal
   verminous
   wall of
   windsock
   worm
aneurysmal bone cyst (ABC)
angel wing sign

AngeLase combined mapping-laser probe
Angelchik ring prosthesis
Anger gamma camera
Anger-type scintillation camera
Anghelescu sign
angiocardiogram
angiocardiographically
angiocardiography (see *angiography*)
angiocatheter (see also *catheter*)
   Angiocath PRN flexible
   Deseret
   Eppendorf
   Mikro-tip
Angio-Conray contrast medium
angiodysplastic lesion
Angiografin contrast medium
angiogram
angiographically confirmed
angiographically occult intracranial vascular malformation (AOIVM)
angiographically occult vessel
angiographic catheter
angiographic finding
angiographic gap at site of injury
angiographic targeting
angiographic variceal embolization
angiography (also angiocardiogram)
   adrenal
   ambulatory equilibrium
   aortic root
   balloon occlusion pulmonary
   biplane
   biplane left ventricular
   biplane orthogonal
   black blood magnetic resonance
   blood-pool radionuclide
   blush of dye on
   Brown-Dodge method for
   cardiac
   cardiac gated MR
   carotid

**angiography**

angiography *(cont.)*
  celiac
  cerebral
  cine
  computed tomographic (CTA)
  computerized tomographic hepatic
    (CTHA)
  contrast
  coronary
  cystic duct
  diagnostic
  digital subtraction (DSA)
  digital subtraction cerebral
  digital subtraction pulmonary
  digital subtraction rotational
  directional color (DCA)
  dobutamine thallium
  DSA (digital subtraction)
  dynamic tagging MR
  ECG-synchronized digital subtraction
  elastic subtraction spiral CT
  electrocardiogram-synchronized
    digital subtraction
  Epistar subtraction
  equilibrium radionuclide
  first-pass nuclide rest and exercise
  first-pass radionuclide exercise
  fluorescein
  FluoroPlus
  four-vessel cerebral
  gated blood pool
  gated equilibrium radionuclide
  gated nuclear
  gated radionuclide
  IDIS (intraoperative digital
    subtraction)
  indocyanine green
  innominate
  intercostal artery
  internal carotid
  intra-arterial digital subtraction
    (IADSA)

angiography *(cont.)*
  intra-arterial DSA (digital
    subtraction)
  intravenous DSA (digital subtraction)
  intravenous fluorescein (IVFA)
  Judkins coronary
  left ventricular
  magnetic resonance (MRA)
  mesenteric
  nonselective
  nontriggered phase-contrast MR
  pancreatic
  phase-contrast
  postangioplasty
  postembolization
  postoperative
  post-tourniquet occlusion
  preoperative
  PTCA coronary
  pulmonary
  pulmonary artery wedge
  pulmonary vein wedge
  pulmonary wedge
  radionuclide (RNA)
  renal
  rest and exercise gated nuclear
  RI (resistive index)
  segmented k-space time-of-flight
    MR
  Seldinger
  selective
  selective coronary cine
  selective presaturation MR
  shaded-surface display (SSD) CT
  single plane
  SIR
  sitting-up view
  small angle-double incidence
    (SADIA)
  spinal
  STAR
  stereotactic cerebral

angiography *(cont.)*
  superselective
  three-compartment wrist
  three-dimensional (3D)
    3DFT magnetic resonance
    3D gadolinium-enhanced MR
    3D inflow MR
    3D phase contrast MR (3D-PCA)
    3D gadolinium-enhanced MR
    3D helical CT
    3D phase-contrast MR
  time-of-flight (TOF)
  transseptal
  transvenous digital subtraction
  tumor blush on
  ventricular
  vertebral
  visceral
  velocity encoding on brain MR
angiogram suite
angiography suite
angiolipoma, spinal
angioma
  arteriovenous
  cavernous
  cutaneous
  intracranial cavernous
  intradermal
  venous
Angiomat 6000 contrast delivery system
Angiomedics catheter
angiomyolipoma, multifocal
angioparalytic blockade
angioplastic meningioma
angioplasty
  balloon
  boot-strap two-vessel
  color duplex US-guided
    percutaneous transluminal
  coronary artery
  coronary balloon

angioplasty *(cont.)*
  Dotter-Judkins technique for
    percutaneous transluminal
  femoropopliteal
  Grüntzig balloon catheter
  iliac artery
  LAIS excimer laser for coronary
  laser
  laser balloon
  laser thermal
  laser thermal coronary
  laser-assisted balloon (LABA)
  microwave thermal balloon
  multilesion
  multivessel
  one-vessel
  patch
  patch-graft
  percutaneous laser
  percutaneous transluminal (PTA)
  percutaneous transluminal coronary
    (PTCA)
  peripheral
  peripheral laser (PLA)
  single-vessel
  supported
  synthetic patch
  transluminal
  transluminal balloon
  transluminal coronary
  transluminal coronary artery
  vein patch
angioplasty catheter, high-speed
  rotation dynamic
angioplasty laser, Lastec System
angioplasty sheath
angiopneumography
angioreticuloendothelioma of heart
angiosarcoma, cavernous
Angio-Seal hemostatic puncture
  closure device

angiotensin II (AT-II), AT1 receptor imaging
angiotomomyelography
AngioVista angiographic system
Angiovist contrast medium
angle
  acetabular
  acromial
  anorectal
  antegonial
  anteroposterior talocalcaneal (APTC)
  arch
  Bauman
  Beatson combined ankle
  bimalleolar
  blunting of costophrenic
  blunting of costovertebral
  Boehler (Böhler)
  Boehler calcaneal
  Boehler lumbosacral
  Bragg
  C
  calcaneal pitch
  calcaneoplantar
  cardiodiaphragmatic
  cardiohepatic
  cardiophrenic
  carrying
  CE (capital epiphysis)
  central collodiaphysial (CCD)
  cephalic
  cephalometric
  cerebellopontile (CPA)
  cerebellopontine (CPA)
  Citelli
  Clarke arch
  Cobb lumbar
  Cobb scoliosis
  Codman
  condylar
  costal
  costolumbar

angle *(cont.)*
  costophrenic (CP)
  costosternal
  costovertebral (CVA)
  craniofacial
  distal articular
  dorsoplantar talometatarsal
  dorsoplantar talonavicular
  Drennan metaphyseal-epiphyseal
  duodenojejunal
  Ebstein
  epigastric
  fan
  femorotibial (FTA)
  first-fifth intermetatarsal
  first metatarsal
  first-second intermetatarsal
  flip
  foot-progression (FPA)
  Garden
  Gissane
  gonial
  hallux dorsiflexion (DFA)
  hallux interphalangeus
  hallux valgus (HVA)
  hallux valgus interphalangeus
  hepatic-renal
  hepatorenal
  Hibbs metatarsocalcaneal
  Hilgenreiner
  IM (intermetatarsal)
  increased carrying
  infrasternal
  intermetatarsal (IMA)
  Kite
  Konstram
  lateral plantar metatarsal
  lateral talocalcaneal (LATC)
  lateral tarsometatarsal
  Laurin
  Louis
  Ludovici

angle *(cont.)*
  Ludwig
  lumbosacral joint
  mandibular
  Meary metatarsotalar
  mediolateral radiocarpal
  Merchant
  metaphyseal-epiphyseal
  metatarsocalcaneal
  metatarsotalar
  metatarsus adductus
  metatarsus primus
  Mikulicz
  navicular to first metatarsal
  neck shaft
  nutation
  obliterated costophrenic
  occipitocervical
  Pauwel
  pelvic femoral
  phase
  phrenopericardial
  Pirogoff
  plantar metatarsal
  pontine
  proximal articular set (PASA)
  Q
  QRST
  radiocarpal
  Ranke
  resting forefoot supination
  sacrohorizontal
  sacrovertebral
  scapular
  set
  slip
  spinographic
  splenic-renal
  splenorenal
  sternal
  sternoclavicular
  subtalar

angle *(cont.)*
  substernal
  sulcus
  talar-tilt
  talocalcaneal
  talocrural
  talometatarsal
  talonavicular
  tarsometatarsal
  TC
  thigh-foot (TFA)
  tibiofemoral (TFA)
  tibiotalar
  TMA-thigh (transmalleolar axis)
  transmetatarsal (TMA)
  urethrovesical
  valgus
  valgus carrying
  varus
  varus metatarsophalangeal (MTP)
  venous
  vertebrophrenic
  vesicourethral
  wedge isodose
  Wiberg
  Wiltze
  xiphoid
angled pleural tube
angled slice
angle from horizontal plane
angle from vertical plane
angle of anteversion
angle of declination of metatarsal
angle of greatest extension (AGE)
angle of greatest flexion (AGF)
angle of inclination of urethra
angle of incongruity
angstrom
angular frequency
angular gyrus (AG)
angular momentum
angular process of orbit

angularis body
angularis sulcus
angulated fracture
angulation
  anterior
  cephalic
  degrees of valgus
  degrees of varus
  forefoot
  posttraumatic
  spinal
angulus of stomach
anhaustral colonic gas pattern
anisotrophy, curvature
anisotropic diffusion
anisotropic effect
anisotropic 3-D or volume study
ankle
  disk of
  eversion of
  footballer's
  fractured
  fused
  fusion of
  instability of
  inversion injury of
  mortise of
  neuropathic
  sprained
  swelling of
  syndesmosis sprain of the
  synthetic graft bypass to
  tailor's
  transmalleolar
  twisted
ankle joint complex (AJC)
ankle mortise widening
ankle systolic pressure
ankylosing spondylitis
ankylosis (pl. ankyloses)
  bony
  extracapsular

ankylosis *(cont.)*
  false
  fibrous
  intracapsular
  joint
  ligamentous
  shoulder
  spurious
  vertebral
ankyroid cavity (also *ancyroid*)
anlage (pl. anlagen), cartilaginous
ANMR Insta-scan MR scanner
annealing algorithms
annotated imaging
annular abscess
annular array
annular calcification
annular cartilage
annular constriction
annular detector
annular dilatation
annular disruption
annular fibrosis
annular foreshortening
annular fracture
annular hypoplasia
annular ligament
annulus (also anulus) (pl. annuli)
  aortic valve
  atrioventricular
  calcified
  fissure of
  friable
  mitral
  pulmonary valve
  redundant scallop of posterior
  septal tricuspid
  tricuspid valve
  valve
  Vieussens
annulus fibrosus
annulus ovalis

annulus umbilicalis
anococcygeal raphe
anode tube reloading
anomalous insertion
anomalous origin
anomalous pathway
anomalous pulmonary venous
    connection
  partial
  total
anolomous pulmonary venous return
anomalous vein of scimitar syndrome
anomalous vessel
anomaly (pl. anomalies)
  aortic arch
  back-angle
  bell clapper (BCA)
  cardiac
  cloacal
  congenital
  congenital cardiac
  conotruncal congenital
  cranial
  Cruveilhier-Baumgarten
  cutaneous vascular
  Ebstein
  extracardiac
  Freund
  May-Hegglin
  migrational
  multiple congenital (MCA)
  radial ray
  Shone
  Taussig-Bing
  tricuspid valve
  Uhl
  vascular
  vertebral segmentation
  Zahn
anorectal ring
anoxic ischemia
ansa (pl. ansae)

anserinus, pes
antagonist muscle groups
antebrachial fascia
antebrachium
antecolic anastomosis
antecubital approach for cardiac
    catheterization
antecubital fossa
antecubital space
antecubital vein
anteflexion
antegonial angle
antegonial notch
antegrade (forward)
antegrade blood flow
antegrade fast pathway
antegrade filling of vessels
antegrade flow
antegrade imaging
antegrade perfusion
antegrade pyelography
antegrade refractory period
antegrade urography
anterior cardiac vein
anterior cerebellar artery syndrome
anterior colliculus
anterior column of spine
anterior commissure
anterior communicating artery
anterior compartment syndrome
anterior coronary plexus (of heart)
anterior corpus
anterior corticospinal tract
anterior cruciate ligament (ACL)
anterior cusp
anterior descending artery
anterior fascicular block
anterior feet view
anterior fibular ligament
anterior gray column of cord
anterior head region
anterior horns of spinal cord

anterior hypothalamus
anterior inferior cerebellar artery
    (AICA)
anterior inferior cerebral artery
    (AICA)
anterior inferior communicating artery
    (AICA)
anterior inferior iliac spine
anterior intercostal artery
anterior interhemispheric cistern
anterior interhemispheric fissure
anterior internodal pathway
anterior internodal tract of Bachman
anterior interventricular groove
anterior leaflet prolapse
anterior lobe
anterior maxillary spine
anterior mediastinum
anterior motion of posterior mitral
    valve leaflet
anterior papillary muscle
anterior planar image
anterior/posterior (AP)
anterior projection
anterior pulmonary plexus
anterior semilunar valve
anterior septal myocardial infarction
anterior spinal artery
anterior spinocerebellar tract
anterior spinothalamic tract
anterior superior iliac spine (ASIS)
anterior talar dome
anterior talofibular ligament
anterior tibial artery
anterior tibial compartment
anterior tibiofibular ligament
anterior tibiotalar ligament
anterior urethra
anterior wall dyskinesis
anterior wall myocardial infarction
anteroapical wall myocardial infarction
anterofundal placenta

anterograde peristalsis
anterolateral wall
anterolateral white matter of cord
anterolisthesis
anteromedial
anteroposterior (AP) (also anterior-
    posterior)
antetorsion, femoral
anteversion
    angle of
    femoral
    Magilligan technique for measuring
    neutral
anteversion determination, Budin-
    Chandler
anteverted
anthracosilicosis
anthrocotic tuberculosis
anthropoid pelvis
anthropometric imaging
anthropometry, 3D surface
anti-AChR (antiacetylcholine receptor)
    antibody
anti-aliasing techniques
antibody (pl. antibodies) (see also
    *imaging agent*)
    AChR (acetylcholine receptor)
    ACTH
    AE1
    AE3
    anti-ACh receptor
    anti-AChR (antiacetylcholine
        receptor)
    anticardiolipin (aCL)
    antiglioma monoclonal antibody
    antimyosin
    antimyosin monoclonal (with Fab)
    antinuclear (ANA)
    antiphospholipid
    antistriated muscle
    beta-endorphin
    CAM 5.2

**antibody** • **antral**

antibody (cont.)
  carcinoma-specific monoclonal
  cytokeratin
  EMA (epithelial membrane antigen)
  GFAP (glial fibrillary acidic protein)
  glutinin 1
  growth hormone
  heterophile
  IgM anti-human parvovirus
  ImmuRAID (CEA-Tc 99m)
  indium
  indium-labeled antimyosin
  kinase C
  kinase C antiglioma monoclonal
  lectin
  luteinizing hormone
  lym-1 monoclonal
  Mab-170 monoclonal
  MG (myasthenia gravis)
  monoclonal (MOAB, MoAb)
  neuron-specific enolase (NSE)
  neutralization
  NSE (neuron-specific enolase)
  OKT3 monoclonal
  polyclonal anticardiac myosin
  prealbumin
  precipitating
  prolactin hormone
  RCA (Ricinus communis
    agglutinin 1)
  Re-188 labeled
  7E3 monoclonal antiplatelet
  sheep antidigoxin Fab
  S-100 protein
  SS-A (Ro)
  SS-B (La)
  St. Louis encephalitis
  teichoic acid
  thyrotropin hormone
  UE (*Ulex europaeus*)
  vimentin
  VZ (varicella-zoster)
  whole blood monoclonal
antibody-antigen complex
antibody-conjugated paramagnetic
  liposomes (ACPLs)
antibody-labeled circulating
  granulocytes
antibody labeling
anticardiolipin (aCL) antibody
anticoincidence circuit
antifibrin (T2G1s) antibodies F(ab)2
antifibrin antibody imaging
antifibrin-MoAb imaging agent
antifibrin scintigraphy
antigen
  antiproliferating cell nuclear
  *Aspergillus*
  autogenous
  CA 15-3
  carcinoembryonic (CEA)
  epithelial membrane (EMA)
  histocompatibility
  HLA-B27
  human leukocyte, B27
  major histocompatability complex
    class II (MHC-2)
  prostate-specific (PSA)
  serum cryptococcal
anti-estrogen radiologic therapy
antigravity muscles
antimesenteric border of distal ileum
antimesenteric fat pad
antimesocolic side of the cecum
antimony
antimotility drug
antimyosin antibodies
antineoplastic therapy
antinuclear antibody (ANA) test
antiphospholipid anticardiolipin
  antibody
antistreptolysin O (ASO) titer
Antoni-A classification of neurinoma
Anton syndrome
antral edema

antral gastritis
antral stasis
antrum
  cardiac
  gastric
  Malacarne
  prepyloric
  pyloric
  retained
  Willus
anulus (see *annulus*)
anus
anvil bone
anvil sign
Ao, AO (aorta)
AO (aortic opening)
AO/AC (aortic valve opening/aortic valve closing) ratio
AO classification of ankle fracture
AO-Danis-Weber classification of ankle fracture
AOIVM (angiographically occult intracranial vascular malformation)
aorta (Ao, AO)
  abdominal
  aneurysmal widening of
  arch of
  ascending (AA)
  bifurcation of
  biventricular origin of
  biventricular transposed
  calcified
  central
  cervical
  coarctation of
  coarcted
  D-malposition of
  descending
  descending thoracic
  dextroposed
  dextropositioned
  double-barreled

aorta *(cont.)*
  draped
  dynamic
  ectasia of abdominal
  ectasia of thoracic
  elongated
  infrarenal
  infrarenal abdominal
  kinked
  L-malposition
  overriding
  pericardial
  porcelain
  preductal coarctation of
  recoarctation of the
  reconstruction of
  retroesophageal
  root of
  sclerosis of
  small feminine
  stenosis of
  supraceliac
  supradiaphragmatic
  terminal
  thoracic
  thoracoabdominal
  tortuous
  transposed
  unwinding of
  ventral
  wide tortuous
  widening of
aorta-iliac-femoral bypass
aorta-renal bypass
aorta-subclavian-carotid bypass
aorta-to-vein anastomosis
aortic allograft
aortic anastomosis
aortic aneurysm
aortic angiography
aortic annular region
aortic annulus

**aortic**

aortic arch
   congenital interruption of
   double
aortic arch angiography
aortic arch anomaly
aortic arch atresia
aortic arch calcification
aortic arch hypoplasia syndrome
aortic arch interruption
aortic atherosclerosis
   juxtarenal
   pararenal
aortic atresia
aortic bifurcation
aortic bulb
aortic calcification
aortic cannulation
aortic cartilage
aortic chemoreceptors
aortic closure (AC)
aortic coarctation, juxtaductal
aortic configuration of cardiac shadow
aortic cusp
   perforated
   ruptured
aortic cusp separation
aortic diameter (AD)
aortic dilatation
aortic dissection
aortic elongation
aortic flush pigtail catheter
aortic flush straight catheter
aortic hiatus
aortic impedance
aortic incisura
aortic incompetence
aortic insufficiency (AI)
aortic insult
aortic isthmus, hypoplasia of
aortic knob, blurring of
aortic knob contour
aortic knuckle

aortic leaflets, redundant
aortic-left ventricular pressure
   difference
aortic-left ventricular tunnel
aortic nipple sign
aortic notch
aorticopulmonary anastomosis
aorticopulmonary defect
aorticopulmonary fenestration
aorticopulmonary septal defect
aorticopulmonary shunt
aorticopulmonary trunk
aorticopulmonary window
aortic orifice
aortic override
aortic oxygen saturation
aortic paravalvular leak
aortic pressure
aortic pseudoaneurysm
aortic pullback
aortic-pulmonary shunt
aortic regurgitation (AR)
   congenital
   massive
   syphilitic
aortic resection
aortic root angiogram
aortic root dilatation
aortic root homograft
aortic root pressure
aortic root ratio
aortic run-off
aortic rupture
aortic segment
   intradiaphragmatic
   intramuscular
aortic septal defect
aortic shag
aortic sinus aneurysm
aortic sinus to right ventricle fistula
aortic spindle

aortic stenosis (AS)
  calcific
  congenital
  congenital subvalvular
  congenital valvular
  hypercalcemia-supravalvular
  subvalvular
  supravalvular (SAS, SVAS)
  uncomplicated supraclavicular
aortic stiffness
aortic stump blow-out
aortic subvalvular ring
aortic-superior mesenteric bypass
aortic thromboembolism
aortic tract complex hypoplasia
aortic transection, traumatic
aortic tube graft
aortic valve (AVA)
  bicommissural
  bicuspid
  calcified
  composite
  ectatic
  native
  nodules of
  opening of
  prolapse of
  stenosed
  thickened
  unicommissural
aortic valve annulus
aortic valve area
aortic valve atresia
aortic valve calcification
aortic valve endocarditis
aortic valve gradient
aortic valve incompetence
aortic valve insufficiency
aortic valve leaflet prolapse
aortic valve obstruction
aortic valve opening
aortic valve pressure gradient
aortic valve prosthesis
aortic valve regurgitation
aortic valve stenosis
  acquired
  congenital
aortic valve thickening
aortic valvular incompetence
aortic valvular insufficiency
aortic vasa vasorum
aortic vestibule of ventricle
aortic window
aortic window node
aortic wrap
aortobifemoral bypass graft
aortobiprofunda bypass graft
aortocarotid bypass
aortocaval fistula
aortoceliac bypass
aortocoronary valve
aortoduodenal fistula
aortoenteric fistula
aortoesophageal
aortofemoral arteriography with
  run-off views
aortofemoral bypass graft (AFBG)
aortofemoral runoff
aortogastric
aortogram
aortography
  abdominal
  antegrade
  arch
  balloon occlusive
  biplanar
  contrast
  counter-current
  digital subtraction
  digital subtraction supravalvular
  flush
  postangioplasty
  retrograde
  retrograde femoral

aortography *(cont.)*
   retrograde transaxillary
   retrograde transfemoral
   retrograde translumbar
   selective visceral
   supravalvular
   thoracic
   thoracic arch
   translumbar
   ultrasonic
aortogram with distal runoff
aortography (see *aortogram*)
aortoiliac aneurysm
aortoiliac bypass
aortoiliac disease
aortoiliac inflow assessment
aortoiliac obstructive disease (AIOD)
aortoiliac-popliteal bypass
aortoiliac thrombosis
aortoiliofemoral arteries
aortoiliofemoral bypass
aortomegaly, diffuse
aortoplasty
   balloon
   patch-graft
   posterior patch
   subclavian flap
aortoplasty with patch graft
aortopopliteal bypass
aortopulmonary anastomosis
aortopulmonary collaterals
aortopulmonary fistula
aortopulmonary shunt
aortopulmonary window
aortosclerosis
aortoseptal continuity
aortosigmoid fistula
aortovelography, transcutaneous (TAV)
aortoventriculoplasty
AoV (aortic valve)
AOVM (angiographically occult vascular malformation)

AP (anteroposterior or anterior-posterior)
AP film
AP projection
AP supine portable view
AP view
APB (abductor pollicis brevis) muscle
APC-3 collimator
APC-4 collimator
APCLs (antibody-conjugated paramagnetic liposomes)
ape hand (simian griffe)
ape hand of syringomyelia
ape-like hand
aperiodic complex
aperiodic functional MR imaging
aperiodic wave
aperistalsis
aperistaltic distal ureteral segment
Apert disease
aperture
apex (pl. apices)
   cardiac
   displaced left ventricular
   duodenal bulb
   external ring
   head of femur
   head of fibula
   head of patella
   heart
   horn of spinal cord
   Koch triangle
   left ventricular
   lung
   orbital
   petrous
   systolic retraction of
   uptilted cardiac
   ventricular cardiac
apex beat
apex cordis

apex of petrous portion of temporal
 bone
APEX 409 camera
APEX 415 camera
apexcardiogram, apexcardiography
 (ACG)
aphagia
aphalangia
aphtha (pl. aphthae)
apical air space on x-ray
apical and subcostal four-chambered
 view
apical cap
apical cap sign
apical capping
apical corn
apical duodenal ulcer
apical four-chamber view
apical granuloma
apical hypoperfusion on thallium scan
apical impulse
apical infiltrate
apical-lateral wall myocardial
 infarction
apical ligament
apical posterior artery
apical posterolateral region of left
 ventricle
apical scar
apical scarring
apical segment
apical short-axis slice
apical surface of heart
apical thinning
apical tissue
apical two-chamber view
apical view
apical wall
apical window
apices (pl. of apex)
apicoabdominal bypass
apicoposterior bronchi

apiculate waveform
aPL (antiphospholipid) antibody
APL (abductor pollicis longus) muscle
aplasia, cerebellar
aplasia of deep veins
APM (anterior papillary muscle)
Apogee CX 200 echo system
Apogee ultrasound device
A point
aponeurosis
 bicipital
 digital
 epicranial
 external oblique
 internal oblique
 palmar
 plantar
 tendon
aponeurotic band
aponeurotic triangle
aponeurotic troika
apophyseal fracture
apophyseal joint
apophysis of Rau
apophysitis
 calcaneal
 iliac
apoplexy
 Broadbent
 cerebellar
 delayed
 pineal
 pituitary
 postpartum pituitary
 posttraumatic (of Bollinger)
 pulmonary
 pulmonary artery
 pulmonary vein
apotentiality, cerebral
APP (average pixel projection)
appearance
 bat wing
 beading of activity

appearance *(cont.)*
  beaten-silver (of the skull)
  beavertail (of balloon profile)
  blade of grass
  cauliflower
  Christmas tree
  cobblestone
  cobra-head
  cobweb
  coiled spring
  collar-button (in colon)
  corkscrew
  cottage loaf
  distortions of image
  drooping lily
  feathery
  flame
  frog-like
  frondlike
  heterogeneous
  homogeneous
  Honda sign
  isodense
  lobulated saccular
  moth-eaten
  onion peel
  signet ring
  spiral
  string-of-beads
  super scan
  target
  trilaminar
  trilayer
  whorled
appendage
  atrial
  cecal
  epiploic
  left atrial (LAA)
  right atrial (RAA)
  truncated atrial
  vermicular

appendage *(cont.)*
  wide-based blunt-ended
  right-sided atrial
appendiceal abscess
appendiceal stump
appendices or appendixes (pl.)
appendicitis, acute
appendicolithiasis
appendicular skeleton
appendix (pl. appendixes, appendices)
  cecal
  ensiform
  epiploic
  filiform
  Morgagni
  paracecal
  preileal
  retrocecal
  retroileal
  subcecal
  vermiform
  xiphoid
appendolithiasis
apple core lesion
applicator, nucletron
application-specific integrated circuit (ASIC)
appose
apposing articular surfaces
apposition
  bone-to-bone
  close
  fracture in close
  apposition of leaflets
apron
  abdominal
  lead
  quadriceps
APS (air plasma spray) hydroxyapatite
APTC (anteroposterior talocalcaneal)
  angle
apudoma

AquaSens FMS 1000 fluid monitoring system
aqueduct
  cerebral
  forking of sylvian
  gliosis of
  mesencephalon
  midbrain
  Monro
  Sylvius
  ventricular
aqueduct compression
aqueduct occlusion
aqueduct stenosis
aqueous scintillator
AR (aortic regurgitation)
AR (atrial rate)
AR 2 diagnostic guiding catheter
arachnodactyly
arachnoid canal
arachnoid cyst
arachnoid granulation
arachnoid of uncus
arachnoid villi
Aran-Duchenne amyotrophy
Arani double loop guiding catheter
Arantius canal
arborescent
arborization of ducts
arborize
arcade
  collateral
  Frohse ligamentous
  mitral
  septal
  Struthers
  superficialis
Arcelin view
arch
  anterior atlas
  anterior metatarsal
  aortic

arch *(cont.)*
  articular
  atlas
  carpal
  cervical aortic
  coracoacromial
  deep
  distal aortic
  double aortic
  flat
  flattened longitudinal (of foot)
  Hapad metatarsal
  hemal
  high
  Hillock
  hypoplastic
  longitudinal (of foot)
  lung
  mid aortic
  mural
  neural vertebral
  palmar arterial
  plantar
  plantar arterial
  posterior metatarsal
  pubic
  right aortic
  right-sided
  Riolan
  subpubic
  superciliary
  superficial palmar arterial
  tarsal
  transverse (of foot)
  transverse aortic
  vertebral
  Zimmerman
  zygomatic
arch and carotid arteriography
Archer syndrome
archicortex
arch index

arching of mitral valve leaflet
architectural alterations of bone
architecture
  bony
  brain
  foot
  hepatic
  intranodal
  lung
  lobular
  network
Arco classification
arcuate artery
arcuate complex
arcuate eminence
arcuate fasciculus (AF)
arcuate fiber involvement
arcuate ligament
arcuate movement
arcuate nucleus
arcuate vessel
ARDS (adult respiratory distress syndrome)
area (see also *region*)
  anechoic
  aortic
  arrhythmogenic
  artery
  Bamberger
  body surface (BSA)
  Broca
  Brodmann
  callosal (parolfactory nerve)
  cardiac frontal
  cortical motor
  cross-sectional (CSA)
  denervated
  echo-free
  effective balloon dilated (EBDA)
  Erb
  Haeckerman

area *(cont.)*
  hilar
  hot
  hyperechoic
  hypoechoic
  ischemic
  language
  luminal cross-sectional
  midsternal
  mitral valve (MVA)
  olfactory
  parietal association
  parietotemporal
  perihilar
  peroneal
  premotor
  pulmonic
  rarefied
  sclerotic
  septal
  sonolucent
  stenosis
  subglottic
  suprapubic
  tricuspid
  valve
  watershed (of periventricular white matter)
  Wernicke
area-length method for ejection fraction
area of abnormal density
area of denudation
area of increased "radiolabeling"
areola
areolar plane
ARF (acute respiratory failure)
argentaffinoma
argon laser
Argyle Medicut R catheter
A ring, esophageal

arm
  abductor lever
  C-
  flail
  Leyla
  linebacker's
  outrigger
  Popeye
Arnold-Chiari (type II) malformation
array
  annular
  convex
  electrode
  high-density
  linear
  linear electrode
  NMRA quadrature detection
  phased
  symmetrical phased
  voxel
array processor (MRI equipment)
arrest
  anoxic
  asystolic cardiac
  bradyarrhythmic cardiac
  cardiac
  cardiopulmonary
  cardiorespiratory
  circulatory
  electrical circulatory
  epiphyseal
  flow
  heart
  hypothermic
  intermittent sinus
  profound hypothermic circulatory (PHCA)
  recurrent cardiac
  respiratory
  sinus
  transient sinus
  arrested circulation

arrest reaction
arrhenoblastoma
arrhythmia-insensitive flow-sensitive alternating IR
arrhythmogenic area
arrhythmogenic border zone
arrhythmogenic right ventricular dysplasia (ARVD) syndrome
arrhythmogenic ventricular activity (AVA)
Arrow-Berman balloon angioplasty catheter
ArrowFlex sheath
ArrowGard Blue Line catheter
ArrowGard central venous catheter
arrowhead-shaped
Arrow-Howes multilumen catheter
Arrow pulmonary artery catheter
arterial aneurysm
arterial avulsion
arterial blockage
arterial brachiocephalic trunk
arterial calcification
arterial cannula
arterial cannulation
arterial capillary
arterial circulation
arterial cutoff
arterial deficiency pattern
arterial degenerative disease
arterial dilatation and rupture
arterial dissection
arterial flow phase image
arterial graft
arterial hyperemia
arterial intima
arterial lumen
arterial malformation (AM)
arterial obstruction
arterial occlusion
arterial patency
arterial peak systolic pressure

arterial portography
arterial pressure
arterial pulsation artifact
arterial recoil
arterial return
arterial runoff
arterial rupture
arterial sclerosis
arterial segment
arterial sheath
arterial spasm
arterial steal
arterial supply
arterial thrombosis
arterial tonus
arterial topography
arterial tree
arterial varices
arterial wall dynamics
arterial wall thickness
arterialization of venous blood
arterio-arterial anastomosis
arteriocapillary sclerosis
arteriogram
arteriography
  aorta and runoff
  aortofemoral (with run-off views)
  arch and carotid
  balloon occlusion
  biplane pelvic
  biplane quantitative coronary
  brachial
  brachiocephalic
  bronchial
  carotid
  celiac
  cerebral
  cine-
  contrast
  coronary
  CT (computed tomography)
  delayed phase of

arteriography *(cont.)*
  femoral
  four-vessel
  hepatic
  infrahepatic
  intraoperative
  Judkins selective coronary
  left coronary cine-
  longitudinal
  lumbar
  mesenteric
  percutaneous
  percutaneous femoral
  peripheral
  pruned-tree
  pulmonary
  pulmonary artery
  quantitative coronary (QCA)
  renal
  retrograde
  runoff
  selective
  selective cerebral
  selective coronary
  Sones selective coronary
  subclavian
  superior mesenteric
  thrombotic pulmonary (TPA)
  vertebral
  visceral
  wedge
arteriolar sclerosis
arteriole
arterioplasty
arteriorenal
arteriosclerosis
  calcific
  cerebral
  coronary
  generalized
  hyaline
  hypertensive

arteriosclerosis *(cont.)*
   infantile
   intimal
   medial
   Mönckeberg (Moenckeberg)
   obliterative
   peripheral
   presenile
   pulmonary
   senile
arteriosclerosis obliterans (ASO)
arteriosclerotic cardiovascular disease (ASCVD)
arteriosclerotic deposits
arteriosclerotic heart disease (ASHD)
arteriosclerotic intracranial aneurysm
arteriosclerotic peripheral vascular disease
arteriosclerotic plaque
arteriosclerotic thoracoabdominal aortic aneurysm
arteriostenosis
arteriosus, ductus
arteriovenous (AV)
arteriovenous aneurysm
arteriovenous angioma
arteriovenous fistula (AVF)
arteriovenous interhemispheric angioma
arteriovenous malformation (AVM)
arteriovenous pressure gradient
arteriovenous varix
artery (pl. arteries)
   A1-A5 segments of anterior cerebral
   Abbott
   abdominal aorta
   aberrant
   aberrant coronary
   aberrant left pulmonary
   Adamkiewicz (Adamkiewitz)
   aneurysm of internal carotid
   aneurysm of posterior communicating

artery *(cont.)*
   angular MCA (middle cerebral artery)
   anomalous origin of
   anterior cerebral (ACA)
   anterior choroidal (ACA or AChA)
   anterior communicating (ACoA)
   anterior descending branch of left coronary
   anterior inferior cerebellar (AICA)
   anterior inferior cerebral (AICA)
   anterior inferior communicating (AICA)
   anterior spinal
   anterior spinal canal
   anterior temporal branch of posterior cerebral
   aortoiliofemoral
   apical posterior
   arcuate
   ascending frontoparietal (ASFP)
   atrioventricular node
   AV (atrioventricular) nodal
   axillary
   basal perforating
   basilar
   beading of
   bifurcation of anterior communicating
   bifurcation of common carotid
   bifurcation of internal carotid
   bifurcation of middle cerebral
   brachial
   brachiocephalic
   branch of
   calcarine
   calcified
   callosomarginal
   cannulated
   carotid
   celiac
   cerebral

**artery**

artery *(cont.)*
  choroidal branch of internal
    carotid
  choroidal pericallosal
  circumflex (circ, CF, CX)
  circumflex groove
  collateral circulation in
  common carotid (CCA)
  common femoral
  common iliac
  compression of
  C1-C5 segments of internal carotid
  conus
  corduroy
  coronary
  cortical branch of middle cerebral
  costocervical
  course of
  deltoid branch of posterior tibial
  descending septal
  diagonal branch of
  diagonal branch of left anterior
    descending coronary
  diagonal coronary
  dilated
  dissection of
  distal circumflex marginal
  dominant coronary
  dominant left coronary
  dominant right coronary
  dorsal spinal
  Drummond marginal
  dural
  dynamic entrapment of vertebral
  eccentric coronary
  en passage feeder
  epicardial coronary
  external carotid (ECA)
  external iliac
  extracranial vertebral
  extradural
  familial fibromuscular dysplasia of

artery *(cont.)*
  feeder
  femoropopliteal
  first diagonal branch
  first obtuse marginal
  friable
  frontopolar (FPA)
  gastroepiploic
  high left main diagonal
  hilar
  hypogastric
  iliac
  inferior epigastric
  inferior mesenteric
  infragenicular popliteal
  infrageniculate
  innominate
  intercostal
  intermediate coronary
  internal carotid (ICA)
  internal iliac
  internal iliac gluteal
  internal mammary (IMA)
  internal thoracic
  intraacinar pulmonary
  intracavernous internal carotid
  intracranial vertebral
  ipsilateral downstream
  Kugel
  labyrinthine
  LAD (left anterior descending)
  lateral posterior choroidal (LPCh)
  LCA (left coronary)
  LCF or LCX (left circumflex)
  left anterior descending
  left circumflex coronary
  left common femoral
  left coronary (LCA)
  left internal mammary (LIMA)
  left main coronary (LMCA)
  left pulmonary (LPA)
  lenticulostriate

**artery** *(cont.)*
- leptomeningeal
- LIMA (left internal mammary)
- LMCA (left main coronary)
- M1-M5 segments of middle cerebral
- main pulmonary (MPA)
- mainstem coronary
- maintenance of flow in
- mammary
- marginal branch of left circumflex coronary
- marginal branch of right coronary
- marginal circumflex
- medial plantar
- medial posterior choroidal (MPCh)
- median sacral
- meningeal
- meningohypophyseal trunk (MHT)
- mesencephalic
- mesenteric
- middle cerebral (MCA)
- middle meningeal
- musculophrenic
- narrowing of
- native coronary
- nodular induration of temporal
- nutrient
- obtuse marginal (OM) coronary
- occipital branch of external carotid
- occlusion of
- ophthalmic
- overriding great
- paramalleolar
- paramedian thalamopeduncular
- parietal MCA
- parieto-occipital branch of posterior cerebellar
- patency of
- PDA (posterior descending)
- peduncular segment of superior cerebellar

**artery** *(cont.)*
- perforating
- pericallosal
- peripancreatic
- peroneal
- petrous segment of carotid
- phrenic
- pipestem
- plantar metatarsal
- plaque-containing
- P1-P4 segments of posterior cerebral
- pontine
- popliteal
- post-temporal MCA
- posterior cerebral (PCA)
- posterior choroidal
- posterior communicating (PCA)
- posterior descending (PDA)
- posterior descending branch of right coronary
- posterior descending coronary
- posterior inferior cerebellar (PICA)
- posterior inferior communicating (PICA)
- posterior intercostal
- posterior parietal
- posterior spinal
- posterior temporal
- posterior tibial
- posterolateral spinal (PLSA)
- precommunicating segment of anterior cerebral
- primitive trigeminal (PTA)
- profunda femoris
- proximal anterior descending
- proximal digital
- proximal left anterior descending
- proximal popliteal
- pulmonary (PA)
- radial digital
- radicular

**artery • arthrosis**

artery *(cont.)*
   radiculomedullary
   radiculospinal
   ramus intermedius
   ramus medialis
   recurrent (of Heubner)
   renal
   reperfused
   resilient
   retinal
   retroesophageal right subclavian
   right coronary (RCA)
   right femoral
   right inferior epigastric
   right internal iliac
   right pulmonary (RPA)
   right ventricular branch of right coronary
   scalp branch of external carotid
   segmental branch of vertebral
   septal perforator
   SFA (superficial femoral)
   sinoatrial node
   sinus nodal
   splenial branch of posterior cerebral
   splenic
   stenotic coronary
   subclavian
   subcostal
   superficial femoral (SFA)
   superficial temporal (STA)
   superior cerebellar (SCA)
   superior epigastric
   superior genicular
   superior intercostal
   superior mesenteric
   superior thyroid
   supraclinoid carotid
   takeoff of
   temporal
   thalamocaudate

artery *(cont.)*
   thalamogeniculate
   thalamoperforating
   thyrocervical trunk of subclavian
   thyroid
   trifurcation of middle cerebral
   truncal
   twig of
   ulnar
   ulnar digital
   vertebral
   vertebral basilar
   weakened
artery-vein-nerve bundle
arthrempyesis
arthrifluent abscess
arthritic talonavicular changes
arthritis (pl. arthritides), rheumatoid (RA)
arthritis deformans
arthrogram
arthrography
   Brostrom-Gordon
   coronal computed tomographic (CCTA)
   CT (computed tomography)
   double-contrast
   Gordon-Brostrom single-contrast
   indirect MR
   joint
   MR
   saline-enhanced MR
   single-contrast
   temporomandibular joint
arthrophyte
arthropyosis
arthroscintigraphy
arthrosis
   crystal-induced
   degenerative
   IRM spiral
arthrosis deformans

arthrotomography of shoulder, double contrast
articular capsule
articular cartilage
articular cartilage degeneration
articular cartilage volume
articular cortex
articular disk
articular facet
articular fracture
articular fragment
articular gout
articular process
articular rheumatism
articular surfaces
  apposing
  contiguous
articulate
articulating bone ends
articulation
  acromioclavicular
  atlantoaxial
  body contour orbit
  calcaneocuboid
  carpometacarpal
  carporadial
  condylar
  costovertebral
  DIP (distal interphalangeal)
  disturbance of
  humeroradial
  humeroulnar
  intercarpal
  intermetacarpal
  interphalangeal
  metacarpophalangeal (MP)
  occipitocervical
  patellofemoral
  PIP (proximal interphalangeal)
  radiocarpal
  radiohumeral
  radioulnar

articulation *(cont.)*
  sacroiliac
  scapuloclavicular
  subtalar
  talocalcaneal
  talocalcaneonavicular
  talonavicular
  tarsometatarsal
  thorax
  tibiofibular
  zygapophyseal
artifact
  acoustic
  alias
  aliasing (wrap-around ghosting)
  arterial pulsation
  artifactual
  asymmetric
  attenuation
  barium
  baseline
  beam hardening
  black boundary
  "black comets"
  bounce point
  braces
  breast
  breathing
  broadband noise detection error
  bulk susceptibility
  calibration failure
  catheter
  catheter impact
  catheter tip motion
  catheter tip position
  catheter whip
  central point
  chemical shift
  chemical shift phenomena
  clothing
  coin
  construction

**artifact**

artifact *(cont.)*
  corduroy
  crescent
  crinkle
  cross-talk effect
  crown
  CSR fluid flow
  data-clipping detection error
  data spike detection error
  DC (direct current) offset
  developer
  distortion of limitations of image
    reconstruction algorithm
  dog
  double exposure
  double exposure drift
  eddy current
  edge-boundary
  edge misalignment
  edge ringing
  effusion
  end-pressure
  entry slice phenomenon
  equipment
  faulty RF (radiofrequency)
    shielding
  flow effect
  flow-induced
  foreign material
  gaseous oxygen
  geophagia
  ghosting
  Gibbs
  Gibbs phenomenon
  glass eye
  glove phenomenon
  half-moon
  hot spot
  image
  image post-processing errors
  imbalance of phase or gain
  intensifying screen

artifact *(cont.)*
  iron overload
  kink
  kissing-type
  lettering
  linear
  low-attenuation pulsation
  "magic angle" effects
  magnetic susceptibility
  main magnetic field inhomogeneity
  mercury
  mirror image
  mitral regurgitation
    (cineangiography)
  moiré
  moiré fringes
  mosaic
  motion
  movement
  muscle
  overlying attenuation
  pacemaker
  pacing
  paramagnetic
  partial volume effect
  patient motion
  pellet
  phase-encoded motion
  pica
  "pseudofracture"
  quadrature phase detector (QPD)
  radiofrequency (RF) spatial distri-
    bution problem reconstruction
  respiratory motion
  reticulation
  RF (radiofrequency) overflow
  screen craze
  skin crease
  skin fold
  skin lesion
  slice-overlap
  slice profile

artifact *(cont.)*
   stairstep
   stimulated echo
   subcutaneous injection of contrast
   summation shadow
   superimposition
   susceptibility
   swallowing
   swamp-static
   temporal instability
   tree
   truncation
   truncation band
   twinkling
   venetian blind
   voluming
   wheelchair
   wrap-around
   wrap-around ghost (aliasing)
   wrap-around ghosting
   wrinkle
   zebra
   zebra stripes
   zero-fill
   zipper
artifacts mimicking intimal flaps
artifactual
artificial cardiac valve
artificial left ventricular assist device (LVAD)
artificial neural network
artificial pneumothorax
Artoscan MRI system
Arvidsson dimension-length method for ventricular volume
aryepiglottic fold
arytenoid cartilage
arytenoid sparing
AS (aortic stenosis)
asbestos bodies
asbestos exposure
asbestos-induced pleural fibrosis
asbestos pleural plaques
asbestosis
A-scan ultrasound
ascending aorta (AA)
ascending aorta hypoplasia
ascending aortic aneurysm
ascending colon
ascending contrast phlebography
ascending hypoplasia of aorta
ascending phlebography
ascending tract
ascertain, ascertained
Aschoff-Tawara node
ascites
ascitic fluid
ASCVD (arterio- or atherosclerotic cardiovascular disease)
ASD (atrial septal defect)
aseptic myocarditis of newborn
aseptic necrosis
ASFP (ascending frontoparietal) artery
ASH (asymmetric septal hypertrophy)
ASHD (arteriosclerotic heart disease)
Asherson syndrome
Ashhurst fracture classification system
Ashhurst sign
ASIS (anterior superior iliac spine)
ASO (atherosclerosis obliterans)
aspect
   anterior
   anterolateral
   anteroposterior (AP)
   apical
   axial
   dorsal
   dorsilateral
   dorsoplantar
   inferior
   infrapatellar
   lateral
   lordotic
   medial

aspect *(cont.)*
   mediolateral
   posterior
   posterolateral
   proximal
   superior
   superolateral
   ventral
Aspect computer
aspergilloma
aspergillosis
aspergillotic aneurysm
aspergillus bronchiolitis
*Aspergillus* invasion of the nervous system
aspirated debris
aspirated foreign body
aspiration
   air
   blood
   CT-guided
   foreign body
   pulmonary
   tracheal
   transtracheal
   ultrasonic
   ultrasound-guided transthoracic needle
aspiration biopsy
aspiration pneumonia
aspiration pneumonitis
aspiration of ova, ultrasonic guidance for
aspiration-tulip device for in vitro percutaneous removal of rigid clots
Aspire continuous imaging (CI) system
asplenia
ASPVD (atherosclerotic pulmonary vascular disease)
assay
   predictive
   radioisotope clearance

assessment
   activity
   aortoiliac inflow
   invasive
   noninvasive
   quantitative Doppler
   real-time
   regional wall motion
associated sequestrum
association cortex of parietal lobes
asthmatic airways
asthmatic bronchitis
asthmatic crisis
astragalar bone
astragalocalcanean
astragalocrural
astragaloscaphoid bone
astragalotibial
astragalus (talus)
   aviator's
   fracture of
astroblastoma
astrocytic gliosis
astrocytic tumor
astrocytoma
astroglial tumor
asymmetric appearance time
asymmetry
   amplitude
   congestive
   facial
   hypertrophic
   interhemispheric
   limb length
   narrowing
   septal
   skull
   thoracic
asymptomatic
asynchronous transfer mode (ATM)
asynchronous ventricular contraction
asyndetic communication

asynergic myocardium
asynergy
  infarct-localized
  left ventricular
  regional
  segmental
asystole
  Beau
  cardiac
  complete atrial and ventricular
  ventricular
asystolic pauses
AT-II (angiotensin II)
atelectasis
  absorption
  acquired
  acute
  acute massive
  apical
  basilar
  bibasilar discoid
  chronic
  compression
  confluent areas of
  congenital
  congestive
  dependent
  disc-like
  discoid
  initial
  lobar
  lobular
  lower pulmonary lobe
  middle pulmonary lobe
  obstructive
  patchy
  peripheral parenchymal
  perpetuation of
  platelike
  platter-like
  primary
  reabsorption

atelectasis *(cont.)*
  relaxation
  resorption
  secondary
  segmental
  slowly developing
  streaks of
  subsegmental bibasilar
  subsegmental lower lobe
  upper pulmonary lobe
atelectatic lung
ATF (anterior talofibular ligament)
atherectomized vessel
atherectomy
  directional
  directional coronary
  percutaneous coronary rotational
    (PCRA)
  retrograde
  rotational
  rotational coronary
  transcutaneous extraction catheter
atherectomy catheter
atherectomy device
  directional
  extraction
  percutaneous
  PET balloon Simpson
  rotational
atherectomy technique
  double-wire
  kissing
athero-occlusive disease
AtheroCath, Simpson
atheroembolism
atherogenesis
atheroma (pl. atheromata)
  carotid bifurcation
  coral reef
  protruding
atheroma formation, exuberant
atheroma molding

**atheromatous • atresia**

atheromatous cholesterol crystal
   embolization
atheromatous debris
atheromatous degeneration
atheromatous embolism
atheromatous material
atheromatous plaque breakup by
   balloon catheter
atheromatous stenosis
atherosclerosis
   accelerated
   atherosclerotic
   carotid
   coronary
   extracranial carotid artery
   fatty streak
   fibrous plaque
   intimal
   intracranial carotid artery
   juxtarenal aortic
   native
   pararenal aortic
   virulent
atherosclerosis obliterans (ASO)
atherosclerotic aortic ulcer
atherosclerotic cardiovascular disease
   (ASCVD)
atherosclerotic carotid artery disease
   (ACAD)
atherosclerotic debris
atherosclerotic fatty streaks
atherosclerotic gangrene
atherosclerotic narrowing
atherosclerotic occlusive syndrome
atherosclerotic plaque
atherosclerotic stenosis
atherostenosis
atherothrombotic brain infarction
athlete's pseudonephritis
athletic heart
Atkin epiphyseal fracture

ATL (anterior tricuspid leaflet)
ATL Mark 600 real-time sector
   scanner
ATL Neurosector real-time scanner
ATL ultrasound system
atlantoaxial articulation
atlantoaxial fixation
atlantoaxial instability
atlantoaxial interval
atlantoaxial joint
atlantoaxial posterior membrane
atlantoaxial separation
atlantoaxial subluxation
atlantomastoid
atlanto-odontoid
atlanto-occipital fusion
atlanto-occipital junction
atlanto-occipital membrane
atlas (C1, first cervical vertebra)
   arch of
   burst fracture of
   compression fracture of
   transverse ligaments of
Atlas LP PTCA balloon dilatation
   catheter
atlas matching
Atlas ULP balloon dilatation catheter
ATM (asynchronous transfer mode)
atm. (atmospheres)
atonic bladder
atonic esophagus
atonic ureter
atony (atonia)
   gastric
   intestinal
   sphincter
atraumatic occlusion of vessels
atresia
   anal
   aortic
   aortic arch
   aortic valve

atresia *(cont.)*
  biliary
  choanal
  congenital biliary
  congenital laryngeal
  duodenal
  esophageal
  extrahepatic biliary (EBA)
  familial
  infundibular
  intestinal
  intrahepatic (IHA)
  laryngeal
  mitral
  mitral valve
  nasopharyneal
  prepyloric
  pulmonary
  pulmonary valve
  pulmonary vein
  pulmonic
  tricuspid
  valvular
  ventricular
atresic
atria (pl. of atrium)
atrial activation mapping, retrograde
atrial activation time
atrial appendage
atrial arrhythmia
atrial cuff
atrial disk
atrial ectopic automatic tachycardia
atrial ectopy
atrial-femoral bypass
atrial infarction
atrial kick
atrial myxoma
atrial pacing wire, temporary
atrial partition
atrial phasic volumetric function
atrial right-to-left shunting
atrial septal aneurysm
atrial septal defect (ASD)
atrial septal defect occlusion (buttoned device)
atrial septal defect with mitral stenosis
atrial septum
atrial single and double extrastimulation
atrial situs
atrial situs solitus
atrial standstill
atrial systole
atrial thrombosis
atrial transposition
atrialized ventricle
atriocaval junction
atriofascicular tract
atriography
  contrast left
  negative contrast left
atrio-His (atriohisian)
atrio-His bypass tract
atrio-His fiber
atrio-His pathway
atrioseptal defect
atrioventricular (AV)
atrioventricular annulus
atrioventricular canal
atrioventricular groove
atrioventricular nodal bypass tract
atrioventricular node mesothelioma
atrioventricular orifice
atrioventricular ostium
atrioventricular ring
atrioventricular septal defect
atrioventricular septum
atrioventricular sequential pacing
atrioventricular valves (mitral and tricuspid)
atrium (pl. atria)
  common
  giant left
  high right

atrium *(cont.)*
  left (LA)
  low septal right
  nontrabeculated
  oblique vein of left
  pulmonary
  respiratory
  right (RA)
  single
  thin-walled
  trabeculated
  ventricular
atrium cordis
atrium dextrum/sinistrum cordis
atrium pulmonale
atrium sinistrum
atrophic emphysema
atrophic fracture
atrophic gastritis
atrophic lesion
atrophic nonunion
atrophic thrombosis
atrophy
  alveolar
  brachial muscular
  brain
  cerebellar
  cerebral surface
  compensatory
  compression
  cortical
  degenerative
  denervation
  disuse
  divopontocerebellar
  dorsum sellae
  eccentric
  frontotemporal
  gastric
  hemisphere
  interstitial
  kidney

atrophy *(cont.)*
  lesser (of disuse)
  lobar
  lobular lung
  localized muscular
  multiple system (MSA)
  muscle
  neurogenic
  olivopontocerebellar
  parenchymatous
  peroneal muscular
  physiologic
  postneuritic
  primary optic
  progressive neuropathic muscle
  progressive post-polio muscle
    (PPPMA)
  quadriceps
  scapuloperoneal muscular
  spinal muscular (SMA)
  subacute denervation
  subcortical
  Sudeck osteoporotic
  sulcal
  temporal horn
  vascular
  villous
atropine flush
attachment
  capsular
  cerebellar
  commissural
  dural
  fibrous
  Hudson cerebellar
  intimate (of diseased vessel)
  ligamentous
  mesenteric
  Pearson
  peritoneal
  tendinous
  vascular

**attenuate • autosomal**

attenuate
attenuated image
attenuated lumen
attenuating
attenuation
  aortic
  breast
  decreased
  diaphragmatic
  expiratory
  gamma ray
  ground-glass
  hemidiaphragm
  increased
  linear
  photon
  Picker SPECT attenuation
    correction
  tendon
  theophylline
  valve
attenuation artifact
attenuation coefficient on MRI scan
attenuation correction
attenuation effect
attenuation threshold
attenuation scan
attenuation value on MRI scan
attic adhesion
attrition rupture of tendon
ATV (anterior terminal vein)
atypical angina
atypical aortic valve stenosis
atypical chest pain
atypical interstitial pneumonia
atypical subisthmic coarctation
atypical verrucous endocarditis
[198]Au (gold) brachytherapy
Auenbrugger sign
Auerbach mesenteric plexus
Auger electron emitter
augmentation, abnormal

augmented filling of right ventricle
augmented stroke volume
auricle
  left
  right
auricular fissure
Aurora MR (magnetic resonance)
  breast imaging system
Aussies-Isseis unstable scoliosis
autoecholalia
autofusion
autogenous antigen
autologous patch graft
autologous pericardium
autologous vein graft
automated airway tree segmentation
  method
automated angle encoder system
automated border detection by
  echocardiography
automated cardiac flow measurement
  (ACM) ultrasound technology
automated cerebral blood flow analyzer
automated computerized axial
  tomography (ACAT)
automated quantification
automated synthesis
automatic extraction
automatic lumen edge segmentation
automatic motion correction
autonomic denervation
autonomic dysfunction
autonomic hyperventilation
autonomic insufficiency
autonomic nervous system
autonomous nodule
autoprescanning
autoradiograph
autoradiographic localization
autoradiography, calcium-45
autoregulation of cerebral blood flow
autosomal recessive polycystic kidney
  disease

AutoSPECT
autostereoscopic
autotopagnosia
AV (arteriovenous)
AV (atrioventricular)
AVA (aortic valve area)
avascular necrosis (AVN)
avascularity
AVCO aortic balloon
AVD (aortic valvular disease)
AVDO$_2$ (cerebral arteriovenous oxygen content difference)
Avellis syndrome
average pixel projection (APP)
averaging
    partial volume
    spike
    volume
AVF (arteriovenous fistula)
AVG (aortic valve gradient)
aviator's astragalus
AVM (arteriovenous malformation)
AVM radiotherapy
AVN (avascular necrosis)
AV-Paceport thermodilution catheter
AVR (aortic valve replacement)
AVSD (acquired ventricular septal defect)
avulse
avulsed fracture fragment
avulsion
    arterial
    bony
    coracoid tip
    epiphysis
    iatrogenic
    ligament
    nail plate
    spinal nerve root
    traumatic
    venous
avulsion chip fracture
avulsion fracture
avulsion fragment
AVVM (angiographically visualized vascular malformation)
axial compression forces
axial compression fracture
axial compression injury
axial dimension
axial gradient echo image
axial hiatal hernia
axial images, multi-echo
axial manual traction test
axial musculature
axial neuritis
axial plane
axial scan
axial section
axial skeleton
axial slice
axial spin density
axial spinal system
axial transabdominal image
axilla (pl. axillae)
axillary-axillary bypass graft
axillary-brachial bypass graft
axillary-femoral bypass graft
axillary-femorofemoral bypass graft
axillary node
axillary tail of Spence
axillary vein traumatic thrombosis
axillobifemoral bypass graft
axillofemoral approach
axillofemoral bypass graft
Axiom DG balloon angioplasty catheter
axis (C2, second cervical vertebra)
axis (pl. axes)
    anatomic
    ankle mortise
    basibregmatic
    basicranial
    bimalleolar foot

axis *(cont.)*
  bowel
  celiac
  coordinate
  cortical hinge
  craniospinal
  distal reference (DRA)
  eccentric axis of ankle rotation
  enteroinsular
  femoral shaft
  flexion-extension
  hypothalamic-pituitary
  hypothalamic-pituitary-adrenal
  hypothalamoneurohypophyseal (HNA)
  leg
  long
  longitudinal
  mechanical
  metatarsal

axis *(cont.)*
  proximal reference (PRA)
  rotation
  single (on knee prosthesis)
  spinal
  subtalar
  transcondylar (TCA)
  vertical
  weightbearing
  Z-
axis of heart
axoid
axonopathic neurogenic thoracic outlet syndrome
axoplasmic flow and papilledema
Ayerza-Arrillaga disease
azotemic osteodystrophy
azygos blood flow
azygos lobe of lung
azygos vein distension

# B, b

baby formula with ferrous sulfate
   contrast
Baccelli sign of pleural effusion
Bachmann, anterior internodal tract of
bacillary angiomatosis
bacillary embolism
back, arching of
back-angle anomaly
back-bleeding
back crease
backfire fracture
backflow from arterial line
backflow of blood into atria
backflux
background subtraction technique
back manipulation
backrush of blood into left ventricle
backscatter characteristics of blood
backscatter electrons
backscattering
back stroke volume
backup of blood
backward flow
backward heart failure
bacterial meningitis
bacterial pneumonia or pneumonitis
Baffe anastomosis

baffle
   atrial
   construction of intra-atrial
   hemi-Mustard pericardial
   interatrial
   intra-atrial
   intracardiac
   Mustard
   pericardial
   Senning type of intra-atrial
baffled tunnel
baffle leak
bag (see also *pouch*)
   bile
   ostomy
   stomal
bagassosis
bagpipe sign
Baillinger, inner stripe of (in brain)
bailout catheter
Baim pacing catheter
baked brain phenomenon
baker's leg (genu valgum)
balance, mass
balanced ischemia
bald gastric fundus
Balint syndrome

Balkan fracture frame
Balke protocol for cardiac exercise stress testing
Balke-Ware treadmill exercise (stress testing) protocol
ball and seat valve
ball-and-socket joint
ball-bearing, Steinmann pin with
ball-occluder valve
ball of foot
ballism
ballismus
ballistic injury
ballistocardiography
balloon
    ACS SULP II
    AVCO aortic
    Ballobes gastric
    banana-shaped
    barium enema retention
    bifoil
    Blue Max
    esophageal
    Extractor three-lumen retrieval
    Fogarty
    Garren-Edwards
    gastric
    Gau gastric
    Grüntzig (Gruentzig)
    Hartzler angioplasty
    hydrostatic
    intra-aortic (IAB)
    intragastric
    kissing
    Kontron intra-aortic
    LPS
    Mansfield
    mercury-containing
    nondistensible
    Percival gastric
    Percor DL-II (dual-lumen) intra-aortic

balloon *(cont.)*
    Percor-Stat intra-aortic
    PET (positron emission tomography)
    pulsation
    rectal
    Riepe-Bard gastric
    Sci-Med Express Monorail
    scintigraphic
    self-positioning
    slave
    Soto USCI
    Spiegelberg epidural
    Stack autoperfusion balloon
    Taylor gastric
    trefoil
    Tru-Trac high-pressure PTA
    waist in the
    Vas-Cath PTA
    Wilson-Cook gastric
balloon and coil embolization
balloon angioplasty
balloon aortoplasty
balloon catheter fenestration
balloon counterpulsation
balloon decompression
ballooned floor of ventricle
balloon embolization (therapeutic)
balloon-expandable flexible coil stent
balloon-expandable intravascular stent
balloon-expandable metallic stent
balloon-flotation pacing catheter
balloon inflation
    sequential
    simultaneous
ballooning mitral valve prolapse syndrome
balloon occlusion
balloon occlusion arteriography
balloon occlusion pulmonary angiography
Balloon-on-a-Wire catheter

balloon pump
balloon sizing
balloon tamponade
balloon test occlusion
balloon-tipped catheter
ball-valve obstruction
ball valve thrombus
ball-valve tumor
ball-wedge catheter
Baló sclerosis
Bamberger-Marie disease
Bamberger sign
banana sign
band
  alpha
  alpha frequency
  amniotic
  anogenital
  anterior (of colon)
  AO tension
  aponeurotic
  atrioventricular
  Broca diagonal
  calf
  Clado
  constriction
  coronary
  external
  fascial
  fibroelastic
  fibromuscular
  fibrous
  free band of colon
  Gennari
  H
  Harris
  His
  Hunter-Schreger
  iliotibial (IT)
  intercaval
  internal
  Ladd

band *(cont.)*
  Lane
  lateral
  longitudinal
  lucent
  Maissiat
  Marlex
  Meckel
  mesocolic
  metaphyseal
  moderator
  omental
  parenchymal
  Parham
  Parham-Martin
  parietal
  peritoneal
  pretendinous band of hand
  Reil
  RF saturation
  scar
  septal
  septomarginal
  septum
  silicone elastomer
  Simonart
  tendinous
  transverse
banding appearance
bandlike adhesion
bandlike shadow
band of Broca
band of colon
  anterior
  free
band of density
band of Gennari
bands of deossification
band tenodesis
bandwidth limitations
Bannister angioedema disease
Banti disease

bar
    Bill
    bony
    cartilaginous
    congenital
    fibrous
    hyoid
    median
    Passavant
    unsegmented vertebral
bar defect
barber pole sign
barber's chair sign
Barclay niche
Bard CPS system
Bardeen disk
Bard guiding catheter
Bardic cutdown catheter
Bardinet ligament
Baricon contrast medium
barium
    double tracking of
    residual
    retained
barium artifact
barium column, head of
barium enema (BE)
    air contrast
    double contrast
    full-column
    therapeutic
barium enema retention balloon
barium enema through colostomy
barium enema with air contrast
barium esophagram
barium GI series, motor meal
barium-impregnated poppet
barium injection (through colostomy)
barium meal
barium sulfate contrast medium
barium suspension
barium swallow
Barkow ligament
bar-like ventral defect on
    myelography
Barlow hip instability test
Barlow sign
Baro-CAT contrast medium
Baroflave contrast medium
Barosperse contrast medium
barotrauma, pulmonary
Barré-Lieou syndrome
barrel chest
Barrett disease
Barrett esophagus
barrier
    blood-brain (BBB)
    blood-spinal cord
    blood-tumor
Barth hernia
Barton fracture
Bartter syndrome
basal, basally
basal chordae
basal cistern
basal ganglia calcifications
basal ganglia of cerebellum
basal joint of thumb
basal layer
basal movements
basal neck fracture
basal short-axis slice
basal skull fracture
basal tuberculosis
basal vein of Rosenthal
basal zone
base
    cranial
    dorsal spinal cord horn
    Dycal
    lung
    posterior spinal cord horn
    skull
baseball elbow

baseball finger
baseball shoulder
base deficit
baseline
   Reid
   reproducible
   return to
baseline artifact
baseline mammogram
baseline of bulb
baseline standing blood pressure
baseline standing pulse rate
baseline tenting (BLT)
base of brain
base of heart
base of lung
base of metacarpal
base of phalanx
base of skull (BOS)
base of thumb
base of toe
basibregmatic axis
basic blood pressure (BP)
basic cycle length (BCL)
basic drive cycle length (BDCL)
basic rate
basicranial axis
basilar artery insufficiency
basilar artery syndrome
basilar atelectasis
basilar cistern
basilar ectasia
basilar fracture
basilar infiltration
basilar insufficiency
basilar intracerebral hemorrhage
basilar invagination
basilar neck fracture
basilar occlusion
basilar pneumonitis
basilar pneumothorax
basilar region

basilar skull fracture
basilar sulcus
basilar suture
basilar syndrome
basilar-vertebral artery disease
basilar zone infiltration
basilic vein
basioccipital bone
basiocciput tumor
basion
basket, pericardial
basketlike calcification
basocervical fracture
batch-reading of x-rays
Batson plexus
Batson vertebral brain system
Batten disease
bat wing appearance
bat wing distribution
bat wing formation
bat wing shadow
Baudelocque diameter
Bauman angle
bauxite fibrosis of lung
bauxite pneumoconiosis
Baxter catheter
bayesian image estimation (BIE)
Bayes theorem in exercise stress
   testing
Bayliss effect
Bayne classification of radial agenesis
bayonet dislocation
bayonet leg
bayonet position of fracture
Bazin disease
BB (metallic foreign body) shot
BBB (blood-brain barrier)
BBC (biceps, brachialis, coraco-
   brachialis) muscles
B bile
BCA (bell clapper anomaly)
BDA (bile duct adenoma)

BDCL (basic drive cycle length)
BE (barium enema)
beach chair position
beaded appearance of fibromuscular dysplasia
beaded hepatic duct
beaded thickening
beading of artery
beads
   methyl methacrylate
   targeting
beaked cervicomedullary junction
beaking of head of talus
beaking, talonavicular
beaklike osteophyte formation
beak sign of a cortical cyst
beam
   blended
   cobalt-60
   fan
   intensity-modulated photon
   lateral opposed
   lucite
   multifield
   open
   pencil
   radiation
   sound
   wedge-pair
   wedged
beam diffraction
beam dosimetry
   adjacent field x-ray
   four-field x-ray
   large-field x-ray
   single x-ray
beam energy
beam's eye view dosimetry
beam filtration, supplemental
beam hardening artifact
beam intensity
beam linear accelerator, high-energy
   bent

BEAM (brain electrical activity map) (or mapping)
bear claw ulcer
bear's paw hand
beat knee syndrome
beaten silver appearance of skull
Beath view
beats per minute (BPM or bpm)
Beatson combined ankle angle
beat-to-beat variability
Beau disease
Beau line
Beauvais disease
beavertail appearance of balloon profile
Beckenbaugh technique
Beck triad
Beclard hernia
becquerel (Bq)
bed
   bladder
   capillary
   gallbladder
   hepatic
   liver
   monitor
   nail
   portal vascular
   primary tumor
   pulmonary
   pulmonary vascular
   skeletal
   stomach
   tumor
   ulcer
   vascular
beep-o-gram
Beer-Bouguer theory
Beevor sign
Behçet disease
Behr syndrome
Bekhterev arthritis

Bekhterev layer
bell clapper anomaly (BCA)
Bell-Dally cervical dislocation
Bell phenomenon
belly of muscle
bend, hand-shaped
bending fracture
Benedict-Talbot body surface area method
benediction posture (of hand)
benign asbestos related pleural disease
benignity
Benink tarsal index
Bennett basic hand dislocation
Bennett basic hand fracture
Bennett lesion
Bennett fracture
benzamide imaging agent
benzene scintillator
benzodiazepine (BN) receptor
benzodiazepine (GABA) receptor
Berman angiographic catheter
Bernard-Horner syndrome
Berndt-Hardy classification of transchondral fracture
Berndt-Hardy talar lesion staging
Bernstein catheter
berry aneurysm
Bertel position
Bertillon cephalometer
beStent balloon-expandable arterial stent
beta decay
beta particle
beta-ray applicators
beta-spectra shapefactor coefficient
Bethea sign
Bethesda bone
Beuren syndrome
Bevatron accelerator
beveled anastomosis
beveled edge sign

beveled electron beam cone
beveling
bezoar
Biad camera
Biad SPECT imaging system
Bianchi nodules
biatrial myxoma
BIB (biliointestinal bypass)
bibasally
bibasilar atelectasis
bibasilar discoid atelectasis
bibeveled
bicaval cannulation
biceps
    long head of (LHB)
    short head of
biceps femoris muscle
bicerebral infarction
Bichat canal
Bichat fat pad
Bichat membrane
bicipital aponeurosis
bicipital groove
bicipital rib
bicipital tuberosity
bicommissural aortic valve
biconcave
biconcavity
bicondylar fracture
biconvex
bicornuate uterus
bicoronal synostosis
bicortical screw
bicuspid aortic valve
bicuspid atrioventricular valve
bicuspid valvular aortic stenosis
bicycle exercise radionuclide ventriculography
bidirectional cavopulmonary anastomosis
BIE (bayesian image estimation)
Bielschowsky-Jansky disease

bifascicular heart block
bifid precordial impulse
bifida, spina
bifocal manipulation with distraction
bifoil balloon
bifurcate
bifurcation
  aortic
  basilar artery
  carotid
  common bile duct
  common carotid artery
  hepatic duct
  iliac
  middle cerebral artery
  patent
  pulmonary artery
  pulmonary trunk
  tracheal
  ureteral bud
bifurcation graft
bifurcation lesion
bigeminal rhythm
  atrial
  atrioventricular nodal
  bisferious pulse
  escape-capture
  nodal
  reciprocal
  ventricular
bihemispheral insult
bi-ischial diameter
bilateral carotid stenosis
bilateral consolidation
bilaterality of ureteral duplication
bilaterally
Bilbao-Dotter catheter
bile concretion
bile duct
  common (CBD)
  infundibulum of
  interlobular

bile duct *(cont.)*
  preampullary portion of
  sphincter of
bile duct proliferation
bile duct scan
bile flow
bile lake
bile plug
bile stasis
bilharziasis
  cardiopulmonary
  protopulmonary
biliary atresia
biliary duct
biliary-duodenal pressure gradient
biliary dyskinesia
biliary mud
biliary obstruction
biliary passages
biliary radicle
biliary saturation index
biliary sludge
biliary stent
biliary stone
biliary structures
biliary-to-bowel transit
biliary tract
biliary tract imaging
biliary tree
Biligrafin contrast medium
biliointestinal bypass (BIB)
biliopancreatic bypass (BPB)
bilirubin pigment stones (gallstones)
Biliscopin contrast medium
Bilivist contrast medium
Bill bar (bone)
billowing mitral valve prolapse
Billroth I type anastomosis
Billroth II type anastomosis
bilobed mass
bilobed polypoid lesion
bilocular stomach

biloma
Bilopaque contrast medium
Biloptin contrast medium
bimalleolar ankle fracture
binarize
binary image
binding, receptor
Bing-Horton syndrome
binning, projection
binocular acuity change
biocompatibility
biodegradable magnetic microclusters
biodegradable stent
bioeffects algorithms
biologic age
biological half-life
biological osteosynthesis
biological tissue valve
biomagnetometer, Magnes
biomechanical analysis
biomechanical imbalance
biomechanics of limb length
   discrepancy
biometry, longitudinal ultrasonic
biomodulator
bioprosthesis
biopsy (pl. biopsies)
   CT (computed tomography)-guided
   point-in-space stereotactic
   ultrasound-guided
Biosound AU (Advanced
   Ultrasonography) system
Biospec imaging system
biparietal bossing
biparietal diameter (BPD)
biparietotemporal hypometabolism
bipartite patella
bipartite sesamoid
bipartition, facial
bipenniform muscles of hand
biphasic contrast-enhanced helical CT
biphasic CT

biphasic curve
biplanar aortography
biplanar MR imaging guidance
biplane area-length method
   (echocardiography)
biplane fluoroscopy
biplane left ventricular angiogram
biplane orthogonal views
biplane pelvic arteriography
biplane pelvic oblique study
biplane sector probe
biplane transesophageal
   echocardiography (TEE)
bipolar gradient
bipolar hip replacement
bipolar sensing, integrated
bipolar temporary pacemaker catheter
bird-beak configuration or narrowing
bird-beak taper at esophagogastric
   junction
bird breeder's lung
birdcage coils
birdcage splint
bird fancier's lung
bird handler's lung
bird's-eye views
bird's nest filter (or bird nest filter)
birth fracture
Bis-Gd-mesoporphyrine (Bis-Gd-MP)
   imaging agent
bisection, AP malleolar
bishop's nod
Bismuth classification of benign bile
   duct stricture
bispinous diameter
bit-rate allocation
bituberous diameter
bivalve
biventricular assist device (BVAD)
biventricular global systolic
   dysfunction
biventricular hypertrophy

biventricular transposed aorta
biventricularly
BKA (below-knee amputation)
black blood magnetic resonance angiography (MRA)
black blood T2-weighted inversion-recovery MR imaging
black boundary artifact
black comets artifact
black dot heel
black echo writing
Blackfan-Diamond syndrome
black lung disease
bladder
  apex of
  atonic
  automatic
  base of
  centrally uninhibited
  dome of urinary
  exstrophy of
  hypertrophic
  hypotonic
  motor paralytic
  neck of
  neurogenic
  papilloma of
  refluxing spastic neurogenic
  sensory paralytic
  spastic
  thickened
  trigone of
  uninhibited
  urinary
  uvula of
bladder contractility study
bladder diverticula
bladder emptying
  complete
  incomplete
bladder floor
BladderManager ultrasound device
bladder neck contracture
bladder perforation
bladder stasis
blade of grass appearance
blade plate
blanch
bland aortic aneurysm
bland embolism
blast chest
bleb
  emphysematous
  myelin
  ruptured emphysematous
  subpleural
Bleck classification of metatarsus adductus
bleed (noun)
  GI
  herald
bleeding ulcer
blended beam technique
blennorrhagic swelling
blennothorax
blind catheter
blind dimple in floor of left atrium
blind intestine
blind loop syndrome
blind pouch
blind tibial outflow tracts
blister (vesicle)
blister, fracture
blister of bone
blistering distal dactylitis (BDD)
Bloch equation
block
  acquired symptomatic AV
  air
  alveolar-capillary
  anodal
  anterior fascicular
  anterograde
  arborization

**block**

block *(cont.)*
AV (atrioventricular)
AV Wenckebach heart
BBB (bundle branch)
BBBB (bilateral bundle branch)
bifascicular
bifascicular bundle branch
bifascicular heart
bilateral bundle branch (BBBB)
bone
bundle branch (BBB)
bundle branch heart
cerrobend
complete AV (CAVB)
complete congenital heart
complete heart (CHB)
conduction
congenital complete heart
congenital heart
congenital symptomatic AV
custom
deceleration-dependent
divisional
donor heart-lung
entrance
exit
false bundle-branch
familial heart
fascicular
filler
first-degree AV
first-degree heart
fixed third-degree AV
heart
high-grade AV
incomplete atrioventricular (IAVB)
incomplete heart
incomplete left bundle branch (ILBBB)
incomplete right bundle branch (IRBBB)
inflammatory heart

block *(cont.)*
infra-His
intermittent third-degree AV
interventricular
intra-atrial
intra-His
intra-Hisian or intrahisian
intranodal
intravenous (IV)
intraventricular conduction
intraventricular heart
inverted Y
ipsilateral bundle branch
irregular
left anterior fascicular (LAFB)
left anterior hemiblock
left bundle branch (LBBB)
left posterior fascicular (LPFB)
mantle
Mobitz I or II second-degree AV
multiple
paroxysmal AV
partial heart
peri-infarction (PIB)
posterior fascicular
pseudo-AV
retrograde
right bundle branch (RBBB)
second-degree AV
second-degree heart
simple
sinoatrial (SAB)
sinoatrial exit
sinus
sinus exit
sinus node exit
supra-Hisian or suprahisian
third-degree AV
third-degree heart
transient AV
transmission
trifascicular

block *(cont.)*
   unidirectional
   unifascicular
   VA (ventriculoatrial)
   ventricular
   vesicular
   Wenckebach AV
   Wilson
Block right coronary guiding catheter
blockage
   bronchus
   pulmonary artery
blocked APC (atrial premature contraction)
blocked artery
blocked bronchus
blocked pleurisy
blocked vertex field
blocker's exostosis
blocking, alpha
Blom-Singer tracheoesophageal fistula
blood
   arterial
   deoxygenated
   egress of
   epidural
   extravasated
   heparinized
   intraparenchymal
   intraventricular
   occult
   parenchymal
   peripheral
   shunted
   sludged
   subdural
   upstream
   venous
blood-brain barrier (BBB)
   alteration in
   defects in
   intact

blood-brain barrier osmotic disruption
blood clearance half-time
blood clot
blood-clotting mechanism
blood flow
   altered
   antegrade
   azygos
   capillary
   cerebral
   Doppler study of
   microcirculatory
   regional
   regional cerebral
   supratentorial cerebral
blood flow analyzer, automated
   cerebral
blood flow extraction fraction
blood flow in heart at rest
blood flow in heart during exercise
blood flow in microcirculation with high frequency Doppler ultrasound
blood flow on Doppler echocardiogram
blood flow reserve
blood flow response
blood flow study
blood flow to tissue beyond obstruction
blood flow velocity
blood inflow
blood leak
bloodless fluid
blood perfusion
blood perfusion monitor (BPM)
blood plate thrombus
blood pool
   vascular
   white-appearing
blood-pool activity
blood-pool imaging
blood-pool phase image

blood-pool radionuclide angiography
blood-pool radionuclide echocardiography
blood-pool radionuclide scan
blood pressure response
blood speckle
blood-spinal cord barrier
blood stream or bloodstream
blood substitute, oxygenated perfluorocarbon
blood supply
   accessory
   dual
   longitudinal
blood-tumor barrier
blood vessel thermography
blood vessel tumor
blood volume
   central
   circulating
   fractional moving
blood volume per minute (vol./min.)
blooming, signal
Blount disease
blow-in fracture
blow-out, aortic stump
blow-out fracture
blowing pneumothorax
BLT (baseline tenting)
Blue FlexTip catheter
Blue Max triple-lumen catheter
blue rubber-bleb nevus syndrome
Blumenbach clivus
Blumensaat line
Blumer rectal shelf
blunt border of lung
blunt chest trauma
blunted costophrenic angle
blunting of posterior sulci
blunt injury
blunt trauma
blurring of aortic knob

blurring of costophrenic angle
blurring of disk margins
blush
   tumor (on cerebral angiography)
   vascular (of tumor on carotid angiography)
BM (bowel movement)
BMC (bone mineral content)
BMD (bone mineral density)
BMI (body mass indices)
BMIPP SPECT scan
BML (billowing mitral leaflet)
B-mode (B-scan)
   longitudinal
   pseudocolor
B-mode echocardiography
B-mode echography
BMP (bone marrow pressure)
B-19036 chelate
BN receptor
BO field variation
board
   Dome Imaging RX20
   Intel PC Link2
Bochdalek, foramen of
Bochdalek hernia
body (pl. bodies)
   alignment of vertebral
   carotid
   coccygeal
   esophageal
   foreign
   foreign (retained)
   geniculate
   height of vertebral
   intra-articular
   juxtarestiform
   Luys
   mamillary
   navicular
   ossified
   osteochondritic loose

body *(cont.)*
    pacchionian
    pineal
    restiform
    retained foreign
    rhinencephalic mamillary
    rice joint
    scapular
    trapezoid
body background activity
body box plethysmography
body coil
body contour orbit, body artifacts due to
body mass indices (BMI)
body of vertebra
body section radiography
body surface area (BSA)
body surface potential mapping
Boeck sarcoid
Boehler (Böhler) angle
boggy synovitis
boggy synovium
Bogros space
Böhler (see *Boehler*)
Bohr effect
BOLD effect
BOLD image
Boltzmann distribution factor
bolus
    air
    contrast
    dynamic
    electron
    intravenous
    simple
    special
    tracer
    water
bolus challenge test
bolus contrast enhancement
bolus intravenous injection
bolus tracking
bolus transit
bombardment, alpha particle
bonds, wedge
bone
    accessory
    accessory navicular
    acetabular
    acromial
    alar
    Albers-Schönberg (Schoenberg) marble
    Albrecht
    alveolar
    alveolar supporting
    ankle
    anvil
    arch of
    areolae of
    articular lamella of
    articular tubercle of temporal
    astragalar
    astragalus
    astragalocalcanean
    astragalocrural
    astragaloscaphoid
    astragalotibial
    atrophy of
    autogenous
    basal
    basilar
    basioccipital
    basisphenoid
    Bertin
    Bethesda
    bicortical iliac
    blade
    bleeding
    Bonfiglio
    breast
    bregmatic
    Breschet

bone *(cont.)*
  brittle
  bundle
  calcaneal
  calcaneus
  Calcitite
  calvarial
  cancellated
  cancellous
  cannon
  capitate
  carpal
  cartilage
  cavalry
  central
  chalky
  cheek
  chevron (V-shaped)
  coccygeal
  coccyx
  coffin
  collar
  compact
  continuity of
  convoluted
  coronary
  cortical
  cortical cancellous
  costal
  coxal
  cranial
  crest of iliac
  cribriform
  cubital
  cuboid
  cuneiform
  dead
  dense
  dense structure of
  depression of nasal
  dermal
  destruction of

bone *(cont.)*
  devitalized portion of
  diastasis of cranial
  displaced fragment of
  dorsal talonavicular
  eburnated
  elbow
  endochondral
  enetral
  epactal
  epihyal
  epihyoid
  epiphysis
  epipteric
  episternal
  erosion of epiphyseal
  ethmoid
  exercise
  exoccipital
  femoral
  fibular
  first cuneiform
  flank (ilium)
  flat
  Flower
  fourth turbinated
  fracture running length of
  fragile
  fragment of
  frontal
  Goethe
  greater multangular (trapezium)
  hamate
  haunch
  heel
  heterotopic
  highest turbinated
  hip
  hollow
  hooked
  humeral
  hyoid

**bone**

bone *(cont.)*
   hyperplastic
   iliac
   iliac cancellous
   immature
   incarial
   incisive
   incomplete fracture of
   incus
   infected
   inferior turbinated
   inflammation of
   innominate
   intermaxillary
   intermediate cuneiform
   interparietal
   intracartilaginous
   intrachondral
   intramembranous
   irregular
   ischial
   ivory
   ivorylike
   jaw
   knuckle
   lacrimal
   lamellar
   lenticular (of hand)
   lentiform
   lesser multangular (trapezoid)
   lingual
   long
   long axis of
   lunate
   lunocapitate
   luxated
   malar
   malleolar
   malleolus
   marble
   mastoid

bone *(cont.)*
   mature
   maxillary
   maxilloturbinal
   medial cuneiform
   medullary
   membrane of
   metacarpal
   metatarsal
   metastasis to
   metatarsal
   middle cuneiform
   middle turbinate
   morcellized
   mortise of
   multangular
   nasal
   navicular
   necrotic
   neoplasm of
   newly woven
   Nicoll
   occipital
   odontoid
   orbicular
   orbitosphenoidal
   os calcis
   os trapezium
   os trapezoideum
   ossifying fibroma of long
   osteonal
   osteopenic
   osteoporosis of
   osteoporotic
   pagetoid
   palatine
   parietal
   pedal
   pelvic
   perichondral
   perilesional
   periosteal

bone *(cont.)*
  periotic
  peroneal
  petrosal
  petrous
  petrous temporal
  phalangeal
  Pirie
  pisiform
  pneumatic
  porous
  postsphenoid
  post-traumatic atrophy of
  preinterparietal
  premaxillary
  presphenoid
  primitive
  proliferation of
  prominence of
  pterygoid
  pubic
  pyramidal
  quadrilateral
  radial
  refractured
  replacement
  resurrection
  reticulated
  rider's
  Riolan
  rudimentary
  sacral
  scaphoid
  scapular
  sclerotic
  scroll
  second cuneiform
  semilunar
  septal
  sesamoid
  shank
  shin

bone *(cont.)*
  short
  sieve
  sphenoid
  sphenoidal turbinated
  sphenoturbinal
  splintered
  split thickness cranial
  spoke
  spongy
  squamo-occipital
  squamous
  squamous-type
  stirrup
  subchondral
  superior turbinated
  subperiosteal new
  substitution
  supernumerary
  supernumerary sesamoid
  supracollicular spike of cortical
  suprainterparietal
  supraoccipital
  suprapharyngeal
  suprasternal
  supreme turbinate
  sutural
  tail
  talus
  tarsal
  temporal
  thick
  thigh
  thoracic
  three-cornered
  tibia
  trabecular
  trapezium (greater multangular)
  trapezoid (lesser multangular)
  trapezoid of Henle
  trapezoid of Lyser
  triangular

bone *(cont.)*
   triangular wrist
   triquetral
   triquetrum
   tubular
   tuberculosis of
   tumor-bearing
   turbinate
   turbinated
   tympanic
   tympanohyal
   ulnar
   ulnar sesamoid
   unciform
   upper jaw
   vascular
   vesalian
   Vesalius
   vomer
   weightbearing
   wing of sphenoid
   wormian
   woven
   wrist triquetrum
   xiphoid
   yoke
   zygomatic
bone absorption
bone age according to Greulich
   and Pyle
bone age ratio
bone allograft
bone atrophy
bone block
bone cement, Surgical Simplex P
   radiopaque
bone chip
bone core
bone debris
bone demineralization
Bone Densitometer, QDR-1500 or
   QDR-2000
bone density, increased
bone density measurement
bone density study
bone deposits, endochondral
bone destruction, localized
bone destructive process
bone dysplasia
bone ends
bone erosion
bone formation
   new
   sparsity of
   subperiosteal new
bone-forming sarcoma
bone-forming tumor
bone fracture
bone fragment
bone graft
bone growth stimulator
bone imaging
bone implant
bone infarct
bone infection
bone island
bone length study
bonelet
bone marrow embolism
bone marrow scintigraphy
bone mass, loss of
bone maturation
bone metastases, occult
bone "mets" (slang for metastases)
bone mineral content (BMC) study
bone mineral density (BMD)
bone mineralization
bone or joint pathology
bone phase image
bone pinhole
bone plate
bone plug
bone powder
bone remodeling

bone resorption
bone scan (see also *imaging*)
   isotope
   triple phase
   TSPP rectilinear
bone scintigraphy
bone screw
bone sequestrum
bone shaft
bone sliver
bone spicule
bone spur
bone substance
bone survey
bone-tendon exposure
bone window
bony (see also *bone*)
bony abnormality
bony ankylosis
bony apposition
bony architecture
bony avulsion
bony bridging
bony callus formation
bony change
bony decompression
bony defect (acoustic window)
bony deformity
bony deposit
bony destruction
bony disruption
bony eburnation
bony encroachment
bony enlargement
bony erosion
bony excrescence
bony exostosis
bony fracture
bony fragment
bony fusion
bony healing
bony island

bony landmark
bony lysis
bony necrosis and destruction
bony osteophyte
bony overgrowth
bony pelvis
bony proliferation
bony prominence (spur)
bony protuberance
bony rarefaction
bony reabsorption
bony resorption
bony ridge
bony sclerosis
bony skeleton
bony spicule
bony spur
bony spurring
bony stability
bony structures, demineralized
bony thorax
bony tufts of fingers
bony union, solid
"boomerang" ovoid-shaped tendon
Boorman classification of gastric
   cancer
boost
   brachytherapy
   electron beam
   interstitial
boot-shaped heart
boot-top fracture
borborygmus (pl. borborygmi)
border
   alveolar
   anterior
   antimesenteric
   cardiac
   ciliated
   corticated
   crescentic
   heart

border *(cont.)*
   inferior
   interosseous
   lateral
   lower sternal (LSB)
   medial
   mid-left sternal
   posterior
   sternocleidomastoid muscle
   superior
   upper sternal
borderline
border of heart
   anterior
   inferior
   left
   posterior
   right
   superior
border zone
Borg scale of treadmill exertion
Born approximation
Bornholm disease
boron neutron capture
BOS (base of skull)
Bosniak classification
boss
bosselated
bosselation
bossing
   biparietal
   frontal
   occipital
Boston LINAC (linear accelerator)
Bosworth fracture
Botallo duct
Botallo foramen
Botallo ligament
both-bone forearm fracture
bottle sign
bottoming out of prosthetic component
Bouchard disease

Bouchard node
bouche de tapir (tapir's mouth)) in muscular dystrophy
Bouillaud disease
bounce point artifact
bouncing, ligamentous
boundary
   bone marrow
   tumor
Bourneville disease
Bourneville-Pringle disease
boutonnière deformity of finger
Bouveret disease
Bouveret-Hoffmann syndrome
Bowditch effect
Bowditch staircase phenomenon
bowed legs
bowel
   aganglionic
   apple-peel
   dead
   dilated loops of
   distal small
   fluid-filled loop of
   infarcted
   intussuscepted
   irritable
   ischemic
   kinked
   kink in
   large
   multiple loops of small
   proximal small
   small
   strangulated
bowel and bladder dysfunction
bowel contents
bowel continuity
bowel fills and evacuates satisfactorily
bowel follow-through, small (SBFT)
bowel gas
   displacement of
   superimposed

bowel gas displaced by extraperitoneal
   blood and urine
bowel gas pattern
bowel loop
bowel lumen
bowel motion
bowel movement (BM)
bowel obstruction
bowel pattern
bowel peristalsis
bowel prep (preparation)
   Colonlite
   CoLyte
   Dulcolax
   Emulsoil
   Evac-Q-Kit
   Evac-Q-Kwik
   Fleet
   GoLytely
   inadequate
   OCL
   Tridrate
   X-Prep
bowel preparation before barium
   enema
bowel preparation before colonoscopy
bowel rest
bowel series, small
bowel shadows, superimposition of
bowel syndrome
   irritable
   spastic
bowel wall
Bowen disease
bowing deformity
bowing of mitral valve leaflet
bowing of tendons
bowleg (genu varum)
bowler hat sign
bowler's thumb
Bowman angle
Bowman capsule
Bowman space
bowstring sign
bowstring tear
bowstringing
bow-tie sign
box
   anatomic snuff-
   ligamentous
   snuff
   view-
boxer's elbow
boxer's fracture of metacarpal
boxer's punch fracture (of fifth
   metacarpal)
Boyd formula
Boyd-Griffin classification
Boyd type II fracture
Bozzolo sign
BP (arterial blood pressure)
BPB (biliopancreatic bypass)
BPD (biparietal diameter)
BPD (bronchopulmonary dysplasia)
BPM (blood perfusion monitor)
BPS spinal angiographic catheter
Bq (becquerel)
Bracco system
brace, bracing (removed for imaging
   studies)
bracelet, $^{89}$Sr (strontium)
braces artifact
brachial artery compression
brachial artery cuff pressure
brachial artery pulse pressure
brachial-basilar insufficiency
brachial bypass
brachial neuritis
brachial plexus compression
brachial plexus injury
brachial plexus neuritis
brachiocephalic (innominate)
brachiocephalic arterial aneurysm
brachiocephalic artery

brachiocephalic ischemia
brachiocephalic lymph nodes
brachiocephalic trunk of aorta
brachiocephalic vein
brachiocephalic vessel
brachiocubital
brachioradialis muscle
brachium (pl. brachia)
brachium of colliculus
brachycephalic head shape
brachycephaly
brachydactyly
brachymetatarsia
brachytherapy (radiotherapy)
  afterloading
  $^{198}$Au (gold)
  endobronchial
  $^{125}$I (iodine)
  $^{192}$I (iodine)
  interstitial
  intracavitary
  intraluminal
  intraoperative high dose rate (IOHDR)
  $^{103}$Pd (pallidium)
  permanent
  remote afterloading (RAB)
  Syed-Neblett
  volumetric interstitial
  $^{169}$Yb (yterrbium)
brachytherapy boost
Bradbury-Eggleston syndrome
Bradbury-Eggleston triad
Braden flushing reservoir
bradykinin
bradyphemic
bradyphrenia
Bragard sign
Bragg angle
Bragg curve
Bragg ionization peak
Bragg law

Bragg peak photon beam therapy
Bragg peak radiosurgery
braided diagnostic catheter
brain
  architecture of
  atrophic lesion of the
  edematous
  inflammation of
  metastasis to
  split
  unicameral
  Virchow-Robin spaces of the
  water on the
  wet
brain abscess
brain activity
brain anoxia
brain contusion
brain cyst
brain-dead patient
brain death
brain disease, organic (OBD)
brain dysfunction
brain electrical activity map (or mapping) (BEAM)
brain function
brain ischemia
brain laceration
brain lesion, atrophic
brain mantle
brain map
brain mapping
brain mass
brain parenchyma, bleeding into
brain perfusion scintigraphy
brain perfusion SPECT
brain plasticity
brain scan (see *imaging*)
brain stem compression
brain stem demyelination
brain stem disease
brain stem displacement

brain stem glioma tumor
brain stem hemorrhage
brain stem infarct
brain stem infarction
brain stem ischemia
brain stem lesion
brain stem pyramidal tract
brain stem reticular formation
brain stem signs
brain surface matching technique
brain swelling
brain syndrome, organic (OBS)
brain-to-background ratio
brain tumor
brain window
branch (pl. branches) (see also *artery*)
  acute marginal
  anterior cutaneous
  arterial
  AV (atrioventricular) groove
  bifid aortic
  bifurcating
  bronchial
  caudal
  circumflex
  cutaneous lateral
  diagonal
  digital
  distal
  feeding
  first diagonal
  first major diagonal
  first septal perforator
  inferior cardiac
  inferior wall
  large obtuse marginal
  left bundle
  marginal
  midmarginal
  motor
  muscular
  nonlingular

branch *(cont.)*
  obtuse marginal (OMB)
  paired parietal
  paired visceral
  perforating
  phalangeal
  posterior descending
  posterior intercostal
  posterior ventricular
  proper digital nerve
  pudendal
  ramus
  ramus intermedius artery
  ramus medialis
  right bundle
  second diagonal
  segmental
  septal
  septal perforating
  side
  subcostal
  superior phrenic
  unpaired parietal
  unpaired visceral
  ventricular
branched calculus
branches of vein
branching line
branching linear structure
branching, mirror-image brachiocephalic
branching tubular structure
branch of artery
branch point
Branham sign (arteriovenous fistula)
Brasdor method
Braun tumor
bread-and-butter heart
bread-and-butter pericarditis
bread-crumbling movement
"bread-loaf" technique (for obtaining
  tomographic slices)
breakthrough vasodilatation

breakthrough visualization
breast
  accessory
  atrophic
  cystic
  cystic disease of
  fibroadenoma of
  fibrocystic
  shoemaker's
  tail of
breast artifact
breast attenuation
breast bone or breastbone
breast fibrocystic disease stages:
  adenosis
  cystic disease
  mazoplasia
breast localizer
breast mass lesion with poorly defined margins
breast microcalcifications
breast shadow
breaststroker's knee
breast thrombophlebitis
breast tissue, attenuation by
breast ultrasound
breath-hold cine MR
breath-hold contrast-enhanced three-dimensional MR angiography
breath-hold GRE sequences
breath-hold MR imaging
breath-hold T1-weighted MP-GRE MR imaging
breath-hold ungated imaging
breath-hold velocity-encoded cine MR imaging
breathing
  ataxic
  labored
breathing artifact
breathing feedback
breathless when wheezing

breath pentane measurement
breath, shortness of (SOB)
breech presentation
bregma
bregmatic bone
bremsstrahlung scan
Breschet sinus
Brett syndrome
Breuerton x-ray view of hand
bridegroom's palsy
bridge (bridging)
  arteriolovenular
  bone
  bony
  interthalamic
  meniseal
  mucosal
  osseous
  osteophytic
  skin
  ventral
  Wheatstone
bridge autograft
bridged loop-gap resonator
bridging osteophytes
bright contrast enhancement
bright highly mobile echoes
brightly increased renal parenchymal echogenicity
brightness-time curves
bright pixel values
bright red flush
brim sign
B ring of esophagus
Brinton disease
brisement therapy
Brissaud syndrome
Bristol-Myers system
brittle bone
brittle bones failure
broadband noise detection error artifact

broad band of pleural fluid
broadband transducer
broad-based
Broadbent inverted sign
broadening, dipolar
broad maxillary ridge
Broca convolution
Broca diagonal band
Broca motor speech area of the brain
Broca region
Brock middle lobe syndrome
Brockenbrough catheter, modified bipolar
Brockenbrough mapping catheter
Broden view
Brodie abscess
Brodie bursa
Brodie disease
Brodie knee
Brodie ligament
Brodmann cytoarchitectonic fields
Bromine-76 bromospirone
bromodeoxyuridine labeling index
bromophenol blue
bronchi (pl. of bronchus)
bronchial adenoma
bronchial annular cartilage
bronchial arteriography
bronchial artery embolization
bronchial asthma
bronchial branch
bronchial bud
bronchial calculus
bronchial caliber
bronchial cartilage, absent
bronchial collapse on forced expiration
bronchial collateral circulation
bronchial cyst
bronchial dehiscence
bronchial diameter

bronchial distortions
bronchial kinking
bronchial lumen
bronchial mucosa
bronchial mucosal edema
bronchial obstruction
bronchial provocation testing
bronchial reactivity
bronchial septum
bronchial smooth muscle spasm
bronchial spasm
bronchial stenosis
bronchial stricture
bronchial tree
bronchial type B disease
bronchial vessels
bronchiectasis
   acquired
   capillary
   congenital
   cylindrical
   cystic
   dry
   follicular
   fusiform
   Polynesian
   postinfectious
   recurrent
   saccular
   tuberculous
   varicose
bronchiectasis-bronchomalacia syndrome
bronchiectasis-ethmoid sinusitis
bronchiectatic pattern
bronchiolar carcinoma
bronchiolar edema
bronchiolar emphysema
bronchiolar narrowing
bronchiolar obstruction
bronchiolar passages, narrowing of

bronchiole (pl. bronchioli)
   alveolar
   conducting
   lobular
   respiratory
   terminal
bronchiolitis
   constrictive
   diffuse pan-
   exudative
   proliferative
   respiratory
   smoker's
   vesicular
bronchiolitis obliterans with organizing pneumonia (BOOP)
bronchioloalveolar carcinoma
bronchiolocentric abnormalities
bronchiolus (pl. bronchioli)
bronchiospasm
bronchiostenosis
bronchitic
bronchitis
bronchitis obliterans
bronchitis with bronchospasm
bronchoadenitis
bronchoalveolar cell carcinoma
bronchoarterial bundles
bronchocavernous
bronchocele
bronchocentric granulomatosis
bronchocentric inflammatory infiltrate
bronchoconstriction
   exercise-induced
   isocapnic hyperventilation-induced
bronchoconstrictor
bronchocutaneous fistula
bronchodilatation or bronchodilation
bronchogenic carcinoma
bronchogenic cyst
bronchogram
bronchographic

bronchography
   air
   bilateral
   fiberoptic
   fluid-filled
   tantalum
   unilateral
broncholith
broncholithiasis
bronchomalacia
bronchomediastinal lymph trunk
bronchoplegia
bronchopleural fistula with empyema
bronchopleuropneumonia
bronchopneumonia
   bibasilar
   hemorrhagic
   hypostatic
   inhalation
   postoperative
   subacute
   tuberculous
   virus
bronchopneumonitis
bronchopulmonary atelectasis
bronchopulmonary dysplasia (BPD)
bronchopulmonary lymph node
bronchopulmonary segment
bronchoradiography
bronchosinusitis
bronchospasm
   paradoxical
   uncontrolled
bronchospastic effects
bronchostaxis
bronchostenosis
bronchotracheal
bronchovascular bundles
bronchovascular markings
bronchus (pl. bronchi)
   anterior
   anterior basal

bronchus *(cont.)*
  apical
  apicoposterior
  beaded
  branch
  cardiac
  contracted
  dilated
  edematous
  eparterial
  extrapulmonary
  granulomatous inflammation of
  hyparterial
  inferior lobe
  inflamed
  inflammation of
  intermediate
  intrapulmonary
  lateral basal
  left main
  left main stem
  lingular
  lobar
  main stem
  major
  medial
  medial basal
  medium-sized
  middle lobe
  mucoid impaction of
  normal-appearing
  posterior basal
  primary (right and left)
  principal
  right lobe
  right main
  right main stem
  secondary
  secretion-filled
  segmental
  stem
  subapical

bronchus *(cont.)*
  subsegmental
  superior
  superior lobe
  tracheal
Brooker classification of heterotopic
  ossification
Brostrom-Gordon arthrography
Broviac atrial catheter
brown atrophy
Brown-Dodge method for angiography
brown induration of lung
brown lung
brown pulmonary induration
brown tumor (osteoclastoma)
brow presentation
Br-76 bromospiperone
Bruce protocol (exercise stress testing)
  modified
  standard
  treadmill exercise
brucellosis, cerebral
Bruck disease
Bruel-Kjaer ultrasound scanner
Bruker console
Bruker CSI MR system
Bruker NMR spectrometer
Bruker PC-10 relaxometer
Brunner gland adenoma
Brunner gland of duodenum
Brunnstrom-Fugl-Meyer (BFM) arm
  impairment assessment
Bryant sign
BSA (body surface area)
BSA ejection fraction
B-scan (B-mode) ultrasound
B-72.3 labeled with [111]In bubble
bubble
  gastric
  intragastric
bubble ventriculography

bubbly lung syndrome
bubbly opacity
Buchbinder Omniflex catheter
Buchbinder Thruflex catheter
bucket-handle fracture
bucket-handle tear
buckle fracture
buckle, wire-fixation
buckled innominate artery syndrome
buckling of mitral valve, midsystolic
Bucky view
bud
  bronchial
  capillary
  dorsal pancreatic
  end
  vascular
  ventral pancreatic
Budd-Chiari syndrome
Budge, ciliospinal center of
Budin-Chandler anteversion determination
Budlinger-Ludlof-Laewen disease
BUdR (bromodeoxyuridine or broxuridine) radiosensitizer
Buerger-Gruetz disease
Buerger thromboangiitis obliterans disease
buffalo hump
bulb
  aortic
  arterial
  baroreceptor in the carotid
  baseline of
  carotid
  dental
  duodenal
  end
  heart
  high jugular (HJB)
  inferior jugular vein
  internal jugular

bulb *(cont.)*
  jugular
  olfactory
  superior jugular vein
bulbar abnormality
bulbar intracerebral hemorrhage
bulbar septum
bulb of occipital horn of lateral ventricle
bulb of posterior horn of lateral ventricle
bulbosity
bulbous stump
bulbous urethra
bulbus (noun), bulbous (adj.)
bulge
  bilateral anterior chest disk
  late systolic
  palpable presystolic
  parasternal
  precordial
  suprasternal
bulging disk
bulk laxative
bulk, muscle
bulk susceptibility artifact
bull neck appearance
bulla (pl. bullae)
bulla formation
bullet
  hollow-point
  stabilizing
  tri-point
bullous edema
bullous emphysema
bullous lung disease
bull's-eye deformity
bull's-eye images
bull's-eye map
bull's-eye mapping
bull's-eye polar map

bull's-eye sign
bump
  hip
  inion
  runner's
bumper fracture
bunamiodyl contrast medium
bundle
  aberrant
  artery-vein-nerve
  AV (atrioventricular)
  Bachmann
  bronchoarterial
  bronchovascular
  common
  fascicular
  Flechsig bundle in cerebellum
  Gierke respiratory
  Gowers bundle in cerebellum
  His
  intercostal
  intercostal neuromuscular
  James
  Keith sinoatrial
  Kent
  Kent-His
  maculoneural
  Mahaim
  main
  neurovascular
  Pick
  Schultze
  sinoatrial
  Thorel
  vascular
bundle bone
bundle branch block (BBB) (on EKG)
bundle branch reentry (BBR)
bundle function
bundle of His
bundle of Kent accessory bypass
  fibers
bundle of Stanley Kent
bundle of Vicq d'Azyr
bunk bed fracture
Burdach, column of
Burke syndrome
burned-out tabes
burning
  selective hole
  substernal
Burns space
bursa (pl. bursae)
  Achilles
  adventitious
  anserine
  bicipitoradial
  Brodie
  calcaneal
  Fleischmann
  flexor
  intermediate
  intermetatarsophalangeal
  ischiogluteal
  Luschka
  Monro
  olecranon
  omental
  plantar
  popliteal
  prepatellar
  radial
  retrocalcaneal
  subacromial
  subdeltoid
  suprapatellar
  trochanteric
  ulnar
bursal adhesion
  subacromial
  subdeltoid
bursal flap
bursal fluid
bursal sac

bursitis (pl. bursitides)
　anserine
　bicipital
　calcaneal
　chronic retrocalcaneal
　infracalcaneal
　intermetatarsophalangeal
　intertubercular
　ischiogluteal
　olecranon
　patellar
　pigmented villonodular (PVB)
　postcalcaneal (posterior calcaneal bursitis)
　posterior calcaneal
　prepatellar
　radiohumeral
　retrocalcaneal
　septic
　subacromial
　subdeltoid
　Tornwaldt
　trochanteric
bursography
bursolith
burst (compression) fracture of the atlas
burst fracture of spiral column
bursting fracture
Burton sign
Burwell-Charnley classification of fracture reduction
Busquet disease
butterfly flap
butterfly fracture fragment
butterfly pattern of infiltrates
butterfly shadow
butterfly-type glioma
buttock sign
button
　aortic
　duodenal

button (cont.)
　patellar
　subdural
button toe amputation
buttonhole fracture
buttonhole opening
buttonhole rupture
buttonhole stenosis
buttress plate
buttressing
BVAD (biventricular assist device)
BVR (basal vein of Rosenthal)
BVS (biventricular support system)
BV2 needle
bypass
　aorta-iliac-femoral
　aorta-renal
　aorta-subclavian-carotid
　aorta-subclavian-carotid-axillo-axillary
　aorta to first obtuse marginal branch
　aorta to LAD
　aorta to marginal branch
　aorta to posterior descending
　aortic-femoral
　aortic-superior mesenteric
　aortobifemoral
　aortocarotid
　aortoceliac
　aortocoronary
　aortocoronary-saphenous vein
　aortofemoral
　aortofemoral-thoracic
　aortoiliac
　aortoiliac-popliteal
　aortoiliofemoral
　aortopopliteal
　aortorenal
　apico-abdominal
　atrial-femoral artery
　axillary

**bypass** *(cont.)*
- axillary-brachial
- axillary-femoral
- axilloaxillary
- axillobifemoral
- axillofemoral
- axillopopliteal
- brachial
- cardiopulmonary (CPB)
- carotid-axillary
- carotid-carotid
- carotid-subclavian
- common hepatic-common iliac-renal
- coronary
- coronary artery (CAB)
- cross femoral-femoral
- crossover
- distal arterial
- dorsal pedal
- DTAF-F (descending thoracic aortofemoral-femoral)
- EC-IC (extracranial-intracranial)
- extended tibial in situ
- extra-anatomic
- extracranial-intracranial (EC-IC)
- fem-fem (femoral-femoral)
- femoral-above-knee popliteal
- femoral crossover
- femoral distal popliteal
- femoral-femoral
- femoral to tibial
- femoral vein-femoral artery
- femoral venoarterial
- femoral-popliteal
- femoral-tibial-peroneal
- femoroaxillary
- femorodistal
- femorofemoral
- femorofemoral crossover
- femorofemoropopliteal
- femoroperoneal

**bypass** *(cont.)*
- femoropopliteal
- femoropopliteal saphenous vein
- femorotibial
- "fem-pop" (femoral-popliteal)
- heart-lung
- hepatorenal saphenous vein
- hypothermic cardiopulmonary
- iliac-renal
- iliofemoral
- iliopopliteal
- ilioprofunda
- infracubital
- infrainguinal stenosis
- in situ
- intracranial arterial
- ipsilateral nonreversed greater saphenous vein
- left atrium to distal arterial aortic
- left heart
- lesser saphenous vein in situ
- Litwak left atrial-aortic
- mammary-coronary artery
- marginal circumflex
- microscope-aided pedal
- nonreversed translocated vein
- normothermic cardiopulmonary
- obtuse marginal
- partial
- partial cardiopulmonary
- percutaneous femoral-femoral cardiopulmonary
- popliteal
- popliteal in situ
- popliteal to distal in situ
- pulsatile cardiopulmonary
- renal artery-reverse saphenous vein
- reversed
- right heart
- saphenous vein
- sequential in situ
- subclavian-carotid

bypass *(cont.)*
  subclavian-subclavian
  superior mesenteric artery
  supraceliac aortofemoral
  temporary aortic shunt
  thoracic aorta-femoral artery
  tibial in situ
  total cardiopulmonary
  upper extremity in situ
bypass circuit
bypass graft
bypass tract
  atrio-Hisian or atriohisian
  AV (atrioventricular) nodal
  concealed
  fasiculoventricular bypass
  nodo-Hisian
  nodoventricular
  right ventricular
byte mode

# C, c

C (carbon)
CA (coronary artery)
"cabbage" (CABG)
CABG (coronary artery bypass graft)
CABS (coronary artery bypass surgery)
Cacchione syndrome
cachexia, lymphatic
CAD (computer-aided [or assisted] design [or diagnostics])
CAD (coronary artery disease)
cadmium iodide detector
caecum (cecum)
CAEP (chronotropic assessment exercise protocol)
Caffey disease
CA15-3 antigen radioimmunoassay imaging agent
cage
  bony thoracic
  osseocartilaginous thoracic
CAH (congenital adrenal hyperplasia)
calamus scriptorius
calcaneal bone
calcaneal fracture
calcaneal spur
calcaneocavus (clubfoot)
  talipes calcaneus
  talipes cavus
calcaneoclavicular ligament
calcaneocuboid joint
calcaneocuboid ligament
calcaneofibular (CF) ligament
calcaneonavicular coalition
calcaneoplantar angle
calcaneotibial fusion
calcaneovalgocavus
calcaneovalgus flatfoot
calcaneovalgus, pes
calcaneus
  pes
  sulcus
  talipes
calcaneus altus
calcar avis
calcar femorale
calcar pedis
calcar, pivot of
calcareous deposits
calcarine cortex
calcarine fissure
calcarine sulcus
calcific aortic stenosis

**calcific • calcinosis**

calcific arteriosclerosis
calcific artery
calcification
  aneurysmal wall
  annular
  aortic
  aortic valve
  arterial
  artery
  basal ganglia
  basketlike
  cartilage
  cerebral
  choroid plexus
  coarse vascular
  conglomerate
  coronary artery
  costal cartilage
  curvilinear
  dentate nuclei
  dural
  dystrophic
  eggshell
  falx
  fine
  focal
  foci of
  free body
  glial tumor
  granulomatous
  gyriform
  idiopathic pleural
  intervertebral cartilage
  intervertebral disk
  intracardiac
  intracranial
  irregular
  laminated
  ligamentous
  linear
  lymph node
  medial collateral ligament

calcification *(cont.)*
  metastatic
  mitral annular
  mitral ring
  mitral valve
  Mönckeberg (Moenckeberg)
  mottled
  multiple
  myocardial
  node
  normal
  parietal pericardial
  Pellegrini-Stieda
  periarticular
  pericardial
  pericardium
  periductal
  periventricular
  pineal gland
  plaque
  plaquing
  popcorn
  premature
  renal mass
  secondary
  sella turcica
  soft tissue
  stippled
  subannular
  target
  thrombus
  thyroid adenoma
  tramline cortex
  valve
  valvular leaflet
  visceral pericardial
calcific matrix
calcific plaque
calcific round body
calcific spur
calcifying
calcinosis circumscripta

calcinosis, tumoral
calcis, os
calcium deposit
calcium deposition
calcium-45 imaging agent (autoradiography)
calcium hydroxyapatite
calcium, intracardiac
calcium layering
calculated clearance time
calculation
   bayesian
   Cerenkov
   gap
   Monte Carlo
   multiplane dosage
   radiation dosimetry
   spectrophotometric
   volume implant
calculus (pl. calculi)
   alvine
   articular
   biliary
   branched
   bronchial
   cat's eye (in common bile duct)
   decubitus
   echogenic
   encysted
   fibrin
   gallbladder
   gastric
   hemic
   hepatic
   impacted
   intestinal
   joint
   lacteal
   lucent
   lung
   mammary
   metabolic

calculus *(cont.)*
   mulberry
   nephritic
   nonopaque
   opaque
   pancreatic
   primary vesical
   pocketed
   prostatic
   radiopaque
   renal
   salivary
   spermatic
   staghorn
   stomach
   stonelike
   ureteral
   urinary tract
Caldani ligament
Caldwell occipitofrontal view
calf muscle pump (anatomical)
calf vein thrombus
caliber
   bronchus
   internal
   luminal
   medium
   modest
   narrow
   tracheal
   vessel
   wide
calibration, absolute-peak efficiency
calibration failure artifact
calibration method
calibrator
caliceal blunting
caliceal clubbing
caliceal dilatation
caliceal system
caliectasia (or caliectasis)
California disease (coccidioidomycosis)

calix (pl. calices) (also calyx, calyces)
   major
   minor
   renal
callosal dysgenesis
callosal formation
callosal gyrus
callosal lesion
callosal sulcus
callosomarginal artery
callosum, corpus
callous (adj.)
callus
   bony
   bridging
   central
   definitive
   ensheathing
   external
   florid
   fracture
   intermediate
   permanent
   provisional
callus distraction
callus formation (*not* callous)
callus weld
calvarial bone
calvarium (pl. calvaria)
Calvé-Perthes disease
calyx (see *calix*)
CAM 5.2 antibody
camelback sign
camera
   ADAC gamma
   Anger gamma
   Anger-type scintillation
   APEX 409
   APEX 415
   Biad
   CeraSPECT
   CID

camera *(cont.)*
   Cidtech
   Digirad gamma
   DSI
   dual-head gamma
   Elscint
   Elscint dual-detector cardiac
   four-head
   gamma
   GE gamma
   GE single-detector SPECT-capable
   GE Starcam
   GE Starcam single-crystal tomographic
   Haifa
   Helix
   Israel
   MEDX gamma
   multicrystal
   multicrystal gamma
   Picker
   Pixsys FlashPoint
   R&F
   rotating gamma
   scintillation
   Siemens gamma
   slip-ring
   SP6
   Starcam
   Technicare
   three-head
   Trionix
   Vertex
   Vision
cameral fistula
Camper chiasma
camptocormia
camptodactyly
Camurati-Engelmann disease
CAMV (congenital anomaly of mitral valve)

**canal**
- abdominal
- accessory
- adductor
- Alcock
- alimentary
- alveolar
- alveolodental
- ampulla of semicircular
- anal
- anterior condyloid
- anterior semicircular
- arachnoid
- Arantius
- archenteric
- Arnold
- arterial
- atrial
- atrioventricular (AV)
- auditory
- basipharyngeal
- Bernard
- Bichat
- biliary
- birth
- bony semicircular
- Böttcher
- Braune
- Breschet
- calciferous
- carotid
- caroticotympanic
- carotid
- carpal
- caudal
- central
- central spinal
- cerebrospinal
- cervical (of uterus)
- cervical axillary
- cervicoaxillary
- ciliary

**canal** *(cont.)*
- Civinini
- Cloquet
- cochlear
- common atrioventricular
- complex atrioventricular
- condylar
- condyloid
- connecting
- Corti
- Cotunnius
- craniopharyngeal
- crural
- Cuvier
- deferent
- dental
- dental root
- dentinal
- diploic
- Dorello
- Dupuytren
- endocervical
- endodermal
- ethmoid
- ethmoidal
- eustachian
- external auditory
- facial
- facial nerve
- fallopian
- femoral
- femoral medullary
- Ferrein
- flexor
- Fontana
- galactophorous
- ganglionic
- Gartner
- gastric
- genital
- greater palatine
- gubernacular

canal *(cont.)*
Guyon
gynecophoric
Hannover
haversian
hemal
Henle
Hensen
Hering
hernial
Hirschfeld
His
Huguier
Hunter
Huschke
hyaloid
hydrops
hypoglossal
iliac
incisive
incisor
inferior dental
infraorbital
inguinal
inioendineal
interdental
interfacial
intersacral
intestinal
intramedullary
Jacobson
lacrimal
lateral
lateral semicircular
Löwenberg (Loewenberg)
lumbar
mandibular
marrow
mastoid
maxillary
medullary
mental

canal *(cont.)*
Müller (Mueller)
musculotubal
narrowing of spinal
nasal
nasolacrimal
nasopalatine
neural
neurenteric
notochordal
Nuck
nutrient
obstetric
obturator
olfactory
optic
orbital
palatine
palatomaxillary
palatovaginal
paraurethral
parturient
pelvic
pericardioperitoneal
perivascular
persistent atrioventricular
persistent common atrioventricular
petrous carotid
pharyngeal
pleural
pleuropericardial
pleuroperitoneal
portal
posterior semicircular
principal artery of pterygoid
pterygoid
pterygopalatine
pudendal
pulmoaortic
pulp
pyloric
recurrent

canal *(cont.)*
  Reichert
  Richet tibio-astragalocalcaneal
  Rivinus
  root (of tooth)
  Rosenthal
  sacculocochlear
  sacculoutricular
  sacral
  Santorini
  Schlemm
  scleral
  semicircular
  sheathing
  small (of chorda tympani)
  Sondermann
  sphenopalatine
  sphenopharyngeal
  spinal
  spinal cord
  Stensen
  Stilling
  subsartorial
  Sucquet-Hoyer
  supraorbital
  tarsal
  temporal
  Theile
  tibial medullary
  tibio-astragalocalcaneal of Richet
  tight spinal
  Tourtual
  tubal
  tubotympanic
  tympanic
  umbilical
  uniting
  urogenital
  uterine
  uterocervical
  uterovaginal
  utriculosaccular

canal *(cont.)*
  vaginal
  Van Hoorne
  ventricular
  Verneuil
  vertebral
  vesicourethral
  vestibular
  vidian
  Volkmann
  vomerine
  vomerorostral
  vomerovaginal
  vulvouterine
  zygomaticofacial
  zygomaticotemporal
canal decompression
Canale-Kelly classification of talar
  neck fracture
canaliculus (pl. canaliculi)
  apical
  auricular
  bile
  bone
  cochlear
  haversian
  innominate
canalization
Canavan disease
Canavan-van Bogaert-Bertrand disease
cancellated bone
cancellous bone
cancellous tissue
cancellus
cancer (see *carcinoma, sarcoma, tumor*)
  aniline
  betel
  chimney-sweep's
  clay pipe
  contact
  cystic

cancer *(cont.)*
    dendritic
    dye worker's
    hereditary
    latent
    melanotic
    mule-spinner's
    oat cell
    occult
    paraffin
    pitch worker's
    swamp
    tar
    tubular
cancer embolus
candle wax appearance of bone
C angle
Cannon-Boehm point
Cannon point
Cannon ring
Cannon segmentation
cannula (pl. cannulae, cannulas)
    double-lumen
    femoral artery
    high-flow
    inflow
    infusion
    inlet
    internal jugular venous
    intra-arterial
    intraventricular
    large-bore inflow
    large-egress
    LV (left ventricular) apex
    metallic tip
    needle
    outlet
    perfusion
    peripheral
    single-bore
    small-egress
    two-stage

cannula *(cont.)*
    vena cava
    venous
    ventricular
    washout
cannulation
    aortic
    arterial
    atrial
    bicaval
    direct caval
    left atrial
    ostial
    retrograde
    selective
    single-cannula atrial
    two-stage venous
    venoarterial
    venous
    venovenous
cannulation catheter
cannulization
    selective
    subselective
Canon scanner
Cantelli sign
cap
    duodenal
    fibrous
    hilar
    knee
    phrygian
    pleural
    thin
capacious veins
capacitator, MOS
capacity
    bladder
    closing
    cranial
    functional bladder
    lung

capacity *(cont.)*
  respiratory
  vasodilatory
capillary (pl. capillaries)
  arterial
  bile
  continuous
  lymph
  Meigs
  sinusoidal
  venous
capillary bed
capillary blood volume
capillary bud
capillary congestion
capillary density
capillary embolism
capillary filling, compensatory
capillary filling time
capillary fracture
capillary hydrostatic pressure
capillary hyperpermeability
capillary leak (or leakage)
capillary-lymphatic malformation (CLM)
capillary malformation (CM)
capillary permeability
capillary pneumonia
capillary pressure
capillary pulsation
capillary refill
capillary resistance test
capillary-venous malformation (CVM)
capillary walls
capillary wedge pressure, pulmonary
capital epiphysis (CE) angle
capital extension
capital flexor
capital fragment
capital mover
capitate bone
capitellum

capitolunate joint
capitular epiphysis
capitulum costae
capitulum fibulae
capitulum humeri
capitulum mandibulae
capitulum radii
capitulum ulnae
Caplan syndrome
capsular imbrication
capsular ligament rupture
capsular plane
capsular reefing
capsular thrombosis
capsule
  adrenal
  articular
  auditory
  Bowman
  cartilage
  cricoarytenoid articular
  cricothyroid articular
  dorsal
  external
  facet
  fatty renal
  fibrous
  fibrous renal
  Gerota
  Glisson
  hepatic
  internal
  joint
  limb of anterior metatarsophalangeal (MTP) joint
  liver
  organ
  plantar
  posterolateral
  redundant
  renal
  rim of

capsule (cont.)
   splenic
   suprasellar
   talonavicular
   thyroid
   tumor
   wrist
capsulocaudate infarction
capsulolabral complex
capsuloperiosteal envelope
capsuloputaminal infarction
capsuloputaminocaudate infarction
Captopril renal scan
capture, boron neutron
caput medusae
Carabello sign (rise in arterial blood pressure; do not confuse with *Carabelli dental sign*)
carbogen radiosensitizer imaging agent
carbon (C)
   $^{11}$C acetate
   $^{11}$C butanol
   $^{11}$C carbon monoxide
   $^{11}$C carfentanil
   $^{11}$C deoxyglucose
   $^{11}$C FLU
   $^{11}$C flumazenil
   $^{11}$C imaging agent
   $^{11}$C labeled cocaine
   $^{11}$C labeled fatty acids
   $^{11}$C L-159
   $^{11}$C L-884
   $^{11}$C L-methylmethionine
   $^{11}$C lumazenil
   $^{11}$C methionine
   $^{11}$C methoxystauro-sporine
   $^{11}$C N-methylspiperone
   $^{11}$C N-methylspiroperidol (NMS)
   $^{11}$C nomifensine
   $^{11}$C palmitate
   $^{11}$C palmitic acid radioactive

carbon (cont.)
   $^{11}$C raclopride
   $^{11}$C thymidine
   carbon dioxide (see $CO_2$)
   carbon dioxide laser
   carbon-loaded thermoluminescent dosimeter
carcinoid syndrome
carcinoma (also *cancer, sarcoma, tumor*)
   acinous cell
   adenocystic
   adenosquamous
   adnexal
   adrenocortical
   aldosterone-producing
   aldosterone-secreting
   alveolar
   alveolar cell
   ameloblastic
   anaplastic (of thyroid gland)
   apocrine
   basal cell
      alveolar
      comedo
      cystic
      multicentric
      nodulo-ulcerative
      pigmented
      sclerosing
      superficial
   basaloid
   basosquamous cell
   bile duct
   bilharzial
   bladder
   breast
   bronchioalveolar
   bronchiolar
   bronchogenic
   cavitary squamous cell

carcinoma *(cont.)*
  cavitating
  cerebriform
  cervical
  cholangio-
  cholangiocellular
  chorionic
  choroid plexus
  clear cell
  colloid
  colon
  colorectal
  comedo
  corpus
  cortisol-producing
  cribriform
  cylindrical
  ductal
  duct cell
  eccrine
  embryonal
  embryonal cell
  endobronchial
  endometrial
  epidermal
  epidermoid
  esophageal
  exophytic
  extrahepatic bile duct
  fibrolamellar hepatocellular
  FIGO stage
  fibrolamellar
  follicular
  gallbladder
  gastric
  gelatinous
  genital
  giant cell (of thyroid gland)
  glandular
  glans
  granulosa cell
  hepatic

carcinoma *(cont.)*
  hepatocellular
  Hürthle cell
  hypernephroid
  infantile embryonal
  infiltrating ductal
  infiltrating lobular
  inflammatory
  intraductal
  intraepidermal
  intraepithelial
  invasive
  invasive lobular
  juvenile embryonal
  Kulchitzky cell
  large cell
  lenticular
  leptomeningeal
  lobular
  lung
  medullary
  melanotic
  meningeal
  Merkel cell
  metastatic
  metatypical
  microinvasive
  micropapillary
  moderately well-differentiated
  mucinous
  mucoepidermoid
  mucous
  nasopharyngeal
  neuroendocrine
  noninfiltrating lobular
  non-small cell
  oat cell
  osteoid
  ovarian
  Paget
  pancreatic
  papillary

carcinoma *(cont.)*
  perforated
  periampullary
  polypoid
  poorly differentiated
  preinvasive
  prickle cell
  primary
  primary intraosseous
  pulmonary
  rectal
  rectosigmoid
  renal
  renal pelvic urothelial
  residual
  retinoblastoma hereditary human
  scar
  schistosomal bladder
  schneiderian
  scirrhous
  sclerosing hepatic (SHC)
  sebaceous
  sessile nodular
  sigmoid
  signet-ring
  small cell
  small cell lung (SCLC)
  small round cell
  spindle cell
  squamous cell (SCC)
  string cell
  superficial depressed
  superficial
  terminal
  thyroid
  tonsillar
  transitional cell (TCC)
  tubular
  undifferentiated
  undifferentiated squamous cell
  uterine cervix
  uterine corpus

carcinoma *(cont.)*
  vaginal
  verrucous
  villous
  well-differentiated
carcinoma de novo
carcinoma en cuirasse
carcinoma ex pleomorphic adenoma
carcinoma in situ
  ductal (DCIS)
  lobular (LCIS)
carcinoma-specific monoclonal antibody
carcinomatosis
carcinomatous meningitis
carcinosis
card, Intel Plink Ethernet
Cardarelli sign
cardia
  crescent of
  gastric
  patulous
cardiac antrum
cardiac apex
cardiac atrial shunt
cardiac blood pool imaging, gated equilibrium
cardiac border
cardiac branch
cardiac catheter
cardiac catheterization
cardiac compensation
cardiac compression
cardiac contractility
cardiac contraction
cardiac creep
cardiac cycle
cardiac death, sudden
cardiac decompensation
cardiac decompression
cardiac denervation
cardiac dilatation

cardiac dynamics
cardiac effusion
cardiac enlargement
cardiac failure
cardiac fibroma
cardiac fibrosarcoma
cardiac filling pressure
cardiac fossa
cardiac ganglion, Wrisberg
cardiac gated MRA
cardiac gated PGSE sequence
cardiac gated respiration
cardiac gating
cardiac hamartoma
cardiac hemangioma
cardiac hypertrophy
cardiac impression on liver
cardiac index (CI)
cardiac infarct
cardiac insufficiency
cardiac irritability
cardiac laminography
cardiac lipoma
cardiac long axis view
cardiac lung
cardiac lymphangioma
cardiac MRI
cardiac mapping
cardiac margins
cardiac monitor
cardiac muscle fibers
cardiac myxoma
cardiac node
cardiac notch
cardiac output (CO)
cardiac output = stroke volume x heart rate (vol./min.)
cardiac overload (or overloading)
cardiac perforation
cardiac positron emission tomography (PET)
cardiac pumping ability
cardiac radiation syndrome
cardiac radiography
cardiac recovery
cardiac reserve
cardiac rhabdomyoma
cardiac rhabdomyosarcoma
cardiac rupture
cardiac sarcoma
cardiac scan
cardiac series
cardiac shadow
cardiac shape
cardiac short axis view
cardiac shunt
cardiac silhouette
cardiac sling
cardiac standstill
cardiac steady state
cardiac stomach
cardiac tamponade
cardiac teratoma
cardiac thrombosis
cardiac tumor embolization
cardiac valve
cardiac valve mucoid degeneration
cardiac vasculature
cardiac vein, great
cardiac waist
cardiac wall motion
cardinal sign
cardioangiography
CardioCamera imaging system
cardiochalasia
CardioCoil self-expanding coronary stent
cardiocutaneous syndrome
Cardio Data MK3 Holter scanner
cardiodilator
cardiodynia
cardioesophageal (CE) junction
cardiofacial syndrome
cardiogenesis

cardiogenic embolic stroke
cardiogenic embolism
cardiogenic pulmonary edema
cardiogenic shock
Cardiografin imaging agent
cardiogram
cardiography
  apex (ACG)
  esophageal
  precordial
  ultrasonic (UCG)
  vector
cardiohepatic
cardiohepatomegaly
cardiointegram (CIG)
cardiokymography (CKG)
Cardiolite ($^{99m}$Tc sestamibi) imaging agent
cardiology, invasive
cardiomegaly
  alcoholic
  borderline
  familial
  globular
  hypertensive
  iatrogenic
  idiopathic
  postoperative
cardiomotility
cardiomyopathy
  alcoholic dilated
  amyloidotic
  apical hypertrophic (AHC)
  arrhythmogenic right ventricular
  beer-drinker's
  beriberi
  concentric hypertrophic
  congenital dilated
  congestive
  constrictive
  diabetic
  diffuse symmetric hypertrophic
cardiomyopathy *(cont.)*
  dilated (DCM)
  end-stage
  familial hypertrophic (FHC)
  Friedreich ataxic
  hypertrophic (HCM)
  hypertrophic obstructive (HOC or HOCM)
  idiopathic
  idiopathic dilated (IDC)
  idiopathic restrictive
  infantile
  infectious
  infiltrative
  ischemic
  ischemic congestive
  left ventricular
  metabolic
  mucopolysaccharidosis
  myotonia atrophica
  noncoronary
  nonischemic congestive
  nonobstructive
  obliterative
  obscure
  obstructive
  obstructive hypertrophic
  peripartum
  peripartum dilated
  postmyocarditis dilated
  postpartum
  primary
  restrictive (RCM)
  right ventricular
  right-sided
  secondary
  tachycardia-induced
  thyrotoxicotic
  toxic
cardionecrosis
cardionephric
cardioneural

cardiopathy
  hypertensive
  infarctoid
  obscure
cardiophrenic angle
cardiophrenic junction
cardioplegic needle
cardiopneumatic
cardioptosis, Wenckebach
cardiopulmonary arrest
cardiopulmonary bilharziasis
cardiopulmonary bypass (CPB)
cardiopulmonary deterioration
cardiopulmonary insufficiency
cardiopulmonary obesity
cardiopulmonary support system (CPS)
cardiopuncture
cardiopyloric
cardiorenal disease
cardiorespiratory sign
cardiorrhexis
cardiosclerosis
cardioselective agent
cardiospasm
Cardio Tactilaze peripheral angioplasty laser catheter
CardioTec ($^{99m}$Tc teboroxime) imaging agent
cardiotherapy
cardiothoracic index
cardiothoracic ratio (CTR)
Cardio3DScope imaging system
cardiothyrotoxicosis
cardiotocograph
cardiotocography
cardiovalvular
cardiovascular accident (CVA)
cardiovascular anomalies
cardiovascular renal disease
cardiovascular shunt
carina of trachea
Carleton spots

C-arm digital fluoroscopy
C-arm fluoroscopy
C-arm portable x-ray unit
Carney syndrome
Caroli disease
caroticocavernous fistula
carotid angiography
carotid artery
  kinking of
  redundant
carotid artery aneurysm
carotid artery-cavernous sinus fistula
carotid atherosclerotic disease
carotid bifurcation
carotid blowout syndrome
carotid bulb baroreceptor
carotid-carotid venous bypass graft
carotid cavernous fistula occlusion
carotid distribution TIA (transient ischemic attack)
carotid duplex study
carotid ejection time
carotid occlusive disease
carotid phonoangiography
carotid plexus
carotid pulse peak
carotid pulse tracing
carotid pulse upstroke
carotid shudder
carotid sinus hypersensitivity (CSH)
carotid sinus massage
carotid sinus syncope
carotid sinus syndrome
carotid siphon
carotid stenosis
carotid string sign
carotid-subclavian bypass
carotid vein
carpal arch
carpal bone
carpal deviation

carpal-metacarpal (see *carpometacarpal*)
carpal navicular
carpal row
carpal scaphoid bone fracture
carpal tunnel release (CTR)
carpal tunnel syndrome (CTS)
carpal tunnel view
Carpenter syndrome
carpometacarpal (CMC) joint
carpophalangeal joint
carporadial articulation
carpus
Carrel, triangulation of
carrier
    GABA uptake
    radionuclide
carrier-free separation
Carr-Purcell-Meiboom-Gill sequence
carrying angle
Carswell grapes
Carter equation
Carter-Rowe view
Cartesian reference coordinate voxel array
cartilage
    accessory
    accessory nasal
    alar
    arthrodial
    articular
    annular
    arytenoid
    auditory
    auricular
    basilar
    branchial
    calcified
    cariniform
    ciliary
    circumferential
    conchal

cartilage *(cont.)*
    connecting
    corniculate
    costal
    cricoid
    cuneiform
    elastic
    ensiform
    epiglottic
    epiphyseal
    falciform
    fibroelastic
    fibrous
    floating
    hyaline
    hyaline articular
    interarticular
    loss of elasticity of
    physeal
    pitted
    quadrangle
    roughened
    scored
    semilunar
    thinned
    thyroid
    tracheal
    triradial
    yellow
cartilage articulation
cartilage bone
cartilage joint
    primary
    secondary
    symphysis
cartilage joint space
cartilaginous ring
cartographic projection
cartwheel fracture
Carvallo sign in tricuspid regurgitation
CAS (coronary artery scan)

cascade (pl. cascades)
   abdominal
   diagnostic
cascade stomach
Castellani disease
Castellino sign
Castillo catheter
Castleman disease
CAT-CAM conversion
cat's eye calculi in common bile duct
cathartic colon
catheter
   Abramson
   Accu-Flo ventricular
   ACE
   Achiever balloon dilatation
   Ackrad balloon-bearing
   ACS (Advanced Catheter or
      Cardiac Systems) balloon
   ACS Endura coronary dilation
   ACSJL4
   ACS mini
   ACS RX coronary dilatation
   AL1 or AL-1
   Alzate
   Amplatz
   Angiocath PRN flexible
   angiographic balloon occlusion
   Angio-Kit
   Angiomedics
   angiopigtail
   angioplasty balloon
   angled balloon
   angulated
   Anthron heparinized
      antithrombogenic
   aortic flush pigtail
   aortic flush straight
   aortogram
   Arani double loop guiding
   Argyle Medicut R
   Arrow pulmonary artery

catheter *(cont.)*
   Arrow Twin Cath multilumen
      peripheral
   Arrow-Berman balloon
   ArrowGard Blue Line
   ArrowGard central venous
   Arrow-Howes multilumen
   arterial embolectomy
   AR-2 diagnostic guiding
   atherectomy
   AtheroCath
   Atlas LP PTCA balloon dilatation
   Atlas ULP balloon dilatation
   Atri-pace I bipolar-flared pacing
   Auth atherectomy
   AV-Paceport thermodilution
   Axiom DG balloon angioplasty
   bail-out
   Baim pacing
   Baim-Turi monitor/pacing
   balloon
   balloon biliary
   balloon dilatation
   balloon dilating
   balloon embolectomy
   balloon flotation
   balloon-flotation pacing
   balloon-tipped angiographic
   balloon-tipped end-hole
   ball-wedge
   Bard
   bat-wing
   Baxter
   Berman angiographic
   Bernstein
   bifoil balloon
   Bilbao-Dotter
   biliary
   bipolar pacing electrode
   bipolar temporary pacemaker
   blind
      Block right coronary guiding

catheter *(cont.)*
    Blue FlexTip
    Blue Max triple-lumen
    BPS spinal angiographic
    braided diagnostic
    Brockenbrough transseptal
    bronchial
    Bronchitrac L
    bronchospirometric
    Broviac
    Buchbinder Omniflex
    Buchbinder Thruflex
    Buerhenne steerable
    Camino ICP (intracranial pressure)
    cannulation
    Cardio Tactilaze peripheral angioplasty laser
    Cardiomarker
    Castillo
    Cath-Finder
    Cath-Track
    central venous (CVC)
    Chemo-Port
    cholangiographic
    cholangiography
    Cloverleaf
    coaxial
    coaxial Tracker
    Cobra and Cobra 2
    cobra-shaped
    coil-tipped
    Comfort Cath I and II
    conductance
    Cook arterial
    Cook pigtail
    Cope loop
    Cordis Brite Tip guiding
    Cordis Ducor I, II, and III coronary
    Cordis Ducor pigtail
    Cordis Son-II
    coronary sinus thermodilution
    corset balloon

catheter *(cont.)*
    coudé
    Councill
    Cournand cardiac
    CR Bard
    Critikon
    CVP (central venous pressure)
    Dacron
    Datascope DL-II percutaneous translucent balloon
    decapolar
    deflectable quadripolar
    diagnostic
    Diasonics
    dilatation balloon
    DLP cardioplegic
    Doppler coronary
    Dormia stone basket
    Dorros infusion/probing
    Dotter caged balloon
    Double J
    double-lumen
    Dow-Corning ileal pouch
    drainage
    Ducor balloon
    DVI Simpson atherocath
    EAC (expandable access catheter)
    EchoMark angiographic
    Edwards diagnostic
    eight-lumen esophageal manometry
    Elecath thermodilution
    electrode
    El Gamal coronary bypass
    Elite
    embolectomy
    end-hole
    Endosound endoscopic ultrasound
    Endotak C lead
    enhanced torque guiding
    epidural
    Eppendorf

catheter *(cont.)*
 ERCP (endoscopic retrograde cholangiopancreatography)
 Erythroflex hydromer-coated central venous
 expandable access (EAC)
 Express PTCA
 extraction
 extrusion balloon
 Faraday
 FAST (flow-assisted, short-term) balloon
 Finesse large-lumen guiding
 Flexguard Tip
 flotation
 flow-directed microcatheter
 flow-oximetry
 fluid-filled
 Fogarty balloon
 Fogarty balloon biliary
 Fogarty-Chin extrusion balloon
 Fogarty embolectomy
 Foley
 Foltz
 Force balloon dilatation
 French mushroom tip
 Ganz-Edwards coronary infusion
 Gensini coronary
 Gentle-Flo suction
 Goodale-Lubin cardiac
 Gorlin pacing
 Gould PentaCath 5-lumen thermodilution
 graft-seeking
 Grollman pigtail
 Groshong double-lumen
 Groshong tunneled
 Grüntzig (Gruentzig)
 Grüntzig balloon
 Grüntzig Dilaca
 guide
 guiding

catheter *(cont.)*
 Guidezilla guiding
 Halo
 Hanafee
 Hartzler ACX-II and RX-014 balloon
 Hartzler LPS dilatation
 Hartzler Micro II and Micro XT
 headhunter
 helical-tip Halo
 helium-filled balloon
 HemoCath hemodialysis
 Heplock
 hexapolar
 Hickman indwelling
 Hickman tunneled
 Hidalgo
 Hieshima coaxial
 high-fidelity microtipped
 high-flow
 high-pressure
 high-speed rotation dynamic angioplasty
 HNB angiographic
 H-1-H (headhunter)
 hot-tip
 H/S (hysterosalpingography)
 HydraCross TLC PTCA
 Hydrolyser micro-
 hydrophilic-coated
 hydrostatic balloon
 hyperthermia
 IAB (intra-aortic balloon)
 ICP (intracranial pressure)
 Illumen-8 guiding
 ILUS (intraluminal ultrasound)
 indwelling
 Infiniti
 Infuse-a-port
 Inoue balloon
 internal-external drainage
 interstitial

**catheter**

catheter *(cont.)*
  intra-aortic balloon double-lumen
  intra-arterial
  intra-arterial chemotherapy
  Intracath
  intracoronary
  intrahepatic biliary drainage
  intratumoral
  intravascular ultrasound
  intravenous pacing
  intraventricular
  intrepid PTCA angioplasty
  ITC radiopaque balloon
  Jackman orthogonal
  Jackson-Pratt
  JB1
  JB3
  JCL 3.5 guiding
  Jelco intravenous
  JL4 (Judkins left 4 cm curve)
  JR5 (Judkins right 5 cm)
  Judkins USCI
  jugular
  KDF-2.3
  Kensey atherectomy
  Kifa
  King multipurpose coronary graft
  Kinsey atherectomy
  Kontron balloon
  large-bore
  large-caliber
  large-lumen
  laser
  left coronary
  left heart
  left ventricular sump
  Lehman ventriculography
  LeVeen
  Lo-Profile balloon and Lo-Profile
    II balloon
  Longdwel Teflon
  low-pressure

catheter *(cont.)*
  low-speed rotation angioplasty
  LPS
  Lumaguide
  Malecot
  Mallinckrodt angiographic
  Mani
  manometer-tipped cardiac
  manometric
  Mansfield Atri-Pace 1
  Mansfield orthogonal electrode
  Mansfield Scientific dilatation
    balloon
  Marathon guiding
  Match 35 PTA
  Max Force
  McGoon coronary perfusion
  McIntosh double-lumen
  Medicut
  Medi-Tech balloon
  medium-pressure
  Medtronic balloon
  Memory-Vu angiographic
  Micro-Guide
  micromanometer-tip
  Microvasive Rigiflex TTS balloon
  midstream aortogram
  Mikro-tip micromanometer-tipped
  Millar MPC-500
  Millenia balloon
  Mini-Profile dilatation
  Mirage over-the-wire balloon
  Mitsubishi angioscopic
  Molina needle
  Monorail balloon
  MPF
  MS Classique
  Mullins transseptal
  multi-electrode impedance
  Multi-Med triple-lumen infusion
  multifiber
  multilumen

**catheter** *(cont.)*
- multipolar impedance
- Multipurpose-SM
- mushroom
- MVP
- Mylar
- nasobiliary
- NBIH
- Neuhaus implantable port
- NIH (National Institutes of Health) left ventriculography
- nontraumatizing
- NoProfile balloon
- Nycore angiography
- octapolar
- Omniflex balloon
- one-hole angiographic
- Optiscope
- Oracle Focus PTCA
- Oracle Megasonics
- Oracle Micro Plus
- Orion balloon
- over-the-wire balloon
- oximetric
- Paceport
- Pacewedge dual-pressure bipolar pacing
- pacing
- Pathfinder
- PA Watch position-monitoring
- PE Plus II balloon dilatation
- Percor DL and DL-II balloon
- Percor-Stat-DL
- percutaneous
- percutaneous transhepatic biliary drainage (PTBD)
- percutaneous transhepatic pigtail
- perfusion
- peripheral atherectomy
- peripherally inserted central (PICC)
- peritoneal

**catheter** *(cont.)*
- peritoneal dialysis
- pervenous
- Pezzer
- Phantom V Plus
- PIBC (percutaneous intra-aortic balloon counterpulsation)
- pigtail
- pigtail angiographic
- polyethylene
- Polystan venous return
- portal
- Portnoy ventricular
- Positrol II
- preformed
- preshaped
- pressure
- probing
- Profile Plus dilatation
- Proflex 5 dilatation
- Pro-Flo
- Pruitt-Inahara balloon-tipped perfusion
- PTBD (percutaneous transhepatic biliary drainage)
- PTCA (percutaneous transluminal coronary angioplasty)
- Pudenz peritoneal
- pulmonary artery
- pulmonary flotation
- pusher
- quadripolar steerable electrode
- Quanticor
- Quinton Mahurkar dual-lumen peritoneal
- Raaf Cath vascular
- Raimondi spring
- Raimondi ventricular
- Ranfac LAP-013 cholangiographic
- Ranfac ORC-B cholangiographic
- Ranfac XL-11 cholangiographic
- Rashkind septostomy balloon

**catheter**

catheter *(cont.)*
   recessed balloon septostomy
   Reddick cystic duct cholangiogram
   RediFurl TaperSeal IAB
   red Robinson
   red rubber
   Rentrop infusion
   retroperfusion
   RF (radiofrequency-generated thermal) balloon
   right coronary
   right heart
   Rigiflex TTS balloon
   Ring-McLean
   Robinson
   Rodriguez-Alvarez
   Rosch
   rotatable pigtail
   Royal Flush angiographic flush
   Rsch-Uchida transjugular liver access needle-
   Rumel
   Sarns wire-reinforced
   Schneider-Shiley
   Schoonmaker multipurpose
   Schwarten balloon dilatation
   Sci-Med SSC "Skinny"
   Scott silicone ventricular
   Seldinger
   Seldinger cystic duct
   Seletz nonrigid ventricular
   sensing
   serrated
   shaver
   Shaw
   Sheldon
   Shiley-Ionescu
   SHJR4s (side-hole Judkins right, curve 4, short)
   short-arm Grollman
   side-hole
   sidewinder

catheter *(cont.)*
   Silastic
   silicone rubber Dacron-cuffed
   Silicore
   Simmons 1, 2, and 3
   Simplus PE/t dilatation
   Simpson peripheral AtheroCath
   Simpson Ultra Lo-Profile II balloon
   single-stage
   Skinny
   sliding rail
   Smec balloon
   snare
   Softip arteriography
   Softouch guiding
   Soft-Vu angiographic
   Soft-Vu Omni flush
   solid-state manometry
   SoloPass
   Sones Cardio-Marker
   Sones Hi-Flow
   Sones Positrol
   special steering
   Speedy balloon
   split sheath
   Squibb
   Stack perfusion coronary dilatation
   Stamey-Malecot
   standard Lehman
   steerable electrode
   steering
   Steerocath
   Stertzer guiding
   stimulating
   straight flush percutaneous
   subarachnoid
   subclavian
   subcutaneous ventricular reservoir
   subdural drainage
   SULP II
   sump

**catheter** *(cont.)*
- Swan-Ganz Guidewire TD
- Swan-Ganz Pacing TD
- Swan-Ganz thermodilution
- swan-neck
- TAC atherectomy
- Taut cystic duct
- TEC (transluminal endarterectomy)
- Teflon
- temporary pacing
- Tenckhoff peritoneal
- Tennis Racquet angiographic
- tetrapolar esophageal
- thermistor
- thermodilution
- thrombectomy
- thrombosuction
- Thruflex PTCA balloon
- toposcopic
- Torcon NB selective angiographic
- Total-Cross PTA
- Tracker
- transcutaneous extraction
- transducer-tipped
- transluminal endarterectomy (TEC)
- transluminal extraction (TEC)
- transseptal
- transvenous pacemaker
- trefoil balloon
- Triguide
- triple thermistor coronary sinus
- triple-lumen
- tripolar
- TTS (through-the-scope)
- tunneled
- Tygon
- ULP (ultra-low profile)
- UltraLite flow-directed micro-
- ultrasonographic
- umbilical
- UMI
- Ureflex

**catheter** *(cont.)*
- ureteral
- UroLume flow-directed micro-
- USCI Bard
- USCI Mini-Profile balloon dilatation
- valvuloplasty balloon
- Van Andel
- Van Tassel pigtail
- Variflex
- Vas-Cath PTA balloon
- venous
- venting
- Ventra PTA
- ventricular
- ventriculography
- VIPER PTA
- Vitalcor venous
- Voda
- Vygon Nutricath S
- Wanderer micro-
- Was-Cath
- washing
- water-infusion esophageal manometry
- Webster coronary sinus
- Webster orthogonal electrode
- Wexler
- Williams L-R guiding
- Wilton-Webster coronary sinus
- Wishard
- Witzel enterostomy
- Z-Med balloon
- Zucker

catheter advanced under fluoroscopic guidance
catheter artifact
catheter-borne transducer
catheter damping
catheter deployment
catheter exchanged over guide wire
catheter impact artifact

catheter-induced coronary artery
   spasm
catheterization
   cardiac
   Mullins modification of transseptal
   retrograde
   right heart
   selective
   simultaneous right and left heart
   superselective
   transnasal
   transseptal
catheter kinking
catheter mapping
catheter migration
catheter sheath
catheter-skin interface
catheter tip hockey-stick appearance
catheter tip motion artifact
catheter-tipped manometer
catheter-tissue contact
catheter with preformed curves
catheter whip artifact
CathTrack catheter locator system
CAT scan (computerized [or computed] axial tomography)
   enhanced
   nonenhanced
CAT scan cradle
CAT scan gantry
cat scratch disease
Catterall classification
cauda equina compression syndrome
caudad
caudal branch
caudal collaterals
caudal-cranial angulation
caudal regression
caudal tilt
caudal view
caudate nucleus
caudothalamic groove

cauliflower appearance
cauliflower-shaped filling defect
cava, juxtarenal
caval-atrial (or cavoatrial) junction
caval-pulmonary artery anastomosis
caval snare
caval tourniquet
CAVB (complete atrioventricular block)
cavernous angioma
cavernous angiosarcoma
cavernous sinus meningioma
cavitary mass
cavitary squamous cell carcinoma
cavitary tuberculosis
cavitating carcinoma
cavitating pattern
cavitation
cavity
   abdominal
   abdominopelvic
   absorption
   air
   amniotic
   ancyroid (also ankyroid)
   axillary
   body
   buccal
   chest
   cleavage
   coexistent
   cotyloid
   cranial
   crown
   endometrial
   epamniotic
   epidural
   funnel-shaped
   glenoid
   lung
   joint
   marrow

cavity *(cont.)*
　Meckel
　medullary
　oral
　pericardial
　peritoneal
　pleural
　popliteal
　pulmonary
　retroperitoneal
　saclike
　septum pellucidum
　sigmoid
　subarachnoid
　subdural
　synovial
　syringomyelic
　syrinx
　thoracic
　trigeminal
　tubular
　uterine
cavoatrial (caval-atrial) junction
cavogram
cavography
cavovalgus
　pes
　talipes
cavovarus
　pes
　talipes
cavovarus deformity
cavus
　global
　local
　pes
　post-traumatic
　talipes
cavus deformity
Cayler syndrome
CBF (cerebral blood flow)
CBI (convergent beam irradiation)

CBI stereotactic ring
CBT (corticobulbar tract)
CBV (cerebral blood volume)
CBV/CBF ratio
cc (cubic centimeter)
C-C (convexo-concave) heart valve
CCA (common carotid artery)
CCD (central collodiaphyseal) angle
CCD photodetectors
CCF (carotid cavernous fistula)
CCTA (coronal computed tomographic arthrography)
CD (Crohn disease)
CDAI (Crohn disease activity index)
CDC (Crohn disease of colon)
CDCA (chenodeoxycholic acid)
CDE (common duct exploration)
CDH (congenital dislocation [or dysplasia] of hip)
CDI (color Doppler imaging)
CE (capital epiphysis) angle of Wiberg
CE (cardioesophageal) junction
C-E amplitude of mitral valve
CEA (carcinoembryonic antigen)
CEA scan for colorectal carcinoma
cecal appendage
cecal serosa
cecal sphincter
cecal volvulus
cecum (caecum)
　antimesocolic side of
　coned
　mobile
　subhepatic
Cedell fracture of talus
Cedell-Magnusson classification of arthritis on x-ray
Ceelen-Gellerstedt syndrome
Cegka sign
CeI scintillator
celiac and mesenteric arteriography

celiac angiography
celiac artery compression syndrome
celiac axis syndrome
celiac ganglia
celiac plexus
celiac trunk
celiectasia
celioma
CEM (central extensor mechanism)
Cemax/Icon scanner
Cemax PACS platform
cement
   acrylic bone
   hydroxyapatite (HA)
   Implast bone
   methyl methacrylate
   orthopedic
   polymerized
   radiopaque bone
   surface
cementation
cementifying fibroma
cement line
cement mantle
cemento-ossifying fibroma
Cencit surface scanner
center
   anechoic
   ciliospinal center of Budge
   cortical
   diaphyseal
   emetic
   growth center of bone
   ossification
Center of Metabolic and Experimental Imaging
centigray (cGy)
centimeter (cm)
central axis depth dose
central canal
central collodiaphyseal angle (CCD)
central intraluminal saturation stripe
central motor pathways disease
central nervous system (CNS)
central neurogenic hyperventilation
central point artifact
central rays
central splanchnic venous thrombosis (CSVT)
central tegmental tract
central venous pressure (CVP) line
centriciput
centrilobular emphysema
centrilobular region of liver
centrilobular shadow
centroparietal head region
centrum commune
centrum ovale
centrum semiovale
cephalad
cephalic angulation
cephalic index
cephalic presentation of fetus
cephalic vein
cephalization of blood flow
cephalocaudad length
cephalofacial proportionality
cephalohematocele
cephalohematoma, parietal
cephalometry
cephalopelvic disproportion (CPD)
cephalopelvimetry
CeraSPECT camera
cerebellar degeneration
cerebellar disease
cerebellar fiber
cerebellar hemisphere
cerebellar hemorrhage
cerebellar herniation
cerebellar infarction
cerebellar mass
cerebellar pathway
cerebellar peduncle
cerebellar syndrome

cerebellar tonsillar herniation
cerebellar tract
cerebellar vermis
cerebellopontile angle (CPA) tumor
  (also cerebellopontine)
cerebellum
  dentate nucleus of
  midline
  petrosal
cerebral abscess
cerebral aneurysm
cerebral angiography
cerebral aqueduct
cerebral arteries
cerebral arteriography
cerebral arteriovenous fistula
cerebral atrophy
cerebral blood flow (CBF)
cerebral blood volume (CBV)
cerebral blood volume/cerebral blood
  flow ratio
cerebral brain death
cerebral brain flow
cerebral commissure
cerebral contusion
cerebral cortex
cerebral CT venography
cerebral dominance
cerebral dysfunction
cerebral dysrhythmia
cerebral edema
cerebral embolism
cerebral gigantism
cerebral hemidecortication
cerebral hemisphere
cerebral herniation
cerebral hypotension
cerebral infarct (infarction)
cerebral infundibulum
cerebral ischemia
cerebral ischemic event
cerebral mantle

cerebral metabolic rate for glucose
  (CMRglu)
cerebral metabolic rate of oxygen
  (CMRO$_2$)
cerebral metabolism
cerebral nocardiosis
cerebral operculum
cerebral parenchyma
cerebral peduncle
cerebral perfusion SPECT scan
cerebral revascularization
cerebral sign
cerebral SPECT
cerebral steal syndrome
cerebral thrombophlebitis
cerebral Whipple disease
cerebral white matter
cerebri (pl. of cerebrum)
  commotio
  contusio
  falx
  gliomatosis
  pseudotumor
cerebriform
cerebrohepatorenal syndrome
cerebromacular degeneration (CMD)
cerebromeningeal intracerebral
  hemorrhage
cerebropontocerebellar pathway
cerebrospinal fluid (CSF)
cerebrospinal fluid-containing lesion
cerebrospinal fluid fistula
cerebrospinal fluid flow measurement
cerebrospinal fluid leak study
cerebrospinal fluid pathway
cerebrovascular accident (CVA)
cerebrovascular occlusive disease
cerebrum (pl. cerebri)
  central cavity of
  cortex of
  first ventricle of
  great vein of

cerebrum *(cont.)*
　lateral ventricle of
　second ventricle of
　third ventricle of
Cerenkov calculation
Cerenkov measurement
Cerenkov radiation
Cerenkov scintillation analysis
Ceretec imaging agent
cerium silicate imaging agent
cervical aorta syndrome
cervical aortic arch
cervical CT (computed tomography)
cervical disk disease
cervical dorsal outlet syndrome
cervical esophagus
cervical fracture
cervical intervertebral foraminal MR phlebography (CMRP)
cervical mover ligament
cervical musculature
cervical myelogram
cervical myelopathy
cervical nerve root
cervical outlet
cervical pleura
cervical rib
cervical spine (C1 to C7 vertebrae)
cervical spine dens view
cervical spondylosis of the spinal cord
cervical spondylosis, washboard effect on myelography in
cervical triangle
cervicocerebral
cervicography
cervicomedullary junction
cervico-occipital fusion
cervicothoracolumbar
cervicotrochanteric fracture
cervigram
cervix uteri

CES (cauda equina syndrome)
cesium chloride imaging agent
Céstan-Chenais syndrome
cestodic tuberculosis
CF or CX (circumflex) artery
CFR (coronary flow reserve)
CGI (common gateway interface)
CGR biplane angiographic system
cGy (centigray)
Chaddock sign
Chagas disease
chain, obturator nodal
chain of lakes sign
chalasia
chalk (or chalky) bones
challenge
　acetazolamide
　hypotensive
chamber
　cardiac
　false aneurysmal
　infundibular
　ionization
　irradiation
　left atrial
　left ventricular
　right atrial
　right ventricular
　rudimentary outlet
　well-type ionization
　Wilson cloud
chamber compression
chamber dilatation
chamber enlargement
chamber of heart
Chamberlain line
Chamberlain-Towne view
champagne-bottle legs in Charcot-Marie-Tooth disease
Chance spinal fracture
Chandra-Khetarpal syndrome

change (pl. changes)
  cystic
  degenerative
  dystrophic
  ECMO-induced
  fibrotic
  fMRI signal
  focal degenerative
  lytic
  osteoarthritic
  paroxysmal
  pre-slip
  radiation-induced
  residual-limb shape
  spondylitic
  vasomotor
change-coupled device
channel (pl. channels)
  blood
  central
  deep venous
  enlarged vascular
  gastric
  pancreaticobiliary common
  pyloric
Chaput tubercle
character cell terminal
characteristic, echo
charcoal trap
Charcot-Bouchard intracerebral
  microaneurysm
Charcot chondroma
Charcot cirrhosis
Charcot-Marie-Tooth disease
Charcot joint
Charcot triad
charge-coupled device digitizer
charged particles
chauffeur's fracture
Chauffard point
Chausse view
CHD (congenital heart disease)

check-valve sheath
Chédiak-Higashi syndrome
cheek bone
cheese handler's (or washer's) disease
cheiromegaly
cheirospasm
chemically induced dynamic nuclear
  polarization
chemical-selective fat saturation MR
chemical-shift artifact
chemical-shift phenomena artifact
chemical-shift ratio
chemiluminescence
chemodectoma
chemoembolization
  therapeutic
  transcatheter arterial
  transcatheter oily
Chemo-Port catheter
chemoradiation therapy
chemotherapy
  adjuvant
  CT-guided intra-arterial
  intra-arterial
  multiagent
  neoadjuvant
  superselective intra-arterial
Chen-Smith image coder
Cherry keyboard
CHESS method
chest
  alar (flat)
  barrel
  blast
  cobbler's
  cylindrical
  flail
  foveated
  funnel
  globular
  hollow
  keeled

chest *(cont.)*
  paralytic
  phthinoid (flat)
  pigeon
  pounding
  pterygoid (flat)
  symmetrical
  tetrahedron
chest tube
  apically directed
  atelectasis following removal of
chest wall paradoxical motion
chest x-ray (CXR), baseline
Chester disease
chevron bone
CHF (congenital hepatic fibrosis)
CHF (congestive heart failure)
Chiari-Budd syndrome
Chiari-Foix-Nicolesco syndrome
Chiari II malformation
chiasmal compression
chiasm of digits of hand
chicken breast
chicken-fat clot
chickenpox pneumonia
Chilaiditi sign
Child classification of esophageal
    varices
chip
  cancellous bone
  corticocancellous bone
chip fracture
chiropractic x-ray films
chisel fracture
choana cerebri
choanal
cholangiocarcinoma, peripheral (PCC)
Cholangiocath
cholangiocatheter
cholangiofibromatosis
cholangiogram

cholangiography
  balloon
  catheter
  Chiba percutaneous
  common duct
  contrast selective
  cystic duct
  drip infusion (DIC)
  endoscopic retrograde (ERC)
  fine-needle percutaneous
    transhepatic (PTHC)
  fine-needle transhepatic (FNTC)
  HASTE MR
  intraoperative
  intravenous (IVC)
  magnetic resonance (MRC)
  operative
  Oriental
  transhepatic (THC)
  recurrent pyogenic (RPC)
  serial
  single-shot MR
  T-tube (TTC)
  transjugular
cholangiopancreatography
  endoscopic
  magnetic resonance (MR)
  retrograde (ERCP)
cholangiovenous communication
cholangitis
  acute obstructive
  ascending
  chronic nonsuppurative destructive
  fibrous obliterative
  intrahepatic sclerosing
  nonsuppurative
  primary sclerosing (PSC)
  progressive suppurative
  sclerosing
  septic
  suppurative
Cholebrine imaging agent

cholecystectasia
cholecystitis
  acalculous
  acute
  calculous
  chronic
  emphysematous
  gaseous
  perforated
cholecystitis with cholelithiasis
cholecystocholangiogram
cholecystocholangiography
cholecystoduodenal ligament
cholecystogram, oral (OCG)
cholecystography
cholecystokinetic food
cholecystokinin (CCK)
cholecystokinin-pancreozymin (CCK-PZ)
cholecystolithiasis
cholecystopathy
cholecystoptosis
cholecystostomy
  percutaneous transhepatic
  ultrasound-guided percutaneous
choledochal cyst
choledochocele
choledocholithiasis
cholelith
cholelithiasis
cholelithoptysis
cholescintigram
cholescintigraphy, morphine augmented
cholestatic liver disease
cholesteatoma
cholesterol embolization
  diffuse
  disseminated
cholesterolosis of gallbladder
Cholografin meglumine imaging agent
chololith (cholelith)
chondral fragment
chondrification

chondroblastoma
chondrodiastasis
chondrodystrophia calcificans
chondrodystrophia fetalis
chondrofibroma
chondrogenic tumor
chondroid matrix
chondroitin sulfate iron colloid (CSIS) enhanced MRI
chondrolipoma
chondrolysis
chondroma
  Charcot
  juxtacortical
chondromalacia patellae
chondromatosis
  Henderson-Jones
  synovial
chondromatous hamartoma
chondromyofibroma
chondromyxoid fibroma (CMF)
chondromyxoma
chondromyxosarcoma
chondronecrosis
chondro-osteodystrophy
chondrophyte
chondroporosis
chondrosarcoma
chondrosarcomatosis
chondrosteoma
chondrosternal junction
Chopart ankle dislocation
Chopart joint
Choquet fuzzy integral
chorda (pl. chordae)
  basal
  cleft
  commissural
  first order
  second order
  strut
  third order

chorda magna
chorda tympani
chordae tendineae cordis
chordae Willisii
chordal rupture
chordocarcinoma
chordoepithelioma
chordosarcoma
choriocarcinoma
chorionic villus sampling
choroid glomera
choroid plexus papilloma (CPP)
choroidal fissure
choroidal pericallosal artery
Christmas tree appearance on MR
chromatographic separations
chromium (Cr)
    Cr-HIDA chelate
    Cr-HIDA imaging agent
    $^{51}$Cr-labeled red blood cells
chromium-labeled red blood cells
chronologic age
Churg-Strauss syndrome
Ci (curie)
CI (continuous imaging), Aspire
CID camera
Cidtech camera
CIG (cardiointegram)
cigarette smoking, pack-years of
CIIP (chronic idiopathic intestinal pseudo-obstruction)
ciliary ganglion
ciliated border
ciliospinal center of Budge
cineangiocardiography
cineangiogram
cineangiography
    aortic root
    biplane
    coronary
    left anterior oblique (LAO)
    left posterior oblique (LPO)

cineangiography *(cont.)*
    left ventricular (LV)
    radionuclide
    right anterior oblique (RAO)
    right posterior oblique (RPO)
    selective coronary
    Sones technique for
    ventricular
cine-based viewing
cinecardioangiography
cine CT (computed tomography) scanner
cinedefecogram
cine-esophagogram
cinefluorography
cinefluoroscopy
cine gradient-echo MR imaging
cine (high frame-rate) mode
cine-loop
cine magnetic resonance tagging
Cine Memory with color flow Doppler imaging
cine PC imaging
cine projector, Tagarno 3SD (for angiography)
cineradiography
cine view in MUGA (multiple gated acquisition) scan
cineventriculogram
cineventriculography
cingulate gyrus
cingulate herniation
cingulate sulcus
cipher
    product
    transposition
circadian event recorder
circadian periodicity
circle
    arterial
    articular vascular
circle of Vieussens

circle of Weber
circle of Willis
Circon video camera
circuit
  anticoincidence
  application-specific integrated
    (ASIC)
  arrhythmia
  ASIC
  bypass
  coincidence
  doubly broadband triple resonance
    NMR probe
  macroreentrant
  magnetoresistive sensor
  microreentrant
  reentry
  shunting
circular muscles
circular plane
circular syncytium
circulation
  allantoic
  arrested
  assisted
  balanced
  cerebrospinal fluid
  codominant
  collateral
  compensatory
  cutaneous collateral
  derivative
  extracorporeal
  fetal
  greater
  intervillous
  peripheral
  placental
  spider-web
  systemic
  thebesian
circulation time

circulatory collapse
circulatory compromise
circulatory disturbance
circulatory embarrassment
circulatory failure
circulatory hyperkinetic syndrome
circulatory impairment
circulatory shock
circulatory stasis
circumference (of anatomical structure)
circumferential echodense layer
circumferential fracture
circumferentially
circumflex (circ., CF, CX)
circumflex artery
circumflex branches
circumflex coronary artery
circumflex groove artery
circumflex vessels
circumscribed edema
circumscribed infiltrate
circumscribed pleurisy
circumscript aneurysm
cirrhosis
  acholangic biliary
  acute juvenile
  alcoholic
  atrophic
  biliary
  Budd
  calculus
  cardiac
  Charcot
  cholangitic biliary
  congestive
  Cruveilhier-Baumgarten
  cryptogenic
  decompensated alcoholic
  diffuse septal
  end-stage
  fatty
  focal biliary

cirrhosis *(cont.)*
  frank
  glabrous
  Hanot
  hepatic
  hypertrophic
  Indian childhood
  juvenile
  Laënnec
  liver
  lung
  macrolobular
  macronodular
  medionodular
  metabolic
  microlobular
  micronodular
  multilobular
  nutritional
  obstructive biliary
  periportal
  pipe-stem
  portal
  posthepatic
  postnecrotic
  primary biliary (PBC)
  progressive familial
  pulmonary
  secondary biliary
  septal
  stasis
  Todd
  toxic
  unilobular
  vascular
cirrhotic
cirsoid aneurysm
CISS scheme
cistern
  ambient
  basal
  basal arachnoid

cistern *(cont.)*
  basilar
  carotid
  cerebellomedullary
  cerebellopontine
  chiasmatic
  chyle
  crural
  great
  increased basilar
  interpeduncular
  mesencephalic
  opticochiasmatic
  parasellar
  posterior
  prepontine
  quadrigeminal
  subarachnoidal
  trigeminal
cistern of chiasma
cistern of fossa of Sylvius
cistern of lamina terminalis
cistern of lateral fossa of cerebrum
cistern of Pecquet
cistern of Sylvius
cisternogram
cisternography
  air
  indium
  isotope
  metrizamide CT (MCTC)
  oxygen
  radioisotope
  radionuclide
CJD (Creutzfeldt-Jakob disease)
CKG (cardiokymography)
c-Ki-ras mutation
Clado point
Clarke-Hadefield syndrome
classification
  AAOS acetabular abnormalities
  acromioclavicular injury

classification *(cont.)*
Aitken epiphyseal fracture
Allman acromioclavicular injury
American Spinal Cord Injury Association
Anderson-D'Alonzo odontoid fracture
Antoni-A neurinoma
AO ankle fracture
AO-Danis-Weber ankle fracture
Arco
Arthritis Impact Measurement Scales
Bayne radial agenesis
Berndt-Harty talar lesion staging
Bleck metatarsus adductus
Bosniak
Boyd-Griffin trochanteric fracture
Brewlow malignant melanoma
Broders tumor index
Brooker periarticular heterotopic ossification (PHO)
Burwell-Charnley fracture reduction
Butcher staging
Caldwell-Moloy
Canale-Kelly talar neck fracture
Carnesale-Stewart-Barnes hip dislocation
Catterall
Cedell-Magnusson arthritis
Clark malignant melanoma
Colonna hip fracture
Copeland-Kavat metatarsophalangeal dislocation
Danis-Weber ankle fracture
D'Antonio acetabular
DeBakey aortic
Delbet hip fracture
Denis
Dickhaut-DeLee discoid meniscus
Dukes carcinoma

classification *(cont.)*
Essex-Lopresti calcaneal fracture
Evans intertrochanteric fracture
Ficat stage of avascular necrosis
Fielding-Magliato subtrochanteric fracture
FIGO staging of adenocarcinoma of endometrium
Fränkel spinal cord injury
Freeman calcaneal fracture
Fries score for rheumatoid arthritis
Frykman hand fracture
Garden femoral neck fracture
Gartland supracondylar fracture
Gertzbein seat belt injury
Grantham femur fracture
Gumley seat belt injury
Gustilo-Anderson tibial plafond fracture
Hahn-Steinthal capitellum fracture
Hansen fracture
Hardy-Clapham sesamoid
Hawkins talar neck fracture
Herbert-Fisher fracture system
Hohl tibial condylar fracture
Holdsworth spinal fracture
Hughston Clinic injury
Hunt-Hess aneurysm
Hunt-Kosnik
Hyams grading of esthesioneuroblastoma
Ingram-Bachynski hip fracture
Jackson and Parker (of Hodgkin lymphoma)
Jahss dislocation
Jeffery radial fracture
Jewett bladder carcinoma
Jones
Judet epiphyseal fracture
Kalamchi-Dawe congenital tibial deficiency
Kernohan brain tumor

classification *(cont.)*
Key-Conwell pelvic fracture
Kiel non-Hodgkin lymphoma
Kilfoyle condylar fracture
King classification of thoracic scoliosis
Kistler subarachnoid hemorrhage
Klatskin tumor
Kocher-Lorenz capitellum fracture
Kostuik-Errico spinal stability
Kyle fracture
Lauge-Hansen ankle fracture
Lukes-Butler non-Hodgkin lymphoma
Mason radial fracture
Mazur ankle evaluation
McLain-Weinstein spinal tumor
Merland perimedullary arteriovenous fistula
Meyers-McKeever tibial fracture
Milch elbow fracture
Modic
MSTS (Musculoskeletal Tumor Society) staging system
Mueller humerus fracture
multiaxial
Neer shoulder fractures I, II, and III
Neer-Horowitz humerus fracture
Nevaiser frozen shoulder
Newman radial fracture
Nurick spondylosis
NYHA (New York Heart Association) congestive heart failure
O'Brien radial fracture
Ogden epiphyseal fracture
Olerud and Molander fracture
Ovadia-Beals tibial plafond fracture
osteoarthritis grading
Pauwel femoral neck fracture
Pipkin femoral fracture
Poland epiphyseal fracture
Rappaport lymphoma

classification *(cont.)*
Ratliff avascular necrosis
Riordan club hand
Riseborough-Radin intercondylar fracture
Rockwood acromioclavicular injury
Rowe calcaneal fracture
Rowe-Lowell fracture-dislocation
Ruedi-Allgower tibial plafond fracture
Russell-Rubinstein cerebrovascular malformation
Rye Hodgkin disease
Sage-Salvatore acromioclavicular joint injury
Sakellarides calcaneal fracture
Salter-Harris fracture
Salter-Harris-Rang epiphyseal fracture
Schatzker fracture
Seinsheimer femoral fracture
Shelton femur fracture
Smith sesamoid position
Sorbie calcaneal fracture
Steinbrocker rheumatoid arthritis
Steinert epiphyseal fracture
Steward-Milford fracture
talocalcaneal index
Thompson-Epstein femoral fracture
TNM (tumor size, nodal involvement, metastatic progress)
Tronzo intertrochanteric fracture
Trunkey fracture
Vostal radial fracture
Watanabe discoid meniscus
Watson-Jones
Wiberg patellar types
Wilkins radial fracture
Winquist-Hansen femoral fracture
Wolfe breast carcinoma
Zickel fracture
Zlotsky-Ballard acromioclavicular injury

Claude syndrome
clavicle
clavicular head of sternocleidomastoid
clavicular notch
clavipectoral fascia
clawfoot deformity
  pes arcuatus
  pes cavus
claw hand (or clawhand)
clawtoe deformity
Claybrook sign
clay shoveler's fracture
CLC (Clerc-Levy-Cristeco) syndrome
clean shadow
clearance, aerosol
clearance curve
clearance half-time
clear zone
cleavage fracture
cleavage plane, subintimal
cleaving, plaque
Cleeman sign
cleft
  anal
  branchial
  first visceral
  gill
  interinnominoabdominal
  meniscal
  pudendal
  retrosomatic
  synaptic
  ventricular
cleft chordae
cleidocranial dysostosis
Cleland ligament in the hand
clenched fist view
Clerc-Levy-Cristeco (CLC) syndrome
clinical correlation
clinical sequelae
clinicopathological analysis
clinodactyly

clinoid ligament
clip
  aneurysm
  metallic
  surgical
clivus, Blumenbach
clivus meningioma tumor
CLO (congenital lobar overinflation)
cloacal anomaly
clockwise whirlpool sign
clonogen number
clonogenicity
C-loop of duodenum
closed-break fracture
closed dislocation
closed fracture
close-up view
closure
  growth center
  native aortic valve
  physeal
  threatened vessel
  tricuspid valve
  valve
clot
  agonal (or agony)
  blood
  chicken fat
  marantic
  passive
  preformed
  subarachnoid
  subdural
clot-filled lumen
clot lysis
clouding, alveolar
cloudy swelling of heart
Cloverleaf catheter
cloverleaf deformity
cloverleaf-shaped lumen
cloverleaf skull
clubfoot deformity

clubhand deformity
club-shaped (anatomical structure)
clumsy-hand syndrome
cluneal nerve
cluster plots
clustered microcalcifications
clustering algorithm
clusters, K-means
cm (centimeter)
CMD (cerebromacular degeneration)
CMF (chondromyxoid fibroma)
CMR (congenital mitral regurgitation)
CMRglu (cerebral metabolic rate for glucose)
$CMRO_2$ (cerebral metabolic rate of oxygen glucose metabolite)
CMRP (cervical intervertebral foraminal MR phlebography)
CMT (Charcot-Marie-Tooth) disease
CMV (cytomegalovirus)
C/N (contrast-to-noise) ratio
CNS (central nervous system)
$CO_2$ (carbon dioxide)
  $CO_2$ angiography
  $CO_2$ cylinder
  $CO_2$ generator
  $CO_2$ insufflation
  $CO_2$ laser
  $CO_2$ negative contrast media
  $CO_2$ retention
CO (cardiac output) (L/min)
coagulation, disseminated intravascular
coal miner's (also coal worker's) lung
coalesce
coalescence
coalition
  bony
  calcaneonavicular
  carpal
  fibrous
  intercarpal

coalition *(cont.)*
  lunate-triquetral
  Minaar classification of
  osseous
  talocalcaneal
  tarsal
coaptation point
coapted leaflets
coarctation
  aortic
  atypical
  atypical subisthmic
  congenital isthmic
  isthmic
  juxtaductal
coarctation of aorta
  adult-type
  infantile-type
  juxtaductal
  postductal
  preductal
  reversed
coarctation, reversed
coaxial catheter, Hieshima
coaxial steering
coaxial Tracker catheter
cobalt-chromium alloy
cobalt radioactive source
cobalt-60 beam
cobalt-60 gamma knife radiosurgical treatment
cobbler chest syndrome
cobblestone appearance
cobblestone pattern
Cobb scoliosis angle
Cobb syndrome
Cobra (and Cobra 2) catheter
cobra-head appearance
cobra-head effect
Cobra over-the-wire balloon catheter
cobweb appearance
cobweb pattern

coccidioidal granuloma
coccidioidoma
coccidioidomycosis
   desert
   disseminated
   latent
   Posadas-Wernicke
   primary
   progressive
   San Joaquin Valley
   secondary
   valley
coccygeal body
coccygeal bone
coccygeal spine
coccygeopubic diameter
coccyx
Cockayne syndrome
cocking injury
cock-up deformity of toe
Co-Cr-Mo (cobalt-chromium-molybdenum) alloy implant metal
Co-Cr-W-Ni (cobalt-chromium-tungsten-nickel) alloy implant metal
COD (computerized optical densitometry)
coder
   Chen-Smith
   ICS (improved Chen-Smith)
codfish vertebrae
codivilla extension
Codman angle
Codman sign
Codman triangle
codominant circulation
codominant system
codominant vessel
Codonics color printer
coefficient
   absorption
   attenuation
   beta-spectra shapefactor

coefficient *(cont.)*
   curve fit
   diffusion
   linear absorption
   linear attenuation
   mass attenuation
   partition
   stiffness
coeur en cuirasse
coeur en sabot
coffee worker's lung
coherent scattering
coil
   aneurysmal
   birdcage
   birdcage-type head
   body
   collagen-filled interlocking detachable
   crossed
   defibrillation
   detachable
   double breast
   endoanal
   endorectal
   endoscopic quadrature RF
   endovascular
   flexible surface
   GDC (Guglielmi detachable)
   Gianturco occlusion
   Gianturco wool-tufted wire
   Golay
   gradient
   gradient sheet
   Guglielmi detachable (GDC)
   head
   Helmholtz
   immediately detachable
   interlocking detachable
   liver
   Medrad Mrinnervu endorectal colon probe

coil (cont.)
   modified birdcage
   opposed loop-pair quadrature NMR
   orthogonal RF
   platinum
   quadrature RF receiver
   radiofrequency (RF)
   receiver
   RF (radiofrequency)
   right ventricular
   saddle
   sensing
   shim
   solenoid surface
   surface
   three-axis gradient
   torso phased-array (TPAC)
coiled spring appearance of intussuscepted bowel
coil embolization (therapeutic)
coil-tipped catheter
coil-to-vessel diameter
coincidence circuit
coincidence-summing correction
coin lesion
COLD (chronic obstructive lung disease)
cold nodule
cold spot myocardial imaging
colic impression on the liver
Colinet-Caplan syndrome
colitis
   chronic ulcerative (CUC)
   Crohn
   familial ulcerative
   focal
   fulminant
   fulminating ulcerative
   granulomatous transmural
   ischemic
   mucous

colitis (cont.)
   myxomembranous
   pseudomembranous (PMC)
   radiation
   radiation-induced
   regional
   single-stripe (SSC)
   transmural
   ulcerative (UC)
colitis polyposa
colitis ulcerosa gravis
collagen-filled interlocking detachable coils
collagen tissue proliferation
collagen vascular disease
collapse (of anatomical structure)
collar
   implant
   periosteal bone
collar bone
collar-button abscess
collar-button appearance in colon
collateral
   bridging
   porto-azygos
   retrograde
   septal
collateral blood flow
collateral blood supply
collateral branch
collateral channel
collateral circulation
collateral eminence
collateralization
collateral ligament
collateral sulcus
collateral system
collateral vessel
collecting system
collection of contrast material
Colles fracture
Colles ligament

Collet-Sicard syndrome
collicular fracture
colliculus (pl. colliculi)
   facial
   seminal
collimated
collimation
   detector
   dynamic multileaf
   tertiary
collimation CT
collimation scanning
collimation width
collimator
   APC-3
   APC-4
   converging
   diverging
   Eureka
   fan beam
   Leur-par
   long bore
   Machlett
   Micro-CAST
   multileaf
   multirod
   parallel-hole
   pinhole
   slant hole
   Summit LoDose
collimator exchange effect
collimator helmet
collimator plugging pattern
collimator scatter
collision, inelastic
colloid cystic tumor
colloid oncotic pressure (COP)
colloid shift on scan
colocolic anastomosis
colocolic intussusception
colocutaneous fistula
cology, CT

Colombo count
colon
   anterior band of
   ascending
   descending
   distal
   free band of
   giant
   iliac
   inflammation of
   lateral reflection of
   lead-pipe
   left
   mega-
   mesosigmoid
   midsigmoid
   pelvic
   perisigmoid
   right
   sigmoid
   spastic
   transverse
colonic diverticulum
colonic haustra
colonic motility
colonic pit
colonic polyp
Colonlite bowel prep
colonoscopy, virtual
coloptosis
color amplitude imaging
color-coded duplex sonography
color-coded pulmonary blood flow image
color-coded real-time sonography
color correction, multi-illuminant
color Doppler imaging (CDI)
color Doppler ultrasound
color duplex interrogation
color duplex sonography
color duplex ultrasound-guided percutaneous transluminal angioplasty

colorectal (CR) mucosa
color flow Doppler
color flow Doppler real-time 2-D (two-dimensional) blood flow imaging
color flow duplex imaging
color flow mapping
colorimetric color reproduction
color power transcranial Doppler sonography
color reproduction, colorimetric
color space, C-Y
color space conversion
color space interpolator
color ultrasound
colosigmoid resection
colovaginal fistula
colovesical fistula
colpocele
colpoptosis
column
  anal
  anterior gray (of spinal cord)
  Bertin
  branchial efferent
  Clarke
  contrast medium
  Lissauer
  renal
  variceal
  vertebral
column extraction method
columning of dye
column mode sinogram images
column of Burdach
column of dye
column of Morgagni
CoLyte bowel prep
combination flow and pressure loads
combined flexion phenomenon
combined-modality radiation therapy
combined leukocyte-marrow imaging
combined multisection diffuse-weighted and hemodynamically weighted echo planar MR imaging
combined Myoscint/thallium imaging
combined thallium-Tc-HMPAO imaging
comma sign in truncus arteriosus
comminuted bursting fracture
comminuted fracture
commissural attachments
commissural chordae
commissural leaflet
commissural point
commissure
  anterior (AC)
  anteroseptal
  cerebral
  fused
  gray commissure of spinal cord
  posterior (PC)
  scalloped
  tectum
  valve
  vestigial
  white commissure of spinal cord
common bile duct (CBD)
common carotid artery (CCA)
common cavity phenomenon
common duct cholangiogram
common duct stone
common femoral artery
common gateway interface (CGI)
common iliac artery
communicating hydrocephalus
communicating vein
communication
  asyndetic
  interatrial
communis, extensor digitorum
Comolli sign
compact bone

comparison
  histopathologic
    yield
comparison view
compartment
  anterior
  anterior mediastinal
  deep posterior
  extensor
  extradural
  infracolic
  infratentorial
  lateral
  medial
  patellofemoral
  plantar
  posterior
  posterolateral
  posteromedial
  superficial posterior
  supracolic
compartment lesion, posterior
compartment syndrome
Compass stereotactic frame
compatible
compensated composite spin-lock pulse
compensated congestive heart failure
compensation
  cardiac
  cardiac gating
  respiratory
  scatter
  section-select flow
compensator
  scattering foil
  tissue deficit
compensatory emphysema
compensatory enlargement
compensatory hypertrophy
competent valve
competitive adsorption

complete atrioventricular block
complete atrioventricular dissociation
complete bladder emptying
complete dislocation
complete fracture
complete heart block
complex
  ankle joint (AJC)
  anterior communicating artery
  apical
  arcuate
  atrial
  auricular
  capsulolabral
  caudal pharyngeal
  diisocyanide-triisocyanide $^{99m}$Tc
  discoligamentous
  Eisenmenger
  fabellofibular
  foot–ankle
  gadolinium
  gastrocnemius–soleus
  gastroduodenal artery
  Ghon
  hallux valgus–metatarsus primus varus
  hindfoot joint
  hippocampal-amygdaloid
  ligamentous
  MION-gene
  nipple-areola
  oxidized
  primary
  Ranke
  sesamoid
  sling ring
  subluxation
  superior olivary
  syndesmotic ligament
  tibiocalcaneal joint
  triangular fibrocartilage
  vertebrobasilar

complex blocking
complex dynamic pharyngeal and
   speech evaluation by cine recording
complex electron arc therapy
compound dislocation
compound fracture
compression
   aqueduct
   fingerprint image
   image
   interfragmental
   manual
   multiplanar
   nerve root
   plaque
   radicular
   root
   spot
   thermal
   wavelet
compression atelectasis
compression fracture (burst)
compression plate and screws
compression ratio
compression syndrome
compression ultrasonography
compromise
   circulatory
   respiratory
compromised flow
Compton scattering cross-section
Compton suppression spectrometer
Compuscan Hittman computerized
   electrocardioscanner
computed axial tomography (CAT)
   scan
computed ejection fraction
computed radiograph
computed sonography, Acuson
computed tomographic angiography
   (CTA)
computed tomography (see *CT*)
computed tomography angiographic
   portography (CTAP)
computed tomography dose index
   (CTDI)
computed tomography during arterial
   portography (CTAP)
computed tomography scan (see *CT*)
computed transmission tomography
computer-aided design (CAD)
computer-aided diagnosis scheme
computer, Aspect
computer-assisted intracranial navigation
computer-assisted stereotactic resection of deep-seated and superficial
   lesions
computer-assisted volumetric stereotactic resrection
computer-generated images
computerized (or computed)
   tomography (CT)
computerized axial tomography
   (CAT) with contrast
computerized axial tomography
   (CAT) without contrast
computerized cranial tomography
   (CCT)
computerized optical densitometry
   (COD)
computerized tomographic hepatic
   angiography (CTHA)
computerized tomography guidance
   for placement of radiation therapy
   fields
computerized tomography guidance
   for stereotactic localization
computerized tomography-guided
   needle biopsy
computerized transverse axial
   tomography (CTAT)
computer subtraction techniques
conal papillary muscle

concatenation
Concato disease
concave
concavity
concentric hourglass stenosis
concentric hypertrophy
concept, gooseneck
concha (pl. conchae)
concomitant boost radiotherapy
concordant results
concretion
   bile
   fecal
conducting loop, closed
conductive development
conductivity, vascular hydraulic
conduit
   detour
   ileal
conduit valve
condylar fracture
condylar lift-off, fluoroscopy-guided
condyle
   external
   femoral
   lateral
   medial
   occipital
   tibial
condyloid joint
C1-C5 segments of internal carotid artery
C1-C7 cervical vertebrae
cone
   arterial
   bevelled electron beam
cone and socket bone
cone-beam image
cone-beam reconstruction algorithm
cone disk
cone-down (coned-down) view
coned-down appearance of colon

cone view
configuration
   back-to-back
   biventricular
   dome and dart (on cardiac catheterization)
   horizontal dipole
   stellate
   winged
conformal neutron and photon radiotherapy
conformal radiation therapy
congenital absence
congenital anomaly
congestion
   active
   asymmetric pulmonary
   capillary
   cardiac
   centrilobular
   cerebral
   chronic passive
   hepatic
   hypostatic
   intravascular
   passive vascular
   pulmonary vascular
   splenic
   symmetric
   vascular
   venous
congestive atelectasis
congestive cardiomyopathy
congestive cirrhosis
congestive heart failure (CHF)
conglomerate calcification
congruity, joint
conical heart
conjoined
conjugate diameter
conjugate gradients
conjugate overshooting

conjugate, true
Conn syndrome
connection, ISDN (teleradiology)
connective tissue
  areolar
  dense
  peribronchial
  regular
  reticular
  subcutaneous
connective tissue proliferation
connective tissue septa
conoid ligament
conotruncal anomaly, congenital
conoventricular defect
Conrad-Bugg trapping of soft tissue in ankle fracture
Conradi-Hünermann syndrome
Conray imaging agent
Conray-60 imaging agent
Conray-280 imaging agent
consecutive dislocation
console
  Bruker
  SMIS
consolidated infiltrate
consolidation
  air-space
  alveolar
  bilateral
  confluent
  dense
  exudative
  ill-defined
  lobar
  lung parenchyma
  nonhomogeneous
  parenchymal
  patchy air-space
  peripheral
  pulmonary
  segmental
  unilateral

consolidative change
consolidative pneumonia
conspicuity
constant, Planck
constant tilt wave
constellation of findings; symptoms
constitutional symptoms
constriction
  airway
  hourglass
  occult pericardial
  postglomerular arteriolar
  tangential
construction artifact
constriction band syndrome
contact B-scan ultrasound
contents
  abdominal
  bone mineral (BMC)
  bowel
  brain water
  digestive tract
  gastric
  intestinal
contiguous images (in CT scan)
contiguous slices
continuity of bone
continuous imaging (CI), Aspire
continuous wave (CW)
continuous wave Doppler echocardiography
continuous wave Doppler ultrasonography
continuous wave laser system
continuous wave high frequency Doppler ultrasound system
contour
  irregular hazy luminal
  isodose
  S
  scalloping
  undulating

contoured tilting compression
   mammography
contour extraction
contour following algorithm
contour mapping
contracted bladder
contracted gallbladder
contractile function
contraction
   cicatricial
   concentric
   peristaltic
   tertiary
contracture
   Dupuytren
   elbow
   fixed flexion
   flexion-adduction
   gastroc/soleus (gastrocnemius/
      soleus)
   hip flexion
   ischemic
   joint
   knee flexion
   muscle
   myocardial
   myostatic
   scar
   secondary
   soft tissue
   Volkmann ischemic
   web
contralateral
contrast-enhanced color Doppler
contrast-enhanced dynamic snapshot
contrast-enhanced hepatic CT
contrast-enhanced MR
contrast-enhanced power Doppler
contrast-enhanced radiographic
   examination
contrast-enhanced thoracic CT
contrast-enhanced ultrasound

contrast-filled stomach
contrast medium (pl. media) (see
   *imaging agent*)
contrast resolution
contrast-to-noise (C/N) ratio
contrast venography
contrast ventriculography
contrecoup fracture
control
   fluoroscopic
   image
   radiographic
   roentgenographic
contusion
conus arteriosus
conus artery
conus branch ostia
conus, club-shaped
conus ligament
conus medullaris
conus septum
conventionally fractionated stereotactic
   radiation therapy
conventional study
convergence zone
convergent beam irradiation
converging collimator
convergent color Doppler imaging
conversion
   color space
   spontaneous
converter
   analog-to-digital (A-to-D)
   digital-to-analog (D-to-A)
   motion-compensating format
   real-time format
convex linear array
convexity
convexobasia
convolution
   Arnold
   ascending frontal

convolution *(cont.)*
  ascending parietal
  Broca
  cerebral
  Gratiolet
  Heschl
  occipitotemporal
  Zuckerkandl
convolution mask
Cook arterial catheter
Coopernail sign
coordinate axis (pl. axes)
coordinate, Cartesian
coordinates (X, Y, and Z) for target lesion
COPD (chronic obstructive pulmonary disease)
Cope point
coplanar contour points
copper (Cu)
  $^{62}$Cu PTSM imaging agent
  $^{62}$Cu pyruvaldehyde-bis-(4N-thiosemicarbazone) imaging agent
  Cu/Zn (copper-zinc)-SOD
copper filtration
co-precipitation
coprolith
coprostasis
cor (heart)
cor adiposum
cor arteriosum
cor biloculare
cor bovinum
cor dextrum
cor mobile
cor pendulum
cor pulmonale (c. pulmonale)
coracoacromial arch
coracoacromial ligament
coracoacromial process
coracohumeral ligament
coracoid notch
coracoid process
coracoid tuberosity
cord
  condyle
  fibrous
  hepatic
  Lissauer tracts of spinal
  medullary
  pretendinous
  rostral spinal
  sacral spinal
  spermatic
  spinal
  tethered
  vocal
  Weitbrecht
cordate pelvis
cord compression
cord embarrassment
Cordis Brite Tip guiding catheter
Cordis Ducor brachial I, II, and III coronary catheter
Cordis-Ducor-Judkins catheter
Cordis multipurpose access port (MPAP)
Cordis Son-II catheter
Cordis tantalum stent
cordlike mass
Cordonnier ureteroileal loop
corduroy arteries
corduroy artifact
corduroy cloth pattern on myelogram
core biopsy needle
core, bone
coregistration, morphological and physiological image
cork handler's lung disease
corkscrew appearance
corkscrew esophagus
Cornelia de Lange syndrome
Cornell protocol (exercise stress testing)

cornflake esophageal motility study
corn oil and ferric ammonium citrate contrast imaging agent
cornu (pl. cornua)
coronal computed tomographic arthrography (CCTA)
coronal image, multi-echo
coronal maximum-intensity projection (MIPcor)
coronal orientation
coronal plane
coronal projection
coronal section
coronal slab
coronal slice
coronal suture
coronal synostosis
coronal view
coronary angiography
   left (LCA)
   right (RCA)
coronary artery (see *artery*)
coronary artery disease (CAD)
coronary artery ostia
coronary (artery) perfusion pressure (CPP)
cardonary artery scan (CAS)
coronary artery steal syndrome
coronary artery tree
coronary atherosclerosis
coronary balloon angioplasty
coronary bypass graft patency
coronary-cameral fistula
coronary cineangiography
coronary cusp
coronary fistula
coronary flow reserve (CFR)
coronary groove
coronary heart disease (CHD)
coronary sinus (CS)
coronary sinus of Valsalva
coronary spasm
coronary steal phenomenon
coronary steal syndrome
coronary-subclavian steal syndrome
coronary sulcus
coronoid fossa
coronoid process
Coroskop C cardiac imaging system
corpora cavernosography
corpora fornicis
corpora restiformia
corpus callosum
corpus Luysii
corpus sterni
corpus striatum
corpus uteri
correction
   accidental
   automatic motion
   coincidence-summing
   fuzzy logic contrast
   inhomogeneity
   multi-illuminant color
   Picker SPECT attenuation
   summing
   surface variable attenuation
   trend
correlation
   clinical
   functional
   histologic
   histopathologic-CT
   imaging-anatomic
   imaging-pathologic
   in vivo
   mammographic-histopathologic
   morphological
   radiologic-anatomic
   radiologic-pathologic
correlation algorithms (CR)
Correra line
Corrigan sign

corrugated air column
corset balloon catheter
cortex (pl. cortices)
   adrenal
   articular
   auditory
   bilateral orbital frontal
   bone
   calcarine
   cerebellar
   cerebral
   entorhinal
   femoral
   frontal
   lymphatic
   mesial-frontal
   motor
   nonolfactory
   opercular
   orbitofrontal
   ovarian
   parastriate
   parietal
   perirolandic parietal
   peristriate
   perisylvian
   premotor
   primary auditory
   primary visual
   pyriform
   renal
   rolandic
   sensorimotor
   somatosensory
   striate
   visual
cortical activity
cortical adenoma
cortical atrophy
cortical bone
cortical branch
cortical defect
cortical deficit
cortical dysfunction
cortical gray matter
cortical hinge axis
cortical hyperintensity
cortical hyperostosis
cortical infarcts
cortical intracerebral hemorrhage
cortical ischemia
cortical motor area
cortical necrosis
cortical scintigraphy
cortical sign
cortical signet ring shadow
cortical sulci
cortical thumb
cortical tuber
cortical versus cancellous bone
cortical white matter
corticated border
corticocallosal dysgenesis
corticocancellous strut
corticocerebellar connection
corticogram
corticography
corticomedullary junction
corticomedullary phase (CP)
corticospinal motor pathway
Corti organ
corundum smelter's lung
Corvisart syndrome
cosine transform
costa fluctuans decima
costae spuriae
costae verae
costal angle
costal bone
costal cartilage
costal groove
costal interarticular cartilage
costal margin
costal margin syndrome

costal notch
costal pleura
costal pleural reflection
costal process
costal sulcus
costal surface
costal tubercle
costocervical artery
costocervical trunk
costochondral joint
costochondral junction
costochondritis
costoclavicular syndrome; test
costodiaphragmatic recess
costolateral
costomediastinal recess
costophrenic (CP) angle blunting
costophrenic recess
costophrenic septal lines
costophrenic sulcus
costosternal angle
costotransverse joint
costovertebral angle (CVA)
costovertebral articulation
costovertebral joint
costoxiphoid ligament
COSY H-1 MR spectroscopy
cottage loaf appearance
Cotton ankle fracture
Cotton-Berg syndrome
cotyloid cavity
cotyloid notch
couch view
cough fracture of rib
coulomb (C)
Councill catheter
count
    Cerenkov
    direct liquid scintillation
counter
    Geiger
    proportional

counter-current aortography
counter-occluder
counterpulsation
counting, double-label
coup
Cournand cardiac catheter
course (of anatomical structure)
coursing of gas
Courvoisier gallbladder
covered Gianturco stent
coxa adducta
coxa brevis
coxa flexa
coxa magna
coxa plana
coxa saltans
coxa senilis
coxa valga
coxa vara luxans
CP (costophrenic) angle
CPA (cerebellopontile or cerebellopontine angle)
CPAD (chronic peripheral arterial disease)
CPB (cardiopulmonary bypass)
CPD (cephalopelvic disproportion)
CPI (conventional planar imaging)
CPMG sequence
c. pulmonale (cor pulmonale)
Cr (chromium)
CR (colorectal)
CR (computed radiology)
CR Bard catheter
CR-39 nuclear tract detector
crabmeat-like appearance
cranial and caudal angulations
cranial angled view
cranial nerves (12)
    I (olfactory)
    II (optic)
    III (oculomotor)
    IV (trochlear)

cranial nerves *(cont.)*
  V (trigeminal)
  VI (abducens)
  VII (facial)
  VIII (vestibulocochlear)
  IX (glossopharyngeal)
  X (vagus)
  XI (spinal accessory)
  XII (hypoglossal)
cranial nerve involvement
cranial suture
cranial vessel
cranial view
craniocaudad projection
craniocaudal view
craniocervical junction
craniofacial dysjunction fracture
craniomandibular syndrome
cranio-orbital deformity
craniopharyngioma tumor
craniosclerosis
craniospinal axis
craniospinal hemangioblastoma
craniosynostosis
craniovertebral junction
cranium
cranium bifidum occultum
crater, ulcer
creep, periosteal
cremasteric artery
crenulation
crescent artifact
crescentic lumen
crescent-in-doughnut sign (for intussusception)
crescent-shaped fibrocartilaginous disk
crescent sign
crest
  acoustic
  acousticofacial
  alveolar
  ampullary

crest *(cont.)*
  arched
  arcuate
  articular
  basilar
  buccinator
  conchal
  deltoid
  dental
  ethmoidal
  falciform
  frontal
  ganglionic
  gingival
  gyral
  iliac
  infundibuloventricular
  pubic
  sacral
  supraventricular
  terminal (of right atrium)
  tibial
  urethral
Creutzfeldt-Jakob disease
cribriform bone
cribriform plate
cribriform process
cricoarytenoid
cricoid cartilage
cricopharyngeal diverticulum
cricopharyngeal sphincter
cricopharyngeus muscle
cricothyroid cartilage
cricothyroid membrane
crinkle artifact
crinkling, mucosal
crisscross heart
criterion, error sum
CRL (crown-rump length)
Crohn disease (CD)
Crohn ileocolitis
Crohn regional enteritis

Cronkhite-Canada syndrome
cross-aortic
crossbridge cycle (cycling)
cross-collateralization
cross-correlation technique
crossed-coil design
crossed embolism
crossed-fused renal ectopia
crossed sciatica sign
crossed signs
cross-filling
cross ligament
cross-linked polystyrene (PET scan)
crossover of activity
cross-pelvic collateral vessel
cross-section, Compton scattering
cross-sectional image
cross-sectional zone
cross-table lateral film
cross-talk effect artifact
cross-union
Crouzon disease
crowding of bronchovascular markings
Crowe pilot point
crown artifact
crown, halo
crown-rump length (CRL)
CRT (cathode ray tube)
cruciate ligament
crura of diaphragm (left and right)
crus (leg) (pl. crura)
    diaphragmatic
    lateral
    left
    medial
    right
crushing-type injury
Cruveilhier ulcer
crux cordis (crux of heart)
cryolesion
cryomagnet

cryosurgery, map-guided
crypt
    anal
    enamel
    epithelium
    ileal
    Lieberkühn
    Luschka
    Morgagni
crystallography
CS (coronary sinus)
CSA (cross-sectional area)
CSDH (chronic subdural hematoma)
CSF (cerebrospinal fluid)
CSF-suppressed T2-weighted 3D MP-RAGE MR imaging
CSI (coronary stenosis index)
    CSI-enhanced MRI
    CSI spectroscopy
C sign
C-60 teletherapy
CSL (central sacral line)
C-spine (cervical spine)
CSS (carotid sinus syndrome)
CST (contraction stress test)
CST (corticospinal tract)
CT (cardiothoracic) ratio
CT (computed tomography)
    biphasic
    cine
    collimation
    contrast-enhanced
    dual energy
    dual-isotope single-photon
    electron-beam\
    enhanced
    expiratory
    helical
    helical thin-section
    high resolution
    high spatial resolution cine (HSRCCT)

CT (cont.)
  high temporal resolution cine
    (HTRCCT)
  indirect
  lipiodol
  multiphasic
  nonenhanced
  peripheral quantitative (pQCT)
  quantitative spirometrically
    controlled CT angiography with
    volume rendering
  single-photon emission (SPECT)
  sliding-thin-slab maximum intensity
    projection
  slip-ring
  SPECT (single-photon emission)
  spiral
  superselective angio-
  thallium-201 single-photon emission
  thin-section
  thin-slice
  three-dimensional processed
    ultrafast
  transmission
  triphasic spiral
  two-phase helical
  ultrafast
  water-contrast
  Z-dependent
CT arterial portography (CTAP)
CT arteriography
CT arthrography
CT attenuation value
CT bone window photography
CT cisternogram, metrizamide
  (MCTC)
CT colography
CT densitometry
CT-directed hook wire localization
CT fluoroscopy, real-time
CT gantry
CT-guided aspiration
CT-guided intra-arterial chemotherapy
CT-guided needle biopsy
CT-guided percutaneous biopsy
CT-guided PEG (percutaneous endo-
  scopic gastrostomy)
CT-guided stereotactic surgery
CT-guided transsternal core biopsy
CT-guided ultrasound
CT holography (CTH)
CT imaging error
CT laser mammography (CTLM)
CT Max 640 scanner
CT myelography
CT PEG (CT-guided percutaneous
  endoscopic gastrostomy)
CT peritoneography
CT reconstruction image
C-TRAK hand-held gamma detector
CT scan directed needle biopsy
CT scan with contrast
CT scanner (see *scanner*)
CT sialography
CT/SPECT fusion
CT stereotaxic guide
CT with MR, single-photon emission
CT9000 scanner
CT9800 scanner
CTA (computed tomographic
  angiography)
CTA dosimetry
CTA-2 (second scan CT arterial
  portography)
CTAP (computed tomography during
  arterial portography)
CTAP-1 (first scan CT arterial
  portography)
CTAT (computerized transverse axial
  tomography)
CTDI (computed tomography dose
  index)
CTH (computerized tomographic
  holography)

CTHA (computerized tomographic hepatic angiography)
CTI 933/04 ECAT scanner
CTI PET scanner
CTLM (computerized tomographic laser mammography)
CTLV (cross-table lateral view)
CT/MRI-compatible stereotactic head-frame
CT/MRI-defined tumor slice image
CT/MRI-defined tumor volume image
CTR (cardiothoracic ratio)
CTS (carpal tunnel syndrome)
CTT (central tegmental tract)
Cu (copper)
cube vertices
cubic centimeter (cc)
cubic convolution interpolation
cubic packing
cubic voxels
cubital fossa
cubital tunnel syndrome
cubitocarpal
cubitoradial
cubitus valgus
cubitus varus
cuboid bone
cubonavicular joint
cue
  biopsy
  exclusionary
  inclusionary
  preclusionary
cue-based image analysis
cuff
  aortic
  atrial
  inflow
  musculotendinous
  rectal muscle
  right atrial
  rotator
  suprahepatic caval

cuffing, peribronchial
cuff rupture
cul-de-sac
  Douglas
  dural
Cullen sign
culprit lesion
culprit vessel
cumulative effect
cuneiform bone of carpus
cuneiform fracture-dislocation
cuneiform joint
cuneiform mortise
cuneus
cup
  acetabular
  hip replacement
  migration of acetabular prosthesis
  retroversion of acetabular
cup-and-spill stomach
CUP (cancer of unknown primary)
cupula
  diaphragmatic
  pleural
curie (Ci)
Curix Capacity Plus film processing system
Curling ulcer
Curracino-Silverman syndrome
Currarino triad
current
  gradient drive
  pulsing
  tube
curvature (see also *curve*)
  angular
  anterior
  backward
  cervical
  dorsal kyphotic
  flattening of normal lordotic

curvature *(cont.)*
   gingival
   greater
   humpbacked spinal
   kyphotic
   lesser
   lumbar
   normal cervical
   radius of
   stomach
curvature anisotrophy
curvature of stomach
   greater
   lesser
curve (pl. curves)
   biphasic
   Bragg
   brightness-time
   cervical spine
   clearance
   depth-dose
   dilution
   dye dilution
   flattening of normal
   flow-time
   free induction delay
   gaussian
   glow
   isoclosed
   lumbar lordotic
   lung count
   normal lordotic
   pulmonary time activity
   renal flow
   renogram
   sigmoid
   signal intensity time
   spline
   superincumbent spinal
   thoracic spine
   time-attenuation
   time-density

curve *(cont.)*
   time-intensity
   videodensity
   washout
curved vessels
curve fit coefficient
curvilinear calcification
curvilinear defect
curvilinear subpleural lines
Cushing syndrome
Cushing ulcer
cushion defect
cushion, endocardial
Cu (copper)
cusp
   accessory
   anterior
   aortic
   asymmetric closure of
   conjoined
   coronary
   dysplastic
   fibrocalcific
   fishmouth
   fusion of
   intact valve
   left coronary
   left pulmonary
   mitral valve
   noncoronary
   perforated aortic
   posterior
   pulmonary valve
   right coronary
   ruptured aortic
   semilunar valve
   septal
   tricuspid valve
   valve
cusp degenerator
cusp motion
cusp shots (films)

custom block
custom shielding blocks
cut (pl. cuts)
   off-center
   tangential
   tomographic
cut and cine film
cut-film technique
Cuvier, canal of
CVA (cerebrovascular accident)
CVA (costovertebral angle)
CVBS (congenital vascular–bone syndrome)
CVIS imaging device
CVM (congenital vascular malformation)
CVM (cryptic vascular malformation)
CVP (central venous pressure) catheter
CX or CF (circumflex) artery
CX-1 metastases
CXR (chest x-ray), baseline
C wave pressure on right atrial catheterization
cyanocobalamin radioactive agent
cyberradiology
Cyberware system
cycle
   aberrant
   cardiac
   forced
   gastric
cycling, phase
cyclohexane scintillator
cyclotron (see also *scanner*)
   medical
   multiparticle
C-Y color space
cylinder, $CO_2$
cylindrical projection map
cylindroma
cyllosis

Cyriax syndrome
cyst
   acoustic
   adenocarcinoma
   Bartholin
   Blessig
   bone
   branchial
   branchial cleft
   bronchogenic
   calcification of
   cerebral
   corpus luteum
   cortical
   dentigerous
   dermoid
   endometrial
   epidermal
   epidermal inclusion
   epithelial
   fluid-filled
   follicular
   functional ovarian
   ganglion
   hemorrhagic
   hydatid
   inclusion
   joint
   mammary
   meibomian
   mesenteric
   mesothelial
   morgagnian
   mucinous
   mucous
   multilocular
   multiloculated
   myxoid
   nabothian
   neoplastic
   non-neoplastic
   ovarian

cyst *(cont.)*
   ovarian follicular
   pancreatic
   paratubal
   parovarian
   pericardial
   pineal
   pituitary
   primordial
   prostatic
   renal
   retention
   serous
   solitary bone
   tarsal
   testicular
   thin-walled
   thyroglossal duct
   unilocular
   wolffian
cystadenoma
cystic artery
cystic change
cystic duct cholangiogram
cystic duct remnant
cystic duct stump
cystic emphysema
cystic fibrosis
cystic hydroma
cystic hygroma
cystic lysis
cystic mazoplasia
cystic medionecrosis
cystic neoplasm
cystic osteofibromatosis
cystic pulmonary emphysema
cystic sac
cystic tumor
cystic wall
cysto-atrial shunt
cystocele, protrusion of
Cysto-Conray II contrast medium
Cystografin contrast medium
cystogram
cystography
   delayed
   double voiding
   excretory
   postdrainage
   postvoiding
   radionuclide
   retrograde
   stress
   triple voiding
   voiding
cystoscopic urography
cystourethrogram, voiding (VCUG)
cytoarchitectonic abnormality
cytoarchitectonic field, Brodmann
cytokine cascades
cytomegalic inclusion disease
cytomegalovirus pneumonitis
Cytomel suppression test
cytometry
   flow
   multicolor flow

# D, d

D (diaphragmatic)
Dacron catheter
Dacron stent
dacryocystography
DAF (dynamic axial fixator)
Dagradi classification of esophageal
　　varices
DAI (diffuse axonal injury)
DALM (dysplasia with associated
　　lesion or mass)
D'Amato sign in pleural effusion
dammed-up CSF (cerebrospinal fluid)
dampened obstructive pulse
dampened pulsatile flow
dampened wave form
damping of catheter tip pressure
Dance sign
dancer's fracture
Dandy-Walker cyst
Dandy-Walker deformity
Dandy-Walker syndrome
Dane particle
Danis-Weber classification of ankle
　　fractures
D'Antonio classification of acetabular
　　abnormalities
DANTE sequence

DANTE-selective pulses
Dardik Biograft
dark pixel values
dark region
darkroom error
Darrach-Hughston-Milch fracture
DASA (distal articular set angle)
Daseler-Anson classification of
　　plantaris muscle anatomy
data
　　radiology outcomes
　　volumetric image
data acquisition time
data-clipping detection error artifact
data log, ICD
data sets
data spike detection error artifact
Datascope DL-II percutaneous
　　translucent balloon catheter
Datascope System 90 balloon pump
daughter product
Davies-Colley syndrome
Davies endomyocardial fibrosis
Dawbarn sign
DBM (demineralized bone matrix)
DBP (diastolic blood pressure)
DC (direct current) offset artifact

DC (dynamic compression) plate
DCA (directional color angiography)
DCA (directional coronary angioplasty)
DCA (directional coronary atherectomy)
DCBE (double contrast barium enema)
DCIS (ductal carcinoma in situ)
DCP (dynamic compression plate)
DCS (distal coronary sinus)
dD/dt (derived value on apex cardiogram)
DDD (double-dose delay)
DDFP (dodecafluoropentane) imaging agent
DDH (developmental dysplasia of hip)
dead space, anatomical
dead time
death
  brain
  cerebral
debilitation
debris
  aspiration of
  atheromatous
  atherosclerotic
  bone
  calcium
  cholesterol
  extra-articular
  foreign
  gelatinous
  grumous
  intimal
  intra-articular
  joint
  necrotic
  particle
  particulate
  thallium
De Broglie wavelength
Debye-Scherrer photographic technique
decalcification

decalcified dorsum sellae
decannulated
decannulation
decapolar catheter
decay
  beta
  exponential
  free induction
decay series
deceleration time
decelerative injury
dechondrification
decidua
decidual cyst
decidual reaction
decidual sac
deciduous
decimalized variance map
declamping
decoding
  document image (DID)
  Viterbi
decompensated congestive heart failure
decompensation
  cardiac
  chronic respiratory
  end-stage adult cardiac
  end-stage fetal cardiac
  hemodynamic
  respiratory
  ventricular
decompress
decompression
  balloon
  canal
  cardiac
  endoscopic
  gastric
  hydrostatic
  intestinal
  laser-assisted disk (LDD)

decompression *(cont.)*
  microvascular (MVD)
  percutaneous transhepatic (PTD)
  peripheral nerve
  portal
  surgical
  transduodenal endoscopic
  tube
  variceal
decompression tube
deconditioning
deconvolutional analysis
deconvolution, statistical
decortication
  cardiac
  chemical
  heart
  lung
decoupling
decreased attenuation
decryption algorithms
DecThreads software
decubitus film
decubitus position
  dorsal
  lateral
  ventral
decubitus ulcer
decubitus view
decussation
deep arch
deep artery
deep veins
deep cardiac plexus
deep Doppler velocity interrogation
deep hyperthermia treatment
deep lesion
deep respirations
deep-seated lesion
deep-seated tumor
deep-shelled acetabulum
deep vein thrombosis

deep venous aplasia
deep venous channel
deep venous incompetence
deep venous insufficiency (DVI)
deep venous thrombosis (DVT)
deep white matter track
defecation
defecogram
defography
defect (see also *deformity*)
  acquired ventricular septal (AVSD)
  anastomotic
  anteroapical
  aortic septal
  aorticopulmonary
  ASD (atrioseptal defect)
  atrial ostium primum
  atrioseptal (or atrial septal) (ASD)
  atrioventricular canal
  atrioventricular septal
  bar
  bar-like ventral (in myelography)
  birth
  bony
  bridging of
  cardiofacial
  cauliflower-shaped
  chain of lakes filling
  chiasmatic
  chondral
  cold
  concomitant
  congenital
  conoventricular
  contiguous ventricular septal
  cortical
  craniotomy
  crista supraventricularis septal
  curvilinear
  cushion
  developmental
  discoid filling

**defect**

defect *(cont.)*
  endocardial cushion
  extradural
  fibrous cortical
  field
  filling
  fixed
  fixed intracavitary filling
  fixed perfusion
  focal plaquelike
  frondlike filling
  frontal
  fusiform
  global cortical
  hot
  inferoapical
  infracristal septal
  infracristal ventricular septal
  infundibular ventricular septal
  interatrial septal (septum)
  intercalary
  interventricular conduction
  interventricular septal (IVSD)
  intra-atrial conduction
  intra-atrial filling
  intraluminal
  intraluminal filling
  intraventricular conduction
  ischemic
  junctional
  juxta-arterial ventricular septal
  juxtatricuspid ventricular septal
  linear
  lobulated filling
  lucent
  luminal
  luteal phase
  mapping of
  matched V/Q (ventilation-perfusion)
  membranous ventricular septal
  muscular ventricular septal
  myocardial perfusion

defect *(cont.)*
  neural tube
  nonsubperiosteal cortical
  nonuniform rotational (NURD)
  open neural tube
  optic nerve
  osseous
  osteochondral
  ostium primum
  ostium secundum
  partial AV (atrioventricular) canal
  pear-shaped
  perfusion
  peri-infarction conduction (PICD)
  perimembranous ventricular septal
  PG-related
  photopenic
  plication
  polypoid filling
  posteroapical
  postinfarction ventriculoseptal
  postoperative skull
  radial ray
  Rastelli type A, B, or C
    atrioventricular canal
  restrictive ventilatory
  reversible
  reversible ischemic
  reversible perfusion
  scan
  scintigraphic perfusion
  secundum atrial septal
  segmental
  segmental bone
  septal
  sinus venosus
  soft tissue
  spontaneous closure of
  stellar
  subcortical
  subperiosteal cortical
  supracristal septal

defect *(cont.)*
   supracristal ventricular
   supracristal ventriculoseptal
   Swiss cheese ventricular septal
   transient perfusion
   trochlear
   type I (supracristal) ventricular septal
   type II (infracristal) ventricular septal
   type III (canal type) ventricular septal
   type IV (muscular) ventricular septal
   V/Q (ventilation/perfusion)
   valvular
   ventilation
   ventilation/perfusion (V/Q)
   ventral hernia
   ventricular septal or ventriculoseptal (VSD)
   wedge-shaped
   wire-related
defective communication between cardiac chambers
defects in blood-brain barrier
deferential artery
deferens, ductus
defervesce
defervesced
deficit
deficiency
   Aitken femoral
   alpha-1-antitrypsin
   molybdenum cofactor
   pyruvate dehydrogenase complex
deficiency disease
deflectable quadripolar catheter
deflectable-tip catheter
deformans
   osteitis
   osteochondrodystrophia
   Paget osteitis

deformity (also see *defect*)
   Akerlund
   angular
   aortic valve
   Arnold-Chiari
   back-knee
   bell clapper
   biconcave
   bifid thumb
   bone
   bony
   boutonnière (of finger)
   bowing
   bull's-eye
   buttonhole
   calcaneus
   cavovarus
   cavus
   chain of lakes
   Charcot
   checkrein
   clawfoot
   clawhand
   clawtoe
   cloverleaf
   clubhand
   cock-up
   codfish
   compensatory
   congenital
   contracture
   cottage loaf
   coxa vara
   cranio-orbital
   cubitus valgus
   cubitus varus
   curly toe
   Dandy-Walker
   digital
   digitus flexus
   dinner-fork
   DISI (dorsal intercalary segment instability)

**deformity**

deformity *(cont.)*
   duodenal bulb
   equinovalgus
   equinovarus
   equinovarus hindfoot
   equinus
   Erlenmeyer flask-like
   eversion-external rotation
   femoral head
   flatfoot
   flexible spastic equinovarus
   flexion
   forefoot abduction
   funnel-like
   genu valgum
   genu varum
   gibbous
   gooseneck outflow tract
   gunstock
   Haglund
   hallux abductovalgus
   hallux flexus
   hallux malleus
   hallux rigidus
   hallux valgus
   hallux varus
   hammertoe
   hatchet-head
   Hill-Sachs
   hindbrain
   hindfoot
   hockey-stick tricuspid valve
   hourglass
   Ilfeld-Holder
   internal rotation
   intrinsic minus
   intrinsic plus
   J-hook
   J-sella
   joint
   keyhole
   Kirner

deformity *(cont.)*
   lobster-claw
   Madelung
   mallet
   mallet finger
   mermaid
   metatarsus adductocavus
   metatarsus adductovarus
   metatarsus adductus
   metatarsus atavicus
   metatarsus latus
   metatarsus primus varus
   metatarsus varus
   Michel
   mitral valve
   nasal tip
   neuropathic midfoot
   pannus
   parachute mitral valve
   pectus excavatum
   perigastric
   pes cavus
   pes planus
   phrygian cap
   pigeon breast
   planovalgus
   plantar flexion-inversion
   procurvature
   pseudo-Hurler
   pulmonary valve
   recurvatum
   reduction
   rockerbottom foot
   rolled edge
   rotational
   round shoulder
   sabre shin
   scimitar
   seal-fin
   shepherd's crook
   silver-fork
   snowman

**deformity** • **degeneration**

deformity *(cont.)*
  spastic equinovarus
  spastic hindfoot valgus
  splay foot
  split foot
  Sprengel
  static foot
  step-down shoulder
  supination
  supratip nasal tip
  swan-neck
  swan-neck finger
  talus foot
  thumb-in-palm
  torsional
  trefoil
  tricuspid valve
  trigger finger
  triphalangeal thumb
  turned-up pulp
  ulnar drift (motor)
  valgus
  valgus heel
  varus
  Velpeau
  vertical talus foot
  VISI
  Volkmann
  wasp-tail (in Duchenne dystrophy)
  wedging
  whistling
  Whitehead
  windblown
  windswept
defunctionalization
defuzzification algorithm
degeneration
  angiolithic
  articular cartilage
  atheromatous
  atrophic
  ballooning

degeneration *(cont.)*
  bone
  bony
  brain
  breast
  calcareous
  cardiac
  cardiac valve mucoid
  cardiomyopathic
  cartilaginous
  cerebellar
  cerebromacular (CMD)
  cobblestone
  collagen
  colloid
  cortical cerebellar
  corticobasal ganglionic
  corticostriatospinal
  cusp
  cystic
  Doyne familial colloid
  Doyne honeycomb
  dystrophic
  esophageal
  fatty
  fibrinoid
  fibrinous
  fibroid
  gray matter
  heart
  hepatic
  hepatocerebral
  hepatolenticular
  Holmes cerebellar
  Holmes cortical cerebellar
  honeycomb
  hyaline
  hydropic
  hypertensive vascular
  intimal
  lipoid
  lipoidal

degeneration (cont.)
  liquefaction
  malignant
  Menzel olivopontocerebellar
  mitral valve
  Mönckeberg
  mucoid
  mucous
  mural
  muscular
  myocardial
  myocardial cellular
  myocardial fibers
  myxomatous
  olivopontocerebellar
  pancreas
  panceatic
  paraneoplastic cerebellar
  parenchymatous cerebellar
  paving stone
  primary progressive cerebellar
  progressive
  Regnauld-type great toe
  renal tubular
  retinal
  retrograde
  rim
  sclerotic
  secondary
  senile
  spinal
  spinocerebellar
  spongy
  spongy white matter
  subacute combined spinal cord
  testicular
  thyroid
  trabecular
  traumatic
  wear and tear
  Zenker
degenerative atrioventricular node disease
degenerative change
degenerative disease
degenerative disk disease
degenerative joint disease (DJD)
degenerative spurring
DeGimard syndrome
deglutition
deglutition mechanism
deglutition paralysis
deglutition syncope
Degos disease
degradation, image quality
degree, noncircularity
degree of correction
Dehio test
dehiscence
  bronchial
  perivalvular
  prosthesis
de la Camp sign
de Lange syndrome
Delarnette scanner
delay
  developmental
  regrowth
  temporal phase
  time (echo)
delayed excretion of contrast media
delayed films
delayed images
delayed phase
delayed gastric emptying
delayed transport of tracer
delayed traumatic intracerebral hematoma (DTICH)
delayed union
delayed visualization
delay time, echo
Delbet fracture classification
Delbet sign

deleterious effect
delicate crepitation
delivery, timed bolus
Delmege sign of tuberculosis
DELTAmanager MedImage system
deltoid branch of posterior tibial
   artery
deltoid ligament
deltopectoral groove
demagnetization field effect
demand (standby)
demarcate
demarcated
demarcation line
De Martini-Balestra syndrome
dementia
Demianoff sign
demifacets
demilune
demineralization, bone
demineralization from disuse
demineralized bone matrix (DBM)
demodulator
demographic data
Demons-Meigs syndrome
de Musset sign (aortic aneurysm)
de Mussey point or sign (pleurisy)
demyelinating disease
demyelination
   brain stem
   large-fiber
   posterior column
   postinfectious
   segmental
demyelinative disorder
denatured Tc-RBCs
dendritic lesion
denervated area
denervation atrophy
Denis classification of spinal injury
   (A to E)
de novo

dens (odontoid process of axis)
dens fracture
dens view of cervical spine
densitometer
   Achilles+
   bone
   CT
   DEXA (dual-energy x-ray
     absorptiometry)
   DPX-IQ
   dual-photon
   Expert-XL
   Hologic 2000
   Norland bone
   photon
   single-photon
densitometry
density (pl. densities)
   air
   bands of
   bone mineral (BMD)
   calcific
   calcified
   capillary
   diffuse reticular
   discrete perihilar
   double
   echo
   fluid
   ground glass
   hazy
   homogeneous soft tissue
   hydrogen
   ill-defined
   increased
   linear
   metallic
   mottled
   nodular
   patchy
   perihilar
   pleural

density (cont.)
   proton
   pulmonary
   radiographic
   radiolucent
   radiopaque
   retroareolar
   retrocardiac
   ropy
   soft tissue
   spicular
   spin
   tissue
   variations in
   water
   wedge-shaped
density matrix theory
dental cyst
dental scan
DentaScan
dentate fracture
dentate ligament
dentate line
dentate nucleus
dentate suture of skull
dentato-olivary pathway
dentatorubral-pallidoluysian atrophy
dentinogenesis imperfecta
dentoskeletal relationship
denudation, areas of
denude
denuded
denuding
deossification
dependent atelectasis
dependent extracellular fluid accumulation
dependent lung
dephasing gradient
dephasing, signal
depiction, magnetic resonance
depiction of vasculature

deposit, calcium
deposition
   calcium
   callus
   iron
   spontaneous
deposition rate
depressed and compound fracture
depressed fracture
depression
   fragment
   hemidiaphragm
   reciprocal
   sinus node
   spinal cord
depth-dose curves
depth-dose distribution
depth, photon interaction
de Quervain fracture
derangement, internal
derby hat fracture
dermatofibrosarcoma protuberans
dermoid cyst
dermoid tumor
derotate
derotated
derotation
DES (diffuse esophageal spasm)
Desault dislocation
Desault fracture
descending aorta
descending aorta–pulmonary artery shunt
descending colon
descending duodenum
Deseret angiocatheter
desmalgia
desmectasis
desmocytoma
desmodynia
desmoid
desmoma
desmoplasia

desmoplastic
desmosis
desquamative interstitial pneumonia (DIP)
D'Espine sign
destruction, bone (or bony)
destructive lesion
destructive process
destructive tumor
detachable coils
detail
   exquisite
   suboptimal
detecting, collision
detecting module
detection
   magnetic resonance (MR)
   occult
   quadrature
   radioactivity
   radwaste radioactivity
detection and quantification
detection zone
detector
   annular
   cadmium iodide
   CR-39 nuclear tract
   diode
   Doppler blood flow
   GE (General Electric)
   glass track
   HPGe
   passive track
   selenium
   Si (Li)
   sodium detector
   solid state nuclear track
   Wang-Binford edge
detector array
detector collimation
deterioration
   progressive
   uniform

Determann syndrome
determination
   particle size
   void
detour conduit
detritus
deuterium imaging agent
Deutschländer disease
devascularization, paraesophagogastric
developer artifact
development
   conductive
   delayed
   insulative
   interval
developmental delay
Deventer diameter
deviated septum
deviation
   angular
   aortic
   carpal
   fracture
   left axis (LAD)
   mediastinal
   radial
   right axis (RAD)
   rotary
   septal
   tracheal
   ulnar
device-independent (DVI)
device, Navarre interventional radiology
DeVilbiss ultrasound nebulizer
devitalized tissue
devoid of circulation
DEXA (dual-energy x-ray absorptiometry) densitometer (see also *densitometer*)
DEXA scan for bone density determination

Dexter-Grossman classification of
 mitral regurgitation
dextrocardia
dextrocardiac
dextrogastria
dextrogastric
dextroposed
dextroposition
dextrorotatory
dextrorotoscoliosis
dextroscoliosis
dextrotransposition (D-transposition)
 of great arteries
dextrotropic
dextroversion of heart
DFA (hallux dorsiflexion angle)
DFP (diastolic filling pressure)
DGR (duodenogastric reflux)
diabetic gastroparesis
diacondylar fracture
diadochokinesia
diadochokinesis
diagnosis
  clinical
  differential
  empirical
  noninvasive
  pathologic
  postoperative
  preoperative
  presumptive
  radiologic
  remote
  roentgenographic
  sonographic
  tentative
  ultrasound
  working
diagnostic efficacy analysis
diagnostic procedure
diagnostic radiology
diagnostic radiopharmaceutical
diagnostic range ultrasound

diagonal branch of artery
diagonal conjugate diameter
diamagnetic shift
diamagnetic susceptibility
diametaphyseal
diametaphysis
diameter (or dimension)
  anteroposterior (AP)
  aortic (AD)
  aortic root
  artery
  Baudelocque
  bi-ischial
  biparietal (BPD)
  bronchial
  cardiac
  coccygeopubic
  coil-to-vessel
  conjugate
  Deventer
  diagonal conjugate
  gestational sac (GS)
  increased AP (anteroposterior)
  intercristal
  internal conjugate
  intertuberal
  left anterior internal (LAID)
  left ventricular internal (LVID)
  Lohlein
  luminal
  maximum AP (anteroposterior)
  midsagittal (MSD)
  minimal luminal
  narrow anteroposterior
  orthonormal
  pelvic
  right ventricular internal (RVID)
  sacropubic
  spinal cord
  stenosis
  transverse
  valve
  vessel

diamond-shaped anastomosis
diaphanography
diaphragm
  aponeurotic portion of
  arcuate ligaments of
  Bucky
  central tendon
  crus (pl. crura) of
  depressed
  dome of
  duodenal
  elevated
  eventration of
  free air under the
  leaf (or leaves) of
  muscular crus of
  pelvic
  polyarcuate
  Potter-Bucky
  respiratory
  sella turcica
  tenting of
  thoracoabdominal
  twigs to pelvic
  urogenital
diaphragmatic attenuation
diaphragmatic contour
diaphragmatic creep
diaphragmatic crus (pl. crura)
diaphragmatic cupula
diaphragmatic dome
diaphragmatic elevation
diaphragmatic eventration
diaphragmatic hernia
diaphragmatic hiatus
diaphragmatic pericardium
diaphragmatic pleura
diaphyseal cortical mortise
diaphyseal dysplasia
diaphyseal fracture
diaphysis (pl. diaphyses)
diaplasis

diarthrodial joint
diaschisis, crossed cerebellar
Diasonics ultrasound scanner
diastasis
  fracture
  sutural
  syndesmotic
  tibiofibular
diastolic blood pressure (DBP)
diastolic counterpulsation
diastolic depolarization phase
diastolic filling period
diastolic gating
diastolic overload
diastolic perfusion pressure
diastolic pressure-time index (DPTI)
diastolic velocity (cm/sec)
diastrophic dwarfism
diatrizoate meglumine imaging agent
diatrizoate sodium imaging agent
diazepam (used as imaging agent)
DIC (drip infusion cholangiography)
dichromate dosimeter
Dickhaut-DeLee classification of
  discoid meniscus
DICOM (Digital Imaging and
  Communications in Medicine)
  interface
DID (document image decoding)
didactylism
didelphia
diencephalic herniation
diencephalon
DIET fast SE imaging
DIET method of fat suppression
diethylenetriaminepentaacetic acid
  (DTPA) imaging agent
differencing filter
differential diagnosis
differential loading
differentiated
differentiation

diffracting Doppler transducer device
diffraction
  beam
  high resolution
  high temperature
  x-ray
diffraction peak
diffuse axonal injury (DAI)
diffuse esophageal spasm (DES)
diffuse idiopathic sclerosis hyperostosis (DISH)
diffuse idiopathic skeletal hyperostosis (DISH)
diffuse uptake
diffusion
  anisotropic
  spectral
  thermal
diffusion and perfusion magnetic resonance imaging
diffusion coefficient
diffusion magnetic resonance imaging
diffusion pulse sequence
diffusion-weighted pulse sequence
DiGeorge syndrome
digestion
digestive system
digestive tract
Digirad gamma camera
digit (pl. digits)
  accessory
  arthrodesed
  flail
  replanted
  supernumerary
  syndactylization of
digital branches
digital equipment system
digital fluoroscopy, FluoroPlus Roadmapper
digital frequency analysis
digital imaging
Digital Imaging and Communications in Medicine (DICOM) protocol
digital imaging processing (DIP)
digitally fused CT and radiolabeled monoclonal antibody SPECT images
digital mammography
digital radiography
digital rotational angiography (DRA)
digital runoff
digital storage (in cineangiography)
digital subtraction angiography (DSA)
digital subtraction pulmonary angiogram
digital subtraction rotational angiography
digital-to-analog converter
digital unraveling
digital vascular imaging (DVI)
digital videoangiography
digitized slices
digitized spinography
digitizer (see *scanner*)
digitorum
Digitron digital subtraction imaging system
Digitron DVI/DSA computer
digiti manus (fingers)
digiti pedis (toes)
digitus annularis (ring finger)
digitus medius (middle finger)
digitus minimus (little finger)
digiti primus (thumb)
digitus secundus (index finger)
digitus valgus
digitus varus
dihydroxyphenylalanine (DOPA)
diisocyanide-triisocyanide $^{99m}$Tc complexes
dilatation (dilation)
  alveolar
  anal

**dilatation (dilation)** *(cont.)*
  aneurysmal
  annular
  aortic root
  arterial
  artery by balloon catheter
  ascending aorta
  balloon
  bile duct
  biliary
  bowel
  bowel loop
  bronchial
  bronchiolar
  caliceal
  cardiac
  cavitary
  chamber
  colonic
  common duct
  diffuse aortic
  distal ureteral
  ductal
  Eder-Puestow
  endoscopic
  esophageal
  extrahepatic biliary cystic
  fusiform
  gastric
  hepatic web
  idiopathic pulmonary artery
  idiopathic right atrial
  intestinal
  intrahepatic biliary cystic
  intraluminal
  left ventricular
  megacolon
  multiple mural
  myocardial
  percutaneous balloon
  percutaneous transluminal balloon (PTBD)

**dilatation (dilation)** *(cont.)*
  periportal sinusoidal
  pneumatic bag esophageal
  pneumatic balloon catheter
  poststenotic
  probe
  prognathous (or prognathic)
  pulmonary artery
  pulmonary trunk idiopathic
  pulmonary valve stenosis
  rectal
  respiratory bronchiolar
  right ventricular
  sequential
  sulcus
  terminal bronchiolar
  tortuous vein
  transient left ventricular
  ureteral
  ureteric
  vein
  ventricular wall
**dilatation and hypertrophy**
**dilate, dilated**
**dilation** (see *dilatation*)
**dilution curve**
**dilution, isotopic**
**DIMAQ integrated ultrasound workstation**
**dimension**
  absolute artery
  aortic root
  arterial
  axial
  end-systolic
  intraluminal
  intrathoracic
  left atrial
  left ventricular end-diastolic (LVEDD)
  left ventricular end-systolic (LVESD)

dimension *(cont.)*
  left ventricular internal (LVID)
  left ventricular internal diastolic
    (LVIDD)
  left ventricular internal end-diastole
    (LVIDd)
  left ventricular internal end-systole
    (LVIDs)
  left ventricular systolic (LVs)
  luminal
  right ventricular (RVD)
diminished systemic perfusion
diminutive vessel
dimple of bone
dinner-fork deformity
diode detector
diode, infrared light-emitting
diode laser
Diodrast contrast medium
Dionosil contrast medium
DIP (desquamative interstitial
    pneumonia)
DIP (digital imaging processing)
    algorithms
DIP (distal interphalangeal) joint
diplegia spinalis brachialis traumatica
diploic
dipolar broadening
dipolar interaction
diprotrizoate contrast medium
dipyridamole echocardiography test
dipyridamole handgrip test
dipyridamole infusion test
dipyridamole thallium stress test
dipyridamole thallium-201
    scintigraphy
dipyridamole thallium
    ventriculography
dipyridamole tomographic thallium
    stress test
direct caval cannulation
direct current ablation (DCA)

direct current (DC) energy
direct fracture
direct hernia
direct liquid scintillation count
direct puncture phlebography
direct radioiodination
direct visualization
direction, aboral
directional color angiography (DCA)
directional coronary angioplasty
    (DCA)
directional coronary atherectomy
    (DCA)
directly coupled sample changer
    system
director, grooved
dirty shadowing
disarticulate
disarticulation
disc (see *disk*)
discernible findings
discogenic
discogram
discography
diskogram
diskography
discoid atelectasis
discoid lateral meniscus
discoid shadow
discoligamentous complex
discontinuity
discordant nodule
discrepancy, leg length
discreta, porokeratosis plantaris
discrete (separate) (not *discreet*)
discrete bleeding source
discrete lesion
discrete mass
discriminant analysis
discriminate
discrimination
discriminator

discus (disci)
disease (see radiology-related diseases listed alphabetically)
disease-free vessel wall
DISH (diffuse idiopathic sclerosing [or skeletal] hyperostosis)
dishpan fracture
DISI (dorsal intercalary segment instability)
DISIDA (diisopropyliminodiacetic acid) scan
disimpaction
disintegration of plaque by laser pulses
disjointing
disk (also disc)
  acromioclavicular joint
  anal
  articular
  atrial
  Bardeen primitive
  Bowman
  bulge (or bulging)
  cartilaginous (of epiphysis)
  cervical vertebral
  chorionic
  contained
  crescent-shaped fibrocartilaginous
  distal radioulnar joint
  embryonic
  epiphyseal
  extruded
  fibrocartilaginous
  fibrous ring of
  fixation
  frayed
  growth
  H
  hard
  Hensen
  herniated
  herniated cervical

disk *(cont.)*
  herniated intervertebral (HID)
  herniated lumbar
  herniated lumbosacral intervertebral
  herniated sacral
  herniated thoracic intervertebral
  I
  interarticular
  intervertebral
  intra-articular
  isotropic
  locking
  lumbar vertebral
  lumbosacral vertebral
  mandibular
  massive herniated
  Merkel tactile
  midline herniation of
  noncontained
  placental
  protruded (or protruding)
  ruptured
  sequestered
  slipped intervertebral
  soft
  sternoclavicular joint
  tactile
  temporomandibular joint
  thoracic vertebral
  thoracolumbar vertebral
  triangular
  vacuum
  vertebral
disk bulge
disk bulging
disk disease
disk extrusion
disk fragment
disk herniation
disk interspace
disk-like atelectasis
disk margin

**disk • displacement**

disk maturation
diskogram
diskography (discography)
  intranuclear
  intervertebral
diskovertebral infection
disk plication
disk poppet
disk protrusion
disk space height
disk space narrowing
disk-to-magnetic field orientation
disk water signal
dislocate, dislocated
dislocation
  anterior
  anterior-inferior
  Bankart
  bayonet
  Bell-Dally
  Bennett
  boutonnière
  bursting
  central
  Chopart
  chronic recurrent
  closed
  complete
  complicated
  compound
  consecutive
  Desault
  divergent
  facet
  fracture
  frank
  gamekeeper's
  habitual
  Hill-Sachs
  incomplete
  irreducible
  isolated

dislocation *(cont.)*
  Jahss
  Kienböck (Kienboeck)
  Lisfranc
  lunate
  milkmaid's
  Monteggia
  Nélaton
  nonreducible
  nontraumatic
  open
  Otto
  partial
  pathologic
  perilunate
  posterior
  primitive
  recent
  recurrent
  simple
  Smith
  swivel
  traumatic
  volar
dislocation fracture
disobliteration, carotid
disorder
  esophageal motility
  evacuation
  functional
  gastric motor
  intrathoracic lymphoproliferative
  nonspecific esophageal motility
    (NEMD)
  right-left
disparate
disparity
disphenoid extraction
displaced fat pad sign
displacement, Ellis Jones peroneal
displacement field-fitting MR imaging

display
  multiparametric color composite
  pseudocolor B-mode
  real-time
  shaded surface
disproportion
  cephalopelvic (CPD)
  fiber-type
disrupted plaque
disruption, traumatic
dissecans
  osteochondritis (OD)
  osteochondrosis
dissect
dissecting aneurysm
dissecting hematoma
dissection
  aneurysmal
  aortic
  arterial
  descending aorta
  spontaneous
  Stanford type B aortic
disseminated atheromatous
  embolization
disseminated cholesterol embolization
disseminated disease
disseminated intravascular coagulation (DIC)
disseminated sclerosis
disseminated tuberculosis
distal articular set angle (DASA)
distal coronary sinus (CS)
distal interphalangeal (DIP) joint
distal splenorenal shunt (DSRS)
distally
distalward
distance
  interarch
  intercaudate
  interlaminar
  internuclear

distance *(cont.)*
  interopercular
  interorbital
  interpediculate
  interridge
  interslice
  interspinous
  source-skin (SSD)
  surface
distance-based block classification
distant metastases
distend
distended
distensible
distensibility
distention
  abdominal
  bladder
  colonic
  gaseous
  gastric
  intestinal
  neck vein
  pelvicaliceal
  postprandial
  rectal
  ureteral
  vesical
disto-occlusal
distortion
  geometric
  image
  pincushion
  radiographic pincushion
  S
  Y-shaped
distortion of limitations of image reconstruction algorithm artifact
distraction
  callus
  fracture fragment
  hyperflexion injury

distraction (cont.)
  joint
  physeal
  segment
  small-step
  soft tissue
distraction gap
distraction osteogenesis
distribution
  anatomic
  anomalous
  binomial
  Boltzmann
  catecholamine
  centrilobular
  depth-dose
  diffuse
  gaussian
  geometric
  inhomogeneous
  inhomogeneous tracer
  mottled
  peribronchial
  perivascular
  reverse
  rimlike calcium
  spectral noise
  trace element
  uniform
distributive shock
disturbance, functional
disuse
  demineralization from
    lesser atrophy of
disuse atrophy
disuse osteoporosis
diuretic renal scan
dive-bomber discharges
divergent dislocation
diverging collimator
diversion, biliopancreatic
diverticulitis
  acute
  chronic
  colonic
  Meckel
  sigmoid
diverticulosis
diverticulum (pl. diverticula)
  bladder
  colonic
  cricopharyngeal
  epiphrenic
  esophageal
  fallopian tube
  false
  functional
  Ganser
  Graser
  hepatic
  hypopharyngeal
  IDD (intraluminal duodenal)
  intestinal
  intraluminal duodenal (IDD)
  intramural
  inverted Meckel
  juxtapapillary
  Kirchner
  Meckel
  metanephric
  midesophageal
  Nuck
  perforated
  periampullary
  pharyngoesophageal
  pulsion
  Rokitansky
  traction
  urethral
  Vater
  vesical
  Zenker
divisional block

divisionary line (in bipartite sesamoid)
divopontocerebellar atrophy
divot
Dixon method of fat suppression
Dixon method of phase unwrapping
DJD (degenerative joint disease)
DJJ (duodenojejunal junction)
DKS (Damus-Kaye-Stansel) anastomosis
D-loop, ventricular
D-loop ventricular situs
DMA (distal metatarsal angle)
D-malposition of aorta
DMI (Diagnostic Medical Instruments) analyzer
DMI (diaphragmatic myocardial infarction)
DMPE (99mTc-bis-dimethylphosphonoethane)
DMVA (direct mechanical ventricular actuation)
DNA ploidy pattern
DNA-MION
dobutamine echocardiography
dobutamine stress echocardiography
dobutamine thallium angiography
DOBV (double outlet both ventricles)
document image decoding (DID)
document-recognition algorithm
Dodd perforating vein group
dodecafluoropentane (DDFP) imaging agent
Dodge method for ejection fraction
dog artifact
dolichocephaly
dolichocolon
dolichoectasia
dolichoesophagus
dolichosigmoid
dolichostenomelia
DOLV (double outlet left ventricle)
domain, Fourier

dome
  anterior talar
  atrial
  diaphragmatic
  bladder
  liver
  shoulder
  talar
  weightbearing acetabular
dome and dart configuration on cardiac catheterization
Dome Imaging RX20 board
dome-shaped heart
dome-shaped roof of pleural cavity
dominance
  coronary artery
  hemispheric
  mixed
  right ventricular
  shared coronary artery
dominant
  anatomically
  autosomal
dominant hemisphere
dominant left coronary artery
dominant right coronary artery
doming, diastolic
doming of leaflets
doming of valve
D1 (diagonal branch #1)
donut sign (also doughnut)
dopamine D1 agonist
dopamine D2 receptor
dopamine transporter
Doplette monitor
Doppler
  color flow
  continuous wave
  contrast-enhanced color
  contrast-enhanced power
  duplex
  duplex B-mode

Doppler *(cont.)*
  gray-scale
  intraoperative
  pocket
  power
  pulsed wave
  range-gated pulsed
  real-time
  spectral
Doppler blood flow detector
Doppler blood flow monitor
Doppler blood flow velocity signal
Doppler blood pressure
Doppler color flow mapping
Doppler color spectral analysis
Doppler coronary catheter
Doppler-derived stroke distance
Doppler echocardiography
  continuous wave
  pulsed wave
Doppler flow probe study
Doppler flow signal
Doppler flow-imaging system, real-time two-dimensional
Doppler flowmetry
Doppler frequency shift
Doppler imaging
Doppler insonation
Doppler Intra-Dop intraoperative device
Doppler phenomenon
Doppler pulse
Doppler Resistive Index (DRI)
Doppler shift
Doppler shift principle
Doppler signal
Doppler signal enhancers
Doppler spectral analysis
Doppler spectral waveforms
Doppler tissue imaging (DTI)
Doppler ultrasonic blood flow detector
Doppler ultrasonic fetal heart monitor
Doppler ultrasonic velocity detector
Doppler ultrasonography
Doppler ultrasound, high frequency (HFD)
Doppler ultrasound segmental blood pressure testing
Doppler venous examination
Doppler waveform analysis
Dorendorf sign of aortic arch aneurysm
Dormia basket catheter
Dornier scanner
Dorros brachial internal mammary guiding catheter
dorsal branch
dorsal capsule
dorsal decubitus position
dorsal metacarpal ligament
dorsal pedal bypass
dorsal pedal pulse
dorsal position
dorsal ramus of spinal nerve
dorsal recumbent position
dorsal root entry zone (DREZ) lesion
dorsal root ganglia (DRG)
dorsal spine (D1 to D12)
dorsal spinocerebellar tracts
dorsal subaponeurotic space
dorsal subcutaneous space
dorsal wing fracture
dorsal wrist ligament
dorsalis pedis pulse
dorsalward
dorsiflexion
dorsiflexor
dorsoanterior
dorsocephalad
dorsolateral
dorsoplantar talonavicular angle
dorsoplantar view
dorsoposterior
dorsoradial

dorsorostral
dorsum pedis
dorsum sellae
DORV (double outlet right ventricle)
Dos Santos needle for aortography
dose (pl. doses)
  absorbed
  bolus
  divided
  fraction
  fractionated
  incremental
  integral
  iodine
  lethal
  loading
  maintenance
  median lethal
  multiple scan average (MSAD)
  normalized average glandular
  tapering
  titrated
  tracer
dose index, computed tomography (CTDI)
dose-volume histogram
dose-volume relationship
dosimeter
dosimetry
  beam's eye view
  carbon-load thermoluminescent
  CTA
  dichromate
  electron
  EPR
  free-radical
  high-dose film
  LiF thermoluminescence
  therminoluminescent
  transmission
dosimetric penumbra
dosing, titrated

dots, subpleural
Dotter caged balloon catheter
Dotter-Judkins PTA (percutaneous transluminal angioplasty)
double-acting actuator
double aortic arch
double barrel aorta
double barrel lumen
double breast coil
double bubble sign
double camelback sign of knee
double clamping
double contour
double contrast arthrography
double contrast barium enema (DCBE)
double density
double dose delay (DDD)
double dose gadolinium imaging
double echo three-point Dixon method fat suppression
double exposure artifact
double exposure drift artifact
double fracture
double helical CT scan
double helix acquisition on CT scan
double inlet left ventricle/double outlet both ventricles
double inlet ventricles
double label
double label counting
double outflow
double outlet both ventricles (DOBV)
double outlet left ventricle (DOLV)
double outlet right ventricle (DORV)
double outlet right ventricle (I–IV) syndrome
double outline
double phase technetium-99m sestamibi imaging
double photon absorptiometry (DPA)
double-populated detector ring
double spin echo proton spectroscopy

double spiral CT arterial portography
double strand, intracellular DNA
double systolic apical impulse
double tracking of barium
double-walled fibroserous sac
double wire atherectomy technique
doubly broadband triple resonance NMR probe circuit
doughnut (also donut)
doughnut configuration on thallium imaging
doughnut magnet
doughnut sign
Douglas bag method for determining cardiac output
Douglas
  cul-de-sac of
  pouch of
Dow-Corning ileal pouch catheter
dowager's hump
dowel
Dow method for measuring cardiac output
Down syndrome
downscatter
downstream sampling method
downward displacement of apical impulse
downward sloping
dP/dt (upstroke pattern on apex cardiogram), peak
DPA (double [or dual] photon absorptiometry)
D point
DPTI (diastolic pressure-time index)
DPX-IQ densitometer
DRA (digital rotational angiography)
DRA (distal reference axis)
drainage
  aberrent venous
  percutaneous antegrade biliary
  percutaneous transhepatic (PTD)
  transvaginal ultrasound-guided

draining vein pressure (DVP)
draped aorta
DRC (dynamic range control) algorithm used in digital radiography
Drennan metaphyseal-epiphyseal angle
Dressler post-myocardial infarction syndrome
DREZ (dorsal root entry zone) lesion
DRG (dorsal root ganglia)
DRI (Doppler Resistive Index)
drifting wedge pressure
drip infusion cholangiography (DIC)
drooping lily appearance
drop finger
drop foot
dropsy (hydrops)
drop test for pneumoperitoneum
drowned lung
Drummond marginal artery
Drummond sign of aortic aneurysm
dry pleurisy
dry swallow on esophageal manometry
Drystar dry imager
DSA (digital subtraction angiography)
  frameless stereotaxic
  intra-arterial
  intravenous
DSAS (discrete subvalvular aortic stenosis)
DSC (dynamic susceptibility contrast) MR imaging
D-shaped vessel lumen
DSI camera
D signal
DTAF-F (descending thoracic aortofemoral-femoral) bypass
DTI (Doppler tissue imaging)
DTICH (delayed traumatic intracerebral hemorrhage [or hematoma])
D to E slope on echocardiography
DTPA (diethylenetriaminepentaacetic acid)

DTPA renography
DTPA, technetium bound to
D-transposition (dextrotransposition) of great arteries
D2 dopamine receptors
dual atrioventricular node pathway
dual balloon method
dual blood supply
dual contrast study
dual echo DIET fast SE imaging
dual echo sequence
dual energy x-ray absorptiometry (DEXA)
dual GRE pulse sequences
dual head gamma camera system
dual head SPECT
dual isotope scanning
dual isotope single-photon emission CT
dual lookup table algorithm
dual phase scan
dual phase $^{99m}$Tc-sestamibi imaging
dual photon absortiometry (DPA)
dual photon densitometry
dual x-ray absorptiometry (DXA)
Dubin-Johnson syndrome
Dubin-Sprinz disease
Ducor-Cordis pigtail catheter
Ducor HF (high-flow) catheter
duct
  aberrant
  aberrant bile
  accessory hepatic
  accessory pancreatic
  alveolar
  amniotic
  arterial
  Bartholin
  beaded hepatic
  bile
  biliary
  Botallo

duct *(cont.)*
  branchial
  bucconeural
  canalicular
  carotid
  choledochous
  cochlear
  common
  common bile (CBD)
  common gall
  common hepatic
  craniopharyngeal
  cystic
  cystic gall
  deferent
  distal bile
  efferent
  ejaculatory
  endolymphatic
  excretory
  extrahepatic bile
  frontonasal
  fusiform widening of
  galactophorous
  gall
  Gartner
  genital
  hepatic
  Hering
  His
  hypophyseal Rathke
  interlobular bile
  intrahepatic biliary
  involution of
  lacrimal
  lymph
  lymphatic
  main pancreatic (MPD)
  middle extrahepatic bile
  müllerian
  normal caliber
  obstruction of

duct *(cont.)*
  pancreatic
  paramesonephric
  paraurethral
  perilobular
  preampullary portion of bile
  prepapillary bile
  prostatic
  Rathke
  right hepatic
  Santorini
  Stensen
  subvesical
  terminal bile
  thoracic
  thyroglossal
  Vater
  vitelline
  Wirsung
  wolffian
ductal arch
ductal architecture
ductal carcinoma in situ (DCIS)
ductal constriction
ductal dilatation
ductal ectasia
ductal epithelial hyperplasia
ductal hyperplasia
ductal pattern
ductal remnant
ductule
ductular
ductus arteriosus
  patent (PDA)
  persistent
  persistent patency of
  reversed
ductus arteriosus patency
ductus deferens artery
ductus venosus patency
Dulcolax bowel prep
dumb terminal
dumbbell-shaped shadow
dumbbell tumor
dumbbell-type neuroblastoma
dumping syndrome
Dunlop-Shands view
duodenal atresia
duodenal bulb
duodenal cap
duodenal C-loop
duodenal duplication
duodenal impression on liver
duodenal loop
duodenal papilla
duodenal sweep
duodenal terminus
duodenal tumor, periampullary
duodenal ulcer
duodenitis
  chronic atrophic
  erosive
duodenobiliary pressure gradient
duodenogastric reflux
duodenography, hypotonic
duodenojejunal angle
duodenojejunal junction (DJJ)
duodenopancreatic reflux
duodenum
  C-loop of
  curve of
  descending
  distal
  first portion of
  scarified
  second portion of
  supravaterian
  suspensory muscle of
  third portion of
duodenum deformed by scarring
Duografin contrast medium
duplex Doppler scan
duplex Doppler sonography (DS)
duplex Doppler ultrasound

duplex imaging, color-flow
duplex pulsed-Doppler sonography
duplex scan
  color-flow
  renal
duplex screening test
duplex ultrasound
duplicated renal collecting system
DuPont CRONEX x-ray film
DuPont Rare Earth Imaging System
DuPont scanner
Dupuytren contracture
Dupuytren fracture
dura
  attenuated
  bulging
dural arteriovenous malformation
dural attachment(s)
dural fold
dural impingement
dural sac
dural scar
dural sheath
dural sinus thrombosis (DST)
dural tear
dural trail sign
dural venous sinus thrombosis
dura mater of brain
dura mater of spinal cord
Duret lesion
Durham flatfoot
Duroziez mitral stenosis disease
DUS (dynamic ultrasound of shoulder)
Dusard syndrome
Duverney fracture
dV/dt (contractility)
DVI (deep venous insufficiency)
DVI (device-independent)
DVI (digital vascular imaging)
DVI Simpson atherocath
DVP (draining vein pressure)

DVT (deep venous thrombosis)
dwarfism
  achondroplastic
  deprivation
  Lorain-Lévi
  pituitary
  renal
  Russell-Silver
  Walt Disney
dwarf pelvis
DXA (dual x-ray absorptiometry)
$^{166}$Dy (dysprosium) $^{166}$Ho holmium in vivo generator
Dy-DTPA-BMA imaging agent
dye (see *imaging agent*)
dye fluorescence index (DFI)
dye punch fracture
dynamic beat filtration
dynamic bolus
dynamic computerized tomography (CT)
dynamic conformal therapy (irradiation)
dynamic contrast-enhanced subtraction study
dynamic filtering
dynamic lineshape effects
dynamic multileaf collimation
dynamic pedobarography
dynamic radiotherapy
dynamic range control (DRC) algorithm used in digital radiography
dynamic snapshot
Dynamic Spatial Reconstructor (DSR) scanner
dynamic susceptibility contrast (DSC) magnetic resonance imaging
dynamic tagging magnetic resonance angiography
dynamic ultrasound of shoulder (DUS)
dynamic volume-rendered display
dynamic volumetric SPECT

dynamic wedge
Dynarad portable imaging system
dynode
dynograph
dyschezia
dyschondroplasia
dyscollagenosis
dyscrasic fracture
dysfunction
  positional
  swallowing
dysgenesis
  alar
  anorectal
  callosal
  corticocallosal
  epiphyseal
  gonadal
dyshormonogenesis
dyskinesia
  bile duct
  biliary
  regional
  tardive
  anterior wall
  anteroapical
  left ventricular
  segmental wall motion
  wall motion
dysmaturity, pulmonary
dysmotility, esophageal
dysosteogenesis
dysostosis
  cleidocranial
  craniofacial
  metaphyseal
dysostosis multiplex
dyspepsia
dyspeptic
dysphagia
  contractile ring
  esophageal

dysphagia *(cont.)*
  liquid food
  oropharyngeal
  postvagotomy
  pre-esophageal
  progressive
  sideropenic
  soft food
  solid food
  vallecular
dysphagia inflammatoria
dysphagia lusoria
dysphagia nervosa
dysphagia paralytica
dysphagia spastica
dysphagia valsalviana
dysplasia
  acropectorovertebral
  arteriohepatic
  bone
  bronchopulmonary
  cleidocranial
  congenital (of hip) (CDH)
  congenital polyvalvular
  cranioskeletal
  developmental
  diaphyseal
  endocardial
  epiarticular osteochondromatous
  familial arterial fibromuscular
  fibromuscular (FMD)
  fibrous
  foot
  mesomelic
  microscopic cortical
  mammary
  metaphyseal
  Mondini
  monostotic fibrous
  multiple epiphyseal
  Namaqualand hip
  oculoauriculovertebral (OAV)

dysplasia *(cont.)*
   odontoid
   osseous
   perimedial
   polyostotic fibrous
   polypoid
   progressive diaphyseal
   pulmonary valve (PVD)
   retroareolar
   right ventricular
   sheetlike
   Sponastrine
   spondyloepiphyseal
   Streeter
   tricuspid valve
   thymic
   ventricular
   ventriculo-radial
dysplasia with associated lesion or mass (DALM)
dyspnea on exertion
dysprosium analogue
dysprosium ($^{166}$Dy) $^{166}$Ho holmium in vivo generator
dysprosium HP-DO3A imaging agent
dysraphism
   closed spinal
   occult spinal
   spinal
dyssynergia
   biliary
   detrusor-sphincter
   regional
   segmental
dyssynergy
dystocia
   fetal
   shoulder
dystopia
dystopic
dystrophy
dysuria

# E, e

EAC (expandable access catheter)
E:A ratio on echocardiogram
early-phase termination
early venous filling
Eastman Kodak scanner
EBA (extrahepatic biliary atresia)
EBCT (electron beam computed
 tomography)
EBDA (effective balloon dilated area)
Eberth line
EBIORT (electron beam intraoperative
 radiotherapy)
EBRT (external beam radiation
 therapy)
Ebstein sign
eburnation, bony
ECA (external carotid artery)
E-CABG (endarterectomy and
 coronary artery bypass graft)
eccentrically placed lumen
eccentric atherosclerotic plaque
eccentric atrial activation
eccentric axis of rotation of the ankle
eccentric coronary artery
eccentric hypertrophy
eccentricity index
eccentric ledge

eccentric lesion
eccentric plaque disease
eccentric stenosis
eccentric vessel
ecchondroma
eccrine angiomatous hamartoma
ECG (electrocardiogram)
 ECG gating
 ECG-synchronized digital
  subtraction angiography
echo (slang for echocardiogram)
echo (pl. echoes)
 amphoric
 atrial
 bright
 dense
 highly mobile
 internal
 solid
 homogeneous
 inhomogeneous
 linear
 median level
 metallic
 navigator
 shower of
 sonographic

**echo • echocardiography**

echo *(cont.)*
  specular
  spin
  swirling smokelike
  thick
  ultrasonographic
  ultrasound
  ventricular
echocardiogram
echocardiogram adenosine
echocardiographic automated border
echocardiography
  akinesis on
  ambulatory Holter
  A-mode
  anterior left ventricular wall
    motion
  apical
  apical five-chamber view
  apical left ventricular wall motion
    on
  apical two-chamber view
  B bump on anterior mitral valve
    leaflet
  B-mode
  biplane transesophageal
  blood pool radionuclide
  cardiac output
  color flow imaging Doppler
  continuous loop exercise
  continuous wave Doppler
  contrast
  contrast-enhanced
  cross-sectional two-dimensional
  CW (continuous wave) Doppler
  D-to-E slope on
  detection
  dipyridamole
  dobutamine stress
  Doppler
  dyskinesis on
  echo-free space on

echocardiography *(cont.)*
  echo intensity disappearance rate on
  epicardial Doppler
  E point on
  exercise
  Feigenbaum
  fetal (in utero)
  four-chamber
  hypokinesis on
  inferior left ventricular wall
    motion on
  intracardiac (ICE)
  intracoronary contrast
  intraoperative cardioplegic contrast
  late systolic posterior displacement
    on
  lateral left ventricular wall motion
    on
  left ventricular long-axis
  long-axis parasternal view
  loss of an "a" dip on
  MCE (myocardial contrast
    echocardiography)
  M-mode Doppler
  multiplanar transesophageal
  myocardial contrast (MCE)
  myocardial perfusion
  parasternal long-axis view
  parasternal short-axis view
  pharmacologic stress
  postcontrast
  posterior left ventricular wall
    motion on
  postexercise
  postinjection
  postmyocardial infarction
  precontrast
  preinjection
  premyocardial infarction
  pulsed Doppler
  pulsed-wave (PW) Doppler
  real-time

echocardiography *(cont.)*
  resting
  right ventricular short-axis
  sector scan
  septal wall motion on
  short-axis view
  signal averaged
  stress
  subcostal short-axis view
  subxiphoid view of
  three-dimensional (3D or 3-D)
  transesophageal (TEE)
  transthoracic (TTE)
  transthoracic three-dimensional
  two-dimensional (2D or 2-D)
  two-chamber
  ventricular wall motion
echo characteristics on ultrasound
echo contrast
echo delay time (TE)
echo-dense (or echodense)
echo density
echoencephalography
echo FLASH MR
echo-free area
echo-free central zone
echo-free space
Echogen (or EchoGen) imaging agent
echogenic
echogenicity
echogram
echography for placement of radiation therapy fields
echoic
echoicity
echolucent plaque
EchoMark angiographic catheter
echo pattern
  homogeneous
  inhomogeneous
echophonocardiography

echo planar (or echo-planar) imaging (EPI)
  FLAIR
  multi-shot
  one-shot
  MR (magnetic resonance)
  pulse sequence
  sequence
echo reflectivity
echo reverberation
echo signature
echo-tagging technique
echo texture (also echotexture)
echo time (TE)
echo train length (ETL)
Echovar Doppler system
Echovist (SHU 454) imaging agent
ECIC (extracranial-intracranial) arterial bypass
ECHO therapy
ECRB (extensor carpi radialis brevis) muscle
ECRL (extensor carpi radialis longus) muscle
ECT acquisition
ectasia
  alveolar
  annuloaortic
  basilar artery
  coronary artery
  diffuse arterial
  ductal
  mammary
  renal tubular
  tubular
  vascular
ectatic emphysema
ectocardia
ectopic beat
ectopic bone growth in joint
ectopic focus (pl. foci)
ectopic impulse

ectopic pregnancy (EP)
ectopic rest
ectopic thyroid tissue
ectopic ureter
ectopic wall motion abnormality
ectopy
ectrodactyly
ECU (extensor carpi ulnaris) muscle
EDAMS (encephaloduroarteriomyo-
   synangiosis)
EDAS (encephaloduroarterio-
   synangiosis)
EDB (extensor digitorum brevis)
   muscle
EDC (extensor digitorum communis)
   muscle
eddy (pl. eddies)
eddy current artifact
eddy formation
edema
   acute pulmonary
   alveolar
   alveolar pulmonary
   angioneurotic
   antral
   brain
   bronchiolar
   brown
   bullous
   bullous-like
   capillary permeability
   cardiac
   cardiogenic pulmonary
   cardiopulmonary
   cerebral
   chemical pulmonary
   chronic
   circumscribed
   collateral
   compressive
   cyclical
   cyclic idiopathic

edema *(cont.)*
   diffuse
   fingerprint
   focal
   frank pulmonary
   fulminant pulmonary
   generalized pulmonary
   high-altitude pulmonary (HAPE)
   hypervolemic pulmonary
   idiopathic
   ileocecal
   inflammatory
   interstitial
   interstitial pulmonary
   intracompartmental
   laryngeal
   leg
   liver
   local
   localized
   lymphatic
   lymph-
   malignant brain
   massive pulmonary hemorrhagic
   mild
   nephrotic
   nerve root
   neurogenic pulmonary
   noncardiac pulmonary
   noncardiogenic pulmonary
   osmotic
   paroxysmal pulmonary
   passive
   patchy
   pericholecystic
   pericystic
   perihilar
   perineoplastic
   periorbital
   peripheral
   peritumoral
   perivascular

edema *(cont.)*
  plerocephalic
  postoperative pulmonary
  pulmonary
  reexpansion pulmonary
  renal
  solid (of lungs)
  stasis
  subglottic
  supraglottic
  terminal
  thalamic
  trace
  vasogenic
  venous
  vernal (of lung)
  visceral
edema fluid
edema neonatorum
edematous tissues
edentulous
edge
  boundary
  leading
  ligament reflecting
  ligament shelving
  liver
  Poupart ligament shelving
  sawtooth
  shelving
  sternal
  tentorial
  trailing
edge-boundary artifact
edge-detection angiography
edge effect
edge-enhanced error diffusion
  algorithm
edge misalignment artifact
edge profile acutance
edge-region pixel
edge ringing artifact

EDH (epidural hematoma)
EDL (extensor digitorum longus)
  muscle
Edmondson Grading System for
  hepatocellular carcinoma
EDQ (extensor digiti quinti) muscle
EDRT (endothelium-derived relaxant
  factor)
EDSRF spectrome
EDV (end-diastolic volume)
Edwards diagnostic catheter
EDXRF spectrometer
EF (ejection fraction)
EFF (electromagnetic focusing field)
  probe
efface, effacement
  cistern
  cisterna magna
  dural sac
  nerve root sheath
  sulcus
  ventricle
effect
  adverse
  anisotropic
  Anrep
  artifact
  attenuation
  Bayliss
  Bohr
  BOLD
  Bowditch
  bronchodilator
  bronchomotor
  cobra head
  collimator exchange
  Compton
  copper wire
  cumulative
  deleterious
  demagnetization field
  Dotter

effect *(cont.)*
  dottering
  dynamic lineshape
  edge
  flow-related enhancement
  halo
  hemispheral mass
  hemodynamic
  lag
  magnetization transfer
  masquerading
  mass
  neurotoxic
  purse-stringing
  reservoir
  silver wire
  snowplow
  vasodilatory
  Venturi
  washboard
  Wolff-Chaikoff
effective refractory period (ERP)
effective renal plasma flow (ERPF)
efferent arteriolar resistance
efferent digital nerve
efferent view
effervescent agent
efficacious
efficacy
  clinical
  drug therapy
  treatment
efficiency
  absolute-peak
  full energy peak
  valvular
effluent
effort
  inspiratory
  respiratory
  suboptimal
effort-dependent

effort thrombosis
effuse
effused chyle
effusion
  cardiac
  exudative
  free pleural
  hemorrhagic
  inflammatory joint
  ipsilateral pleural
  joint
  layering
  liquid pleural
  loculated
  loculated pleural
  noninflammatory joint
  pericardial (PE)
  pleural
  pleurisy with
  pleuropericardial
  pseudochylous
  serofibrinous pericardial
  subdural
  subpleural
  taut pericardial
  tuberculous
effusion artifact
effusion of blood in pleural cavity
EG (esophagogastric) junction
Egan mammography
Egawa sign
eggshell border of aneurysm
eggshell-like calcification
eggshell nodal calcification
egress of blood
EHL (extensor hallucis longus)
  muscle
EHM (extrahepatic metastasis)
EHT (electrohydrothermo) electrode
eigenvector analysis
eigenvector, principal
8 x 8 pixel-block

eighth nerve tumor
Einthoven triangle
EIP (extensor indicis proprius) muscle
Eisenmenger complex
Eisenmenger syndrome
ejection, accelerated
ejection fraction (EF)
  area-length method for
  basilar half
  blunted
  BSA (body surface area)
  cardiac
  computed
  depressed
  digital
  Dodge method for
  gallbladder
  global
  globally depressed
  interval
  Kennedy method for calculating
  left ventricular (LVEF)
  one-third
  regional
  resting left ventricular
  right ventricular (RVEF)
  systolic
  thermodilution
  well preserved
ejection fraction acoustic quantification, left ventricular
ejection fraction by first-pass technique
ejection phase indices
ejection sound
  palpable aortic
  palpable pulmonic
ejection time
  increased left ventricular
  prolonged
EJV (external jugular vein)
EKG or ECG (electrocardiogram)
EKG-gated multislice
EKG-gated spin-echo
EKG-synchronized digital subtraction angiography
EKG triggered, flow-compensated, gradient echo image
Ektascan laser printer
El Gamal coronary bypass catheter
elaborate
elastic cross-section
elastic recoil of artery
elastic stable intramedullary nailing (ESIN)
elastic subtraction algorithms
elastic subtraction spiral CT angiography
elasticity
elastography, magnetic resonance (MRE)
elastomyofibrosis
elbow
  baseball pitcher's
  boxer's
  floating
  golfer's
  javelin thrower's
  Little Leaguer's
  milkmaid's
  pulled
  reverse tennis
  tennis
  thrower's
  wrestler's
Elecath thermodilution catheter
elective cardiac arrest and subsequent reperfusion
electoplethysmography
electric joint fluoroscopy
electrocardiogram (ECG or EKG)
electrocardiography
electrocardiogram-gated MRI
electrocardiogram-gated SPECT

electrocardiogram tracing
electrocardiographic gating
electrocardiographic variant
electrocardiography, electrocardiogram (ECG or EKG)
electrocardiography-gated echo-planar imaging
electrocardiophonogram
electrocardioscanner, Compuscan Hittman computerized
electrocorticographic evaluation
electrode monitoring
electrogastrogram
electrogastrography
electrolytes
electrolytic
electromagnet, structured coil
electromagnetic blood flow study
electromagnetic interference (EMI)
electromechanical dissociation (EMD) of heart
electrometer
electromyogram
electromyography
electron and x-ray diffraction patterns
electron arc therapy
electron beam boost
electron beam computed tomography (EBCT)
electron beam CT scanner
electron beam intraoperative radiotherapy (EBIORT)
electron bolus
electron dosimetry
electron equilibrium loss
electron linear accelerator
electron microscopy
electron photon field matching
electron production, secondary
electron spin resonance (ESR)
electronic portal imaging
electrons, backscatter

electrophilic radioiodination
electrophoresis
electrostatic potential
electrovectorcardiogram
electrovectorcardiography
element
  posterior
  neoplastic destruction of spinal subluxation of
elevated diaphragms
elevated hemidiaphragms
elimination kinetics
Elite double-loop catheter
Ellestad protocol for treadmill stress test
ellipsoid joint
elliptical
ellipticity index
Ellis-Garland line
Ellis line
Ellis sign
elongated heart
elongation and tortuosity
eloquent areas of brain
ELPIDA architecture
Elscint camera
Elscint dual-detector cardiac camera
Elscint Planar device
Elscint CT scanner
Elscint Twin CT scanner
Elsner syndrome
eluted
elution
elutriation
embarrassment
  circulatory
  cord
  midbrain function
  nerve root
  respiratory
embedding of stent coils
embolectomy, percutaneous balloon

emboli (pl. of embolus), "shower" of
embolic cerebral infarction
embolic event
embolic gangrene
embolic material, nidus of
embolic obstruction
embolic occlusion
embolic phenomenon
embolic shower
embolic stroke
embolism (also embolus)
   air
   amniotic fluid
   arterial
   arterial stenosis
   atheromatous
   bacillary
   bile pulmonary
   bland
   bone marrow
   cancer
   capillary
   cardiogenic
   catheter-induced
   cellular
   cerebral
   cerebral fat
   cholesterol
   coronary artery
   cotton fiber
   crossed
   direct
   fat
   fibrin platelet
   foam
   gas
   gas nitrogen
   hematogenous
   infective
   intracranial
   intraluminal
   lymphogenous

embolism *(cont.)*
   massive
   miliary
   multiple
   obturating
   occluding spring
   oil
   pantaloon
   paradoxical
   peripheral
   plasmodium
   polyurethane foam
   prosthetic valve
   pulmonary (PE)
   pulmonary venous-systemic air
   pyemic
   recurrent
   renal cholesterol
   retinal
   retrograde
   riding
   septic
   septic pulmonary
   silent cerebral
   straddling
   submassive pulmonary
   thrombus
   trichinous
   tumor
   venous
   visceral
embolization
   alcohol
   angiographic variceal
   atheromatous cholesterol crystal
   balloon therapeutic
   balloon and coil
   bronchial artery
   cardiac tumor
   cholesterol
   chronic lung
   coil (of unwanted vessel)

embolization *(cont.)*
  coil (therapeutic)
  diffuse cholesterol
  disseminated atheromatous
  disseminated cholesterol
  endovascular
  flow-directed
  Gelfoam powder
  Ivalon
  massive
  microvascular
  percutaneous transvenous
  selective percutaneous transhepatic
  selective renal artery
  septic
  Silastic bead
  stent
  subsegmental transcatheter arterial (STAE)
  super selective
  therapeutic
  tract
  transarterial
  transcatheter oily chemo-embolization
  transcatheter variceal
  transhepatic (THE)
embolization transcatheter therapy
embolotherapy, catheter
embolus (pl. emboli) (see *embolism*)
embolus trap, Mobin-Uddin
embryonal cell carcinoma
embryonal tumor
embryonal vein
embryonic anastomosis
embryonic aortic arch
embryonic branchial arch
EMED scanner
emergent
emergently
emesis
EMF (endomyocardial fibrosis)
EMI CT scanner
eminence
  arcuate
  articular
  collateral
  cruciate
  cruciform
  deltoid
  facial
  frontal
  genital
  hypothenar
  iliopubic
  iliopectineal
  intercondylar
  intercondyloid
  medial
  median
  occipital
  pyramidal
  thenar
  thyroid
  tibial
emission and transmission data
emission probability
emitter
  alpha-particle
  Auger-electron
emphysema
  alveolar
  alveolar duct
  atrophic
  bronchiolar
  bullous
  centriacinar
  centrilobular
  chronic
  chronic hypertrophic
  chronic obstructive
  chronic tuberculous
  compensating
  compensatory

emphysema *(cont.)*
  congenital lobar
  cystic
  cystic pulmonary
  diffuse
  distal acinar
  distal lobular
  ectatic
  false
  focal-dust
  gangrenous
  generalized
  giant bullous
  glass blower's
  hypoplastic
  idiopathic unilobar
  infantile lobar
  interlobular
  interstitial
  intestinal
  liquefactive
  lobar
  localized obstructive
  lung
  mediastinal
  neck
  necrotizing
  neonatal cystic pulmonary
  obstructive
  oxygen-dependent
  panlobular
  paracicatricial
  paraseptal
  pericicatricial
  postoperative
  postsurgical
  pulmonary
  pulmonary interstitial (PIE)
  pulmonary subcutaneous
    encephalitis
  senile
  skeletal

emphysema *(cont.)*
  small-lunged
  subcutaneous
  substantial
  surgical
  traumatic
  unilateral
  unilateral pulmonary
  vesicular
emphysematous bleb
emphysematous bulla
emphysematous cholecystitis
emphysematous COPD (chronic
  obstructive pulmonary disease)
emphysematous gastritis
emphysematous lungs
emphysematous pyelonephritis
emphysematous type A disease
empirical therapy
emplaced (verb)
empty collapsed lung
emptying time
emptying, tortuous
empty sella syndrome
empyema
  chest
  gallbladder
  interlobar
  latent
  left-sided
  loculated
  metapneumonic
  pericardial
  pleural
  pulsating
  right-sided
  spinal
  subdural
  synpneumonic
  thoracic
  tuberculous
empyema with pachypleuritis

en bloc
encapsulated radioactive "seeds"
encephalitic
encephaloarteriography
encephalocele with cranium bifidum
encephaloclastic lesion
encephalocystocele
encephalodysplasia
encephaloid
encephalolith
encephaloma
encephalomalacia
encephalopathy
encerclage
enchondral ossification
enchondroma
enchondromatosis
encircle
encircled
encircling
encirclement
encoded-Fourier
encoded, wavelet-
encoding gradient
encroachment
   bony
   foraminal
   luminal
encryption algorithms
encryption, scheme
en cuirasse, cor
encysted pleurisy
endarterectomy and coronary artery bypass graft (E-CABG)
end diastole
end-diastolic flow
end-diastolic polar map
end-diastolic pressure
end-diastolic pressure-volume relation
end-diastolic velocity (EDV)
end-diastolic volume (EDV)
end-expiratory lung volume (FRC)

end-expiratory pressure
end-inspiratory pressure
endoanal coil
endoanal sonography
endobrachyesophagus
endobronchial brachytherapy
endobronchial carcinoma
endocardial activation mapping
endocardial catheter mapping
endocardial cushion defect
endocardial fibroelastosis
endocardial fibrosis, Davies
endocardial mapping
endocarditis
endocardium
   disc of
   wafer of
endocavitary applicator system
endochondral bone
endochondral ossification
EndoCoil biliary stent
endocranium
endocrine fracture
endodermal cyst
endoergic reaction
end of atrial systole
endogenous callus formation
endoluminal stent
endolymphatic duct
endolymphatic sac
endometrial echo
endometrial polyp
endometriosis
   colonic involvement of
   sciatic
   studding of
endomyocardial biopsy, ultrasonic guidance for
endomyocardial fibrosis, mural
end-on vessel
endophlebitis
Endo-P-Probe

endoprosthesis
  biliary
  double-lumen
  double-pigtail
  large-bore bile duct
  self-expanding metallic
endorectal coil
endorectal ileal pouch
endorectal ileal pull-through
endorectal ultrasonography
end-organ
endoscopic catheterization
endoscopic quadrature RF coil
endoscopic retrograde cholangiography (ERC)
endoscopic retrograde cholangiopancreatography (ERCP)
endoscopic retrograde pancreatic duct cannulation
endoscopic retrograde parenchymography (ERP)
endoscopic sclerosing therapy
endoscopic ultrasound (EUS)
endoscopic washing pipe
endoscopic water pick
endoscopically
endoscopist
endoscopy, virtual
endoskeleton
EndoSonics IVUS/balloon dilatation catheter
endosonogram
endosonography
endosteal callus
endosteal revascularization
endosteal surface
endosteum
endosystolic volume (ESV)
endotenon
endothelialization of stent
endothelialized vascular grafts
endotheliomatous meningioma
endothelium
  arterial
  pulmonary capillary
  squamous
endothelium-derived contracting factor
endothelium-derived relaxant factor (EDRF)
Endotrac carpal tunnel release system
endotracheal (ET) tube intubation
endovaginal sonography
endovascular aortic graft
endovascular coil
endovascular embolization
endovascular flow wire study
endovascular stent-graft
endovascular therapy
endovascular ultrasonography
endplate
  hyaline-cartilage (of intervertebral disk)
  vertebral body
endpoint, measurable
end-pressure artifact
end-stage rejection
end-stage renal failure
end-systolic polar map
end-systolic pressure-volume relation
end-systolic reversal
end-systolic volume (ESV) indices
end-to-end anastomosis
end-to-side anastomosis
enema
  air
  air contrast barium
  analeptic
  barium (BE)
  blind
  contrast
  Cortenema retention
  double contrast barium (DCBE)
  flatus
  Fleet

enema (cont.)
   full column barium
   Gastrografin
   Harris flush
   hydrocortisone
   hydrogen peroxide
   Kayexalate
   lactulose
   mesalamine
   methylene blue
   nuclear
   phosphate
   phosphosoda
   prednisolone
   retention
   Rowasa
   saline cleansing
   single-contrast barium
   small bowel
   soapsuds (SSE)
   steroid foam
   sulfasalazine
   tap water
   theophylline olamine
   water soluble contrast
enemas administered until clear
energy
   beam
   kinetic
   low photon
   treatment
   variable
energy decays
energy transfer process
en face view
Engel-Recklinghausen disease
Engelmann disease
engorged collecting system
engorged tissues
engorged veins
engorgement
   vascular
   venous

Enhance deblurring method
enhanced imaging
enhancement
   contrast
   Doppler flow signal
   heterogeneous isodense
   isodense
   nodule
   nonhomogeneous
   PALA
   peak
   signal
   vascular MR contrast
enhancement morphology
enhancement pattern
enhancement rate, instantaneous
enhancing lesion
enlargement
   cardiac silhouette
   chamber
   compensatory
   hilar lymph node
   mediastinal lymph node
enophthalmic
en plaque, meningioma
ensiform appendix
ensiform process
ensued, ensuing
enteral alimentation
enteral nutrition (EN)
enterobiliary
enterocele sac
enterococcus
enterocutaneous fistula
enterocystoma
enteroenteral fistula
enteroinsular axis
enterolith
enteroperitoneal abscess
enteroptosis
enterourethral fistula
enterovesical fistula

enthesophytes, subacromial
entrapment
  artery
  gas
  guide-wire
  nerve
  soft tissue
entrapment syndrome
entry slice phenomenon (artifact MRI)
entry zone
enucleated
envelope, soft tissue
environment, fibroblastic
environmental implication
environmental plutonium
enzymes, fluid
EOL (end of life)
EORTC (European Organization for Research and Treatment of Cancer)
EP (ectopic pregnancy)
eparterial bronchus
EPB (extensor pollicis brevis) muscle
EPBF (effective pulmonary blood flow)
ependymoma
  malignant
  myxopapillary
  spinal cord
EPI (echo planar imaging)
epicardial attachment
epicardial Doppler echocardiography
epicardial Doppler flow transducer
epicardial fat pad
epicardial imaging
epicardial implantation
epicardial reflection
epicardial space
epicardial surface
epicardial tension
epicardial vessels, vasorelaxation of
epicardium

epicondylar fracture
epicondyle
epicortical lesion
epicranial aponeurosis
epidermal growth factor
epidermoid cyst
epidermoid tumor
epididymis
  appendix of
  body of
  edema of
  inflammation of
  interstitial congestion of
  ligament of
  lobule of
  sinus of
  tail of
epididymography
epidural blood
epidural catheter
epidural cavity
epidural hematoma
epidural hemorrhage
epidural mass
epidural space
epidural venography
epidurogram
epidurography
epigastric discomfort
epigastric distress
epigastric hernia
epigastrium
epiglottic disruption
epiglottis
epilepsy-causing brain tumors
epileptic focus
epileptogenic foci
epileptogenic zone
epiphrenic diverticulum
epiphyseal arrest
epiphyseal chondroblastic growth
epiphyseal coxa vara

epiphyseal disk
epiphyseal fracture
epiphyseal growth
epiphyseal hyperplasia
epiphyseal plate
epiphyseal (or epiphysial)
epiphysis (pl. epiphyses)
  annular
  atavistic
  capital
  capital femoral
  capitular
  hypertrophy of
  Perthes
  pressure
  slipped
  slipped capital femoral (SCFE)
  slipped upper femoral (SUFE)
  stippled
  tibial
  traction
epiploic
episode, silent ischemic
episodic colic
Epistar subtraction angiography
epistaxis, spontaneous
epitendineum
epithalamus
epithelial malignancy
epithelial membrane antigen (EMA) antibody
epithelial-myoepithelial carcinoma
epithelialization, creeping
epithelioid hemangioendothelioma
epithelioid sarcoma
epitrochlear
EPL (extensor pollicis longus) muscle
E point on apex cardiogram
E point of cardiac apex pulse
E point to septal separation (EPSS)
eponychium
Eppendorf catheter

EPR dosimetry
EPSS (E point to septal separation)
EQP (extensor quinti proprius)
equalization, histogram
equalization of pressure
equalized diastolic pressures
equation
  Bloch
  Kety
  Larmor
  Stewart-Hamilton
equilibrium angiocardiography
equilibrium factor
equilibrium MUGA scan
equilibrium phase
equilibrium point
equilibrium radionuclide angiocardiography
equilibrium radionuclide angiogram
equilibrium view
equinus deformity
equipment artifact
equipment
  interventional
  real-time
equivocal findings
Erb disease
Erb-Duchenne-Klumpke injury to brachial plexus
Erb point (of heart)
ERC (endoscopic retrograde cholangiography)
ERCP (endoscopic retrograde cholangiopancreatography)
ERCP manometry
Erdheim-Chester disease
Erdheim cystic medionecrosis
Erdheim I syndrome
ERE (external rotation in extension)
erect position
erect view
erectile dysfunction

erector spinae
ERF (external rotation in flexion)
ergonovine test
erosion
 articular
 bony
 bronchial
 duodenal
 gastric
 gastric antral
 graft-enteric
 linear
 osteoclastic
 pedicle
 plaque
 salt and pepper duodenal
 tumor
erosion of articular surface
erosive gastritis
ERP (effective refractory period)
ERP (endoscopic retrograde parenchymography)
 atrial
 ventricular
ERPF (effective renal plasma flow)
error
 darkroom
 Hausdorff
 isocenter placement
 magnification
 mean-square
 photoreceptor fractional velocity
 positioning
 raster spacing
 sensing
 size estimation
error diffusion method
error sum criterion
erythema of joint
erythematosus, systemic lupus
escape beat
escape interval

escape mechanism, ventricular
escape of air into lung connective tissue
escape-peak ratio
E sign on x-ray
ESIN (elastic stable intramedullary nailing)
ESOLAN program
EsophaCoil biliary stent
esophageal A ring
esophageal B ring
esophageal fold
esophageal hiatus
esophageal inlet
esophageal motility disorder, nonspecific (NEMD)
esophageal obturator airway
esophageal plexus
esophageal reflux
esophageal spasm
esophageal varices
esophageal web
esophageal window
esophagitis
esophagogastric fat pad
esophagogastric junction
esophagogram
esophagorespiratory fistula
esophagospasm
esophagram
 barium swallow
 contrast
esophagus
 achalasia of
 aperistaltic
 A ring of
 Barrett
 B ring of
 cervical
 columnar-lined
 corkscrew (diffuse esophageal spasm)

esophagus *(cont.)*
   distal
   dysmotile
   nutcracker
   spastic
   thoracic
   tortuous
   upper thoracic
ESP (end-systolic pressure)
ESP/ESV ratio
ESR (electron spin resonance)
ESR measurement
Essex-Lopresti calcaneal fracture
esthesioneuroblastoma
estimated blood loss (EBL)
estimation
   bayesian image (BIE)
   fractional moving blood volume
   MR volume
   volume
estrogen receptor status
ESV (end-systolic volume)
ESVI (end-systolic volume index)
ESWI/ESVI (end-systolic wall stress index/end-systolic volume index)
ESWL (extracorporeal shock wave lithotripsy)
ET (ejection time)
ET (endotracheal) tube
etanidazole
etching, track
ethanol, ethanolism
ethanol injection, percutaneous
ethanol therapy
Ethiodane contrast medium
ethiodized oil
Ethiodol contrast medium
ethmoid bone
ethmoid sinus
ethmoidal canal
ethmoidal foramen
ethmoidal meningoencephalocele

Ethodian (iophendylate) radiopaque contrast medium
etiology undetermined
etiology unknown
ETL (echo train length)
ETL 3D FSE imaging
E to A changes
E-TOF (time of flight) detecting module
E to F slope of valve on echocardiogram
EtOH (ethanol; ethyl alcohol)
EtOH-associated liver disease
ETT (exercise tolerance test)
eukinesis
Eureka collimator
European Organization for Research and Treatment of Cancer (EORTC)
eurysternum
EUS (endoscopic ultrasound)
EUS (endoscopic ultrasonography)
euthyroid sick syndrome
Evac-Q-Kit
Evac-Q-Kwik bowel prep
evacuation
   colonic
   digital rectal
   precipitate
evaluation
   biological
   electrocorticographic
   functional
   in vitro
   initial staging
   noninvasive
evacuation disorder
evaluation of deep veins for patency and valvular reflux
evaluation of glucose metabolism
evanescent
Evans blue imaging agent
Evans fracture classification system

Evans syndrome
EVD (external ventricular drain)
even distribution of echoes in
    ultrasonography
event
    adverse
    atrial sensed (As)
    cardinal
    embolic
    inciting
    ischemic
    morbid
    precipitating
    untoward
    ventricular sensed
event counter
event marker
event recorder
eventration (peaking)
eventration of diaphragms
eversion sprain
evert, everted
evolution, stroke in
evolving stroke
Ewald test meal
Ewart sign
Ewing tumor
ex vacuo, hydrocephalus
ex vivo magnetic resonance imaging
exacerbate, exacerbated
exacerbation, acute
exam (examination)
exametazime imaging agent
exanthematous disease
excavatum, pectus
excellent prognosis
excessive joint play
exchange
    air
    catheter
    coupling
    guide wire
    narrowing

excimer (from "excited dimer") laser
excitation
    TCR rebound
    variable flip angle
    wave of
excitation function measurement
excitation profile
excitation-spoiled fat-suppressed T1-
    weighted SE images
exclusionary cue
exclusion-HPLC technique
exclusion, subtotal gastric
excrescence, bony
excrete
excretory intravenous pyelography
excretory phase
excretory urogram
excursion
exenteration, total pelvic
exercise echocardiography
exercise first-pass LVEF
exercise images
exercise-induced ischemia
exercise intolerance
exercise load (kpm/min)
exercise, modified stage
exercise oximetry
exercise strain gauge venous
    plethysmography
exercise stress-redistribution
    scintigraphy
exercise thallium-201 stress test
exercise thallium-201 tomography
exhalation
exit site of catheter
exit wound
Exner plexus
exocardia
exoccipital bone
exoergic reaction
exogenous obesity
exophytic adenocarcinoma

exostosis (pl. exostoses)
  blocker's
  bony
  epiphyseal
  hereditary multiple
  hypertrophic
  impingement
  marginal
  retrocalcaneal
  tackler's
  traction
  turret
expandable access catheter (EAC)
expanded lung
expanding intracranial mass
expansile lytic lesion
expansion
  complete stent
  emphysematous
  fluid
  lung
  rapid fluid
  stent
Expert-XL densitometer
expiration, quantitative CT during
expiratory chest
expiratory computed tomography
expiratory flow
exploration, common bile duct (CBDE)
exponential decay
exponential shape
exposure, bone-tendon
exposure variation
Express over-the-wire balloon catheter
expression
  acute phase gene
  HER-2 neu oncoprotein
expression vector
exquisite detail
exsanguinate, exsanguinated
exstrophy

extended pattern
extended tibial in situ bypass
extension
  basal
  Buck
  Codivilla
  extraaxial
  hilar
  intracavitary
  medial
  parenchymal
  parietal
  suprasellar
  tumor
extension injury of spine
extensive dissection
extensor
  apparatus
  mechanism
extensor carpi radialis brevis (ECRB) muscle
extensor carpi radialis longus (ECRL) muscle
extensor digitorum communis (EDC) muscle
extensor digitorum longus (EDL) muscle
extensor hallucis longus (EHL) muscle
extensor indicis proprius (EIP) muscle
extensor pollicis brevis (EPB) muscle
extensor pollicis longus (EPL) muscle
extensor quinti proprius (EQP) muscle
extensus, hallux
exteriorization
external beam radiation therapy (EBRT)
external blow over a full bladder
external carotid artery (ECA)
external carotid steal syndrome
external fixation
external heat generating source
external hyperthermia treatment

external iliac artery
external inguinal ring
external jugular vein
external oblique aponeurosis
external ring
external ventricular drain (EVD)
external wire fixation
extirpation of saphenous vein
extra-articular fracture
extra-adrenal chromaffin tissue
extra-adrenal sites
extra-articular resection
extra-axial fluid collection, crescent-shaped
extracapsular dissection
extracapsular fracture
extracardiac anomalies
extracardiac collateral circulation
extracardiac right-to-left shunt
extracavitary-infected graft
extracavitary prosthetic arterial graft
extracerebral intracranial glioneural hamartoma
extracorporeal membrane oxygenation (ECMO) therapy
extracorporeal photochemotherapy
extracorporeal shock wave lithotripsy (ESWL)
extracranial carotid artery atherosclerosis
extracranial carotid occlusive disease
extracranial cerebral circulation
extracranial-intracranial bypass (ECIC)
extracranial vessel
extraction
  automatic
  contour
  disphenoid
  first-pass
  fringe skeleton
  stone
  vascular segmentation and

extraction catheter
  transcutaneous
  transluminal
extraction catheter atherectomy
extraction column
extraction method
extradural artery
extradural compartment
extradural defect
extradural space
extradural tumor
extradural vertebral plexus of veins
extrahepatic bile ducts, dilated
extrahepatic biliary atresia (EBA)
extraintestinal
extraluminal air
extraluminal contrast medium
extraluminal endarterectomy
extramedullary hemangioma
extraneous material
extraovarian mass
extraparenchymal cyst
extrapericardial dissection
extraperitoneal rupture
extrapleural drainage
extrapleural hemorrhage
extrapleural space
extrapolate
extrapolation
extrapulmonary tuberculosis
extrapyramidal tract
extraskeletal osteosarcoma
extrathecal nerve roots
extrathoracic obstruction
extrauterine gestation
extrauterine pregnancy
extravasated blood
extravasated contrast
extravasation
  bile
  blood
  contrast

extravasation *(cont.)*
   dye
   fluid
   intravascular content
   joint fluid
   radiopaque fluid
   urinary
extravascular fluid
extravascular mass
extravascular pressure
extraventricular obstruction
extravesical opacification
extremity (pl. extremities)
   lower (LEs)
   upper (UEs)
extrinsic compression of trachea
extrinsic foot muscles
extrinsic lesion
extrinsic sick sinus syndrome
extrude

extruding
extrusion, disk
extubate, extubation
exuberant atheroma formation
exuberant granulation tissue
exudate
exudation
exudation of fibrin-rich fluid
exudative consolidation
exudative effusion
exudative pericardial fluid
exudative pleurisy
exudative tuberculosis
eye shield
   lead
   tungsten
eye view, beam's
eye-view 3D-CRT
eyelet, rod
E-Z-Paque barium suspension

# F, f

F (fluorine)
FAB (French/American/British)
  classification
Fab (fragment antigen binding)
  fragment
fabella
fabellofibular complex
Fabry disease
face, en
facet (also facette)
  articular
  atlas
  capitate
  clavicular
  corneal
  costal
  flat
  hamate
  inferior
  inferior costal
  inferior medial
  Lenoir
  locked
  lunate
  scaphoid
  squatting
  superior

facet *(cont.)*
  superior articular
  superior costal
  transverse costal
facet capsule disruption
facet dislocation
facet joint
facet joint vacuum
facet surface of vertebra
facet syndrome
facet tropism
facetal imbrication
faceted gallstone
facial bipartition
facial fracture
facial nerve (seventh cranial nerve)
facial nerve canal
facies ossea
facile synthesis
facing of metacarpal heads
facioauriculovertebral (FAV)
  syndrome
faciostenosis
FACScan (fluorescence-activated cell
  sorter) flow cytometer
FACSVantage cell sorter
factitial

factor (pl. factors)
  Boltzmann
  EDRT
  endothelium-derived relaxant (EDRT)
  epidermal growth
  equilibrium
  geometry
  NOMOS correction
  overrelaxation
  prognostic
  recurrent human granulocyte colony stimulating (r-met HuG-CSF)
  technical
  wedge
Fahr-Volhard disease
FAI (functional aerobic impairment)
failed back surgery syndrome (FBSS)
failure
  adrenal
  cardiac
  congestive heart (CHF)
  hepatic
  liver
  heart
  multiple organ
  multisystem
  pituitary
  pulmonary
  renal
  respiratory
  vein graft
  ventricular
Fairbanks changes on x-ray
falciform ligament
falcine region
falcotentorial meningioma
falcula
falcular
fallopian tube
fallopian tube diverticula
fallopian tube occlusion

falloposcopy (with imaging)
Fallot, tetralogy of
fallout, signal
false aneurysm
false channel
false color scale
false diverticulum
false emphysema
false lumen
false sac
falx
  calcification of
  cerebral
falx cerebelli
falx cerebri
falx meningioma
familial adenomatous polyposis (FAP)
familial aortic dissection
familial avascular necrosis of phalangeal epiphysis
familial cardiomegaly
familial cavernous malformation
familial goiter
familial hypophosphatemic rickets
fan angle
fan beam
fan-beam collimator
fan-beam formula
fan-beam projection
fan-beam reconstruction
Fanconi-Hegglin syndrome
fan-shaped view
FAP (femoral artery pressure)
Faraday catheter
Farber disease
Farber syndrome
far field
farmer's lung
fascia
  anal
  antebrachial
  anterior rectus

fascia *(cont.)*
  axillary
  bicipital
  brachial
  broad
  buccopharyngeal
  Camper
  cervical
  clavipectoral
  Cloquet
  Colles
  cremasteric
  crural
  cribriform
  Cruveilhier
  deep
  deltoid
  dentate
  diaphragmatic
  endopelvic
  endothoracic
  extraperitoneal
  Gerota
  iliac
  infraspinous
  investing
  lateral oblique
  lateroconal
  lumbar
  medial geniculate
  obturator
  obturator internus
  palmar
  parietal pelvic
  pelvic
  perineal
  psoas
  quadratus femoris
  renal
  rim of
  Scarpa
  Sibson

fascia *(cont.)*
  subcutaneous
  superficial
  superficial temporalis
  superficial temporoparietal
  thoracolumbar
  visceral pelvic
  fascia lata (but *tensor fasciae latae*)
fascial plane
fascial rent
fascial thickening
fascial tract
fasciculus (pl. fasciculi)
  arcuate
  lenticular
  longitudinal
  longitudinalis medialis
  medial longitudinal (MLF)
fasciogram
FAST (flow-assisted, short-term)
FAST balloon catheter
Fastcard
fast cardiac phase contrast cine imaging
fast dynamic volumetric x-ray CT
fast-FLAIR technique
fast-flow lesions
fast-flow malformation
fast-flow vascular anomaly
fast Fourier spectral analysis
fast Fourier transform (FFT)
fast fractionation
fast GE (Fastcard) sequences
fast low-angle shot (FLASH)
fast multiplanar spoiled gradient-recalled (FMPSPGR) imaging
fast-neutron therapy
fast PC cine MR sequence with echo-planar gradient
fast routine production
fast SE (FSE) imaging
fast SE and fast IR (FMPIR) imaging

fast SE train
fast short tau inversion recovery (fast STIR)
fast spin echo MR imaging
fast spin echo T2-weighted image
fast spoiled gradient-recalled MR imaging
fast STIR (short tau inversion recovery)
fat
  abdominal
  dietary
  digital process of
  extraperitoneal
  ischiorectal pad of
  pericolonic
  perihilar
  perinephric
  perirectal
  perirenal
  preperitoneal
  properitoneal
  protruding
  renal
  subcutaneous
fatal dose of radiation
fatal exsanguination
fatal herniation
fat embolism syndrome (FES)
fat embolus, cerebral
fatigability
fatigue damage
fatigue fracture
fatigue, progressively severe
fat line, subcutaneous
fat metabolism
fat pad
  abdominal
  antimesenteric
  foveal
  heel
  Hoffa

fat pad (cont.)
  intrapatellar
  ischiorectal
  pericardial
  scalene
fat pad sign
fat plane
fat selective presaturation
fat signal intensity
fat-suppressed three-dimensional spoiled gradient-echo FLASH MR imaging
fat suppression, double-echo three-point Dixon method
fat suppression pulse
fat suppression technique
fatty acid metabolism
fatty degeneration
fatty filum terminale
fatty infiltration of liver
fatty liver
fatty meal sonogram (FMS)
fatty streak atherosclerosis
fatty tumor
fat-water interface
fauces (pl. of faux)
  anterior pillar of
  arch of
fault, sagittal plane
faulty colloid preparation with excess aluminum
faulty RF (radiofrequency) shielding in MRI scanner room artifact
faux (see *fauces*)
faveolate
Favre disease
FB (foreign body)
FBP (filtered back-projection) method
FBS (failed back syndrome)
FBSS (failed back surgery syndrome)
FCR (flexor carpi radialis) muscle
FCR 9501HQ high-resolution storage phosphor imaging agent

FCS (full cervical spine) series of x-rays
FCU (flexor carpi ulnaris) muscle
FDC (flexor digitorum communis) muscle
FDG (fluorodeoxyglucose; fludeoxyglucose F-18)
FDG-blood flow mismatch
FDG-labeled positron imaging
FDG myocardial imaging
FDG PET scan
FDG SPECT
FDI (first digital interosseous) muscle
FDI (frequency domain imaging) in ultrasound
FDL (flexor digitorum longus) muscle
FDP (fibrin degradation products) on MRI
FDP (flexor digitorum profundus) muscle
FDQ (flexor digiti quinti) muscle
FDQB (flexor digiti quinti brevis) muscle
FDS (flexor digitorum sublimis) muscle
FDS (flexor digitorum superficialis) muscle
Fe-Ex orogastric tube magnet
feasible alternatives
feathery appearance
fecal impaction
fecal incontinence
fecal material, retained
fecal residue
fecalith
fecaloid
fecaloma
fecaluria
feces
  impacted
  inspissation of
feculence
feculent
Federici sign
feedback
  breathing
  real-time respiratory
feeder arteries
feeder veins
feeding artery to aneurysm
feeding branch of artery
feeding mean arterial pressure (FMAP)
feeding vessel
Feigenbaum echocardiogram
Feiss line
Feldaker syndrome
Feldkamp algorithm
felon
Felty syndrome
fem-pop (slang for femoral-popliteal) bypass
feminine aorta, small
feminizing tumor
femoral above-knee popliteal bypass
femoral anteversion
femoral aortic flush catheter
femoral approach for cardiac catheterization
femoral artery
femoral artery pressure
femoral bone
femoral capital epiphysis
femoral condyle
femoral-femoral bypass graft
femoral-femoral crossover
femoral head and neck
femoral head deformity
femoral head vascularity
femoral hernia
femoral neck
femoral-peroneal in situ vein bypass graft
femoral-popliteal bypass surgery

femoral-popliteal Gore-Tex graft
femoral pulse
femoral tuberosity
femoral vein
femoral vein percutaneous insertion
femoral venoarterial bypass
femoral venous approach
femoral view
femoroaxillary bypass
femorocrural graft
femorodistal bypass
femorodistal popliteal bypass graft
femorofemoral approach
femorofemoral bypass
femorofemoropopliteal
femoroperoneal bypass graft
femoropopliteal angioplasty
femoropopliteal artery
femoropopliteal atheromatous stenosis
femoropopliteal bypass
femoropopliteal thrombosis
femorotibial angle (FTA)
femorotibial bypass graft
femtoliter (fL)
femur (pl. femora)
   apex of
   body of
   greater trochanter of
   head and neck of
   head of
   lesser trochanter of
   neck of
   nutrient artery of
femur length (FL)
fender fracture
fenestra (pl. fenestrae)
fenestration
   aortopulmonary
   apical
   cusp
   interchordal space

fenestration of dissecting aneurysm
Fenwick disease
Feridex contrast medium
ferric ammonium citrate contrast
ferric ammonium citrate-cellulose
   paste
ferric chloride contrast
ferrioxamine methanesulfonate
   contrast
ferrocalcinosis, familial cerebral
ferromagnetic objects creating artifacts
   on imaging studies
   bra underwire
   button
   cigarette lighter
   clothing with metal object
   earring
   hair coloring
   hairpin
   make-up
   metal mesh in toupee or wig
   necklace
   paper clip
   pen
   political button
   probe
   ring
   shunt
   tooth filling
   watch
   zipper
ferromagnetic properties
ferromagnetic relaxation
ferruginous bodies
ferumoxides-enhanced MR imaging
ferumoxsil imaging agent
FES (fat embolism syndrome)
fetal biophysical profile
fetal bradycardia
fetal cardiac anomalies
fetal chromosome abnormality

fetal death
  early
  intermediate
  late
fetal echocardiography in utero
fetal gallbladder
fetal heart
fetal heart failure
fetal hydrops
fetal lobulation
fetal malformation
fetal midface
fetal motion or movement
fetal-pelvic disproportion
fetal-pelvic index
fetal placenta
fetal pole
fetal small parts
fetal sonography
fetal ultrasonography
fetal umbilical vein injection under
  sonographic guidance
fetometry
fetus (pl. fetuses)
  amorphous
  calcified
  growth-retarded
  impacted
  intrauterine
  maturity of
  nonviable
  paper-doll
  parasitic
  placenta of
  presentation of
  previable
  retained dead
  small parts of
  stunted
  tissue of
  umbilical artery in
  viable

fetus papyraceus
FFA (free fatty acid) scintigraphy,
  labeled
FFE sequences
F-4500 Fluorescence Spectrophotometer
FFP (fresh frozen plasma)
FFT (fast Fourier transform) image
FHB (flexor hallucis brevis) muscle
FHC (familial hypertrophic cardiomyopathy)
FHL (flexor hallucis longus) muscle
FI (full-scan with interpolation)
  method/projection
fiber (pl. fibers)
  cardiac muscle
  muscle
  myocardial
  skeletal muscle
  sling muscle
fiberoptic angioscopy
fiberoptic bronchography
fiberoptic light source
fiberoptic tapers
fiberoptic video glasses
fibrillate
fibrin clot
fibrin degradation products (FDP) on
  MRI
fibrin glue, percutaneous
fibrin mass
fibrinogen
  radiolabeled
  technetium $^{99m}$Tc-labeled
fibrinogen degradation
fibrinolytic treatment
fibrinopurulent pleurisy
fibrin sleeve stripping
fibrin split products
fibroadenoma
fibroadipose tissue
fibroblast radiosensitivity

fibroblastic meningioma
fibroblastoma, perineural
fibrocalcific cusps
fibrocalcification
fibrocartilage
  circumferential
  intra-articular plates of
  triangular
fibrocartilaginous disk
fibrocartilaginous plate
fibrocollagenous connective tissue
fibrocystic breast syndrome
fibrocystic residual
fibrodysplasia ossificans progressiva
fibroelastoma of heart valve
fibroelastoma, papillary
fibroid
  calcified
  intramural
  pedunculated
  uterine
fibroid lung
fibroid myocarditis
fibroid uterus
fibrolamellar hepatocarcinoma
fibrolamellar hepatocellular carcinoma
fibrolipoma
fibroma
  aponeurotic
  cementifying
  cemento-ossifying
  chondromyxoid (CMF)
  desmoplastic
  heart
  juvenile ossifying
  meningeal
  nonossifying
  nonosteogenic
  ossifying
  osteogenic
  periosteal
  subcutaneous

fibroma-thecoma tumor of ovary
fibromatosis
fibromuscular dysplasia (FMD)
fibromuscular lesion
fibromuscular ridge
fibromyoma
fibromyxoma, odontogenic
fibronodular
fibro-osseous lesion
fibro-osseous tunnel
fibroretractive
fibrosarcoma
fibrosclerotic
fibrosed muscles
fibroserous pericardial sac
fibrosing inflammatory pseudotumor
fibrosis
  alcoholic
  arachnoid
  basilar
  confluent
  congenital hepatic (CHF)
  cystic
  diffuse interstitial pulmonary
    (DIPF)
  endocardial
  endomyocardial (EMF)
  idiopathic interstitial
  idiopathic pulmonary (IPF)
  interstitial
  interstitial pulmonary
  leptomeningeal
  mediastinal
  meningeal
  myocardial
  nodal
  nodular subepidermal
  noncirrhotic portal (NCPF)
  pericentral
  periductal
  perimuscular
  periportal

fibrosis *(cont.)*
  pipestem
  portal
  portal-to-portal
  postradiation
  progressive perivenular alcoholic (PPAF)
  pulmonary
  radiation-induced
  replacement
  retroperitoneal
  subadventitial
  subintimal
  subserosal
  Symmers
fibrotic cavitating pattern
fibrotic tissue
fibrous dysplasia ossificans progressiva
fibrous goiter
fibrous nonunion
fibrous plaques
fibrous pleural adhesions
fibrous union
fibroxanthoma
fibroxanthosarcoma
fibula
  apex of
  nutrient artery of
fibular bone
fibular notch
fibulotalocalcaneal (FTC) ligament
Ficat-Marcus grading system
Ficat stage of avascular necrosis
Fick equation
Fick method for calculating cardiac output
FID (free induction delay)
fiducial movement
field
  collapsed lung
  disk-to-magnetic

field *(cont.)*
  fringe
  Gibbs random
  high-power
  insonifying wave
  large hinge angle electron
  low-power
  lower lung
  lung
  mantle
  Markov random
  midlung
  near
  oscillating magnetic
  rf or RF (radiofrequency)
  stray neutron
  tangential breast
  tesla (T)
  upper lung
field alignment
field-dependent
field-fitting technique
field gradient
field H of Forel
field lock
field of view (FOV) imaging
field variation, BO
Fielding-Magliato classification of subtrochanteric fracture
fifth compartment
fifth cranial nerve (trigeminal nerve)
fifth intercostal space
fifth left interspace
fifth rib
fighter's fracture
FIGO stage of carcinoma
figure-3 sign
filar lipoma
file transfer protocol, FTP
filiform appendix
filigree pattern
filipuncture

fill and spill of dye (in fallopian
   tubes)
filling
   atrial
   augmented
   capillary
   decreased left ventricular
   left atrial
   left ventricular
   passive
   peak
   rapid
   reduced
   retrograde
   ureteral
   venous
   ventricular
   vessel
filling defect
filling factor
filling phase, rapid
filling pressure
filling rate, peak
film (see also *position, projection, view*)
   Accu-Flo dura
   AP (anteroposterior)
   chest
   chiropractic
   comparison
   cross-table lateral
   decubitus
   digital subtraction
   DuPont Cronex x-ray
   expiratory
   flat plate
   GLP7
   high-contrast
   Knuttsen bending
   lateral
   lateral decubitus
   limited

film *(cont.)*
   low-contrast
   low-dose
   manual subtraction
   oblique
   outside
   overhead
   PA (posteroanterior)
   photo-plotter
   plain
   port
   portable
   postevacuation
   postvoid
   postvoiding
   preliminary
   prone
   radiochromic
   scout
   sequential
   serial
   skull
   spot
   stress
   suboptimal
   subtraction
   supine
   UP7
   upright
   working
film alternator
film-based viewing
film changer, Sanchez-Perez automatic
filmless imaging
film slippage
filter
   bird's nest percutaneous IVC
      (inferior vena cava)
   caval
   differencing
   Gianturco-Roehm bird's nest vena
      caval
   Greenfield vena caval

filter *(cont.)*
   inferior vena caval
   IVC (inferior vena cava)
   Kalman
   Kimray-Greenfield caval
   Mobin-Uddin umbrella
   Mobin-Uddin vena caval
   percutaneous inferior vena cava (IVC)
   prophylactic IVC
   Simon nitinol percutaneous IVC
   Simon nitinol vena cava filter
   translation-invariant
   umbrella
   Venatech percutaneous IVC
   wall
   Wiener
filtered-back projection
filtering, dynamic
filtration
   copper
   dynamic beat
   glomerular
   post beat
filum, fatty
filum terminale, fatty
fimbriated end of fallopian tube
finding (pl. findings)
   angiographic
   auscultatory
   cardinal
   characteristic
   concomitant
   equivocal
   focal
   lateralizing
   no discernible
   ominous
   pathognomonic
   salient physical
   scanty
   specious
   spurious

fine calcification
fine needle
fine-needle biopsy, ultrasound-guided
fine reticular pattern
fine-speckled appearance
Finesse large-lumen guiding catheter
finger
   angle
   baseball
   base of
   bolster
   clubbed
   drop
   fingers
   football
   index
   jammed
   jersey
   little
   long
   mallet
   middle
   pedicle
   pulley of
   pulp of
   replantation of
   replanted
   ring
   sausage
   spade
   speck
   spider
   stoved
   trigger
   webbedb
finger fracture
finger fracture dissection
fingerlike projection
finger of tumor
finger opposition
finger pad
fingerprint image compression

fingertip amputation
fingertip pad
firing of ectopic atrial focus
firing temperature
first-pass effect
first-pass extraction
first-pass imaging
first-pass MUGA
first-pass myocardial perfusion MR
first-pass radionuclide exercise
   angiocardiography
first-pass study
first-pass view
first portion of duodenum
first-trimester nuchal translucency
Fischer sign
fish-flesh appearance
fishmeal worker's lung
fishmouth configuration of mitral
   valve
fishmouth stenosis
fish-scale gallbladder
FISP (gradient echo sequence)
FISP sequence
Fissinger-Rendu syndrome
fission track analysis of urine
fissula
fissuration
fissure
   abdominal
   anal
   anterior median (of cord)
   antitragohelicine
   auricular
   brain
   calcarine
   callosomarginal
   central
   cerebellar
   cerebellopontine or cerebellopontile
   cerebral
   choroidal

fissure *(cont.)*
   chronic
   collateral
   cutaneous
   decidual
   dentate
   displacement of interhemispheric
   glaserian
   hippocampal
   horizontal
   interhemispheric
   lateral
   longitudinal
   lung
   main
   oblique
   occipital
   oral
   palpebral
   portal
   rolandic
   studded
   superior orbital
   supraorbital
   sylvian
   umbilical
fissure fracture
fissure in ano
fissure of Rolando
fissure of Sylvius
fissure sign
fistula
   abdominal
   anal
   anorectal
   aorta-left ventricular
   aorta-right ventricular
   aortic sinus
   aortic sinus to right ventricle
   aortocaval
   aortoduodenal
   aortoenteric

**fistula** *(cont.)*
- aortoesophageal
- aortopulmonary
- aortosigmoid
- AV (arteriovenous)
- biliary
- biliary-cutaneous
- biliary-duodenal
- biliary-enteric
- bilioenteric
- Blom-Singer tracheoesophageal
- branchial
- Brescia-Cimino AV
- bronchobiliary
- bronchocavitary
- bronchocutaneous
- bronchoesophageal
- bronchopleural
- cameral
- carotid artery-cavernous sinus
- carotid cavernous
- carotid-cavernous sinus
- cerebral arteriovenous
- cerebrospinal fluid
- cholecystenteric
- cholecystocholedochal
- cholecystocolonic
- cholecystoduodenal
- cholecystoduodenocolic
- choledochal-colonic
- choledochoduodenal
- chylous
- coil closure of coronary artery
- colocutaneous
- colonic
- colovaginal
- colovesical
- complex anorectal
- congenital
- congenital pulmonary arteriovenous
- coronary
- coronary arteriosystemic

**fistula** *(cont.)*
- coronary arteriovenous
- coronary artery cameral
- coronary artery-pulmonary artery
- coronary artery to right ventricular
- coronary-cameral
- coronary-pulmonary
- CSF (cerebrospinal fluid)
- cystic
- duodenocolic
- dural arteriovenous (AVF)
- durocutaneous
- Eck
- enterocutaneous
- enteroenteral
- enteroenteric
- enterourethral
- enterovaginal
- enterovesical
- esophagorespiratory
- external biliary
- extrasphincteric anal
- fecal
- gastric
- gastrocolic
- gastroduodenal
- gastrojejunal-colic
- gastrojejunocolic
- genitourinary
- graft-enteric
- hepatic
- hepatic arteriovenous
- hepatopleural
- horseshoe
- H-type
- iatrogenic
- ileosigmoid
- intersphincteric anal
- intradural arteriovenous
- intradural retromedullary arteriovenous
- intrahepatic AV

fistula *(cont.)*
  intrapulmonary arteriovenous
  jejunocolic
  Mann-Bollman
  mediastinal
  mesenteric
  microvenoarteriolar
  mucous
  orofacial
  pancreatic
  pancreatic cutaneous
  pancreaticopleural
  paraprosthetic-enteric
  parietal
  perineovaginal
  persistent bronchopleural
  pilonidal
  pleural
  pleurocutaneous
  premedullary arteriovenous
  pulmonary arteriovenous
  radial artery to cephalic vein
  radiation
  rectal
  rectovaginal
  rectovesical
  respiratory-esophageal
  retroperitoneal
  spinal dural arteriovenous
  splanchnic AV
  splenic AV
  suprasphincteric
  thoracic
  tracheobronchial
  tracheoesophageal (TE or TEF)
  transdural
  transsphincteric anal
  trigeminal cavernous
  ureteral
  ureterocutaneous
  ureterovaginal
  urethrovaginal

fistula *(cont.)*
  urinary
  vesical
  vesicovaginal
  vitelline
fistula in ano
fistula tract study
fistulogram
fistulography
fistulous formation
fistulous tract
5-chlorodeoxycytidine
511-keV high-energy imaging
5-iodoacetamidofluorescein imaging
  agent
5-iodo-2-deoxyuridine imaging agent
5 MHz sonography
5 MHz transducer (ultrasound)
5 mm collimation
five-view chest x-ray
fixed airway obstruction
fixed area of narrowing in large
  airway
fixed defect
fixed grid stereologic method
fixed intracavitary filling defect
fixed mass
fixed perfusion defect
fixed pulmonary valvular resistance
fixed segment of bowel
fixed shaped coplanar or nonplanar
  radiation beam bouquet
fL (femtoliter)
FL (femur length)
FL/AC ratio (femur length to
  abdominal circumference)
flabby heart
flaccid
Flack sinoatrial node
flail chest
flail digit
flail foot

flail joint
flail mitral valve
flail shoulder
FLAIR (fluid-attenuated inversion recovery) sequences
FLAIR-FLASH imaging (see *FLASH*)
flake fracture of the hamate
flaking of cartilage in osteoarthritis
flame appearance
flank bone (ilium)
flap
  bone
  entry
  intimal
  liver
  muscle
  necrotic
  osteoplastic
  pedicle
  pericardial
  pleural
  scimitar-shaped
  subclavian
flaplike valves
flap valve ventricular septal defect
flare
  condylar
  metaphyseal
  tibial
  trochanteric
flare phenomenon
FLASH (fast low-angle shot)
  FLASH images
  FLASH 3D sequence
flashlamp-pulsed dye laser
flask, vascular
Flatau-Schilder disease
flat bone
flatfoot deformity
flat-hand test
flat lined (verb)
flat-panel megavoltage imager
flat pelvis
flat plate of abdomen
flattened longitudinal arch of foot
flattening of normal lumbar curve
flat time-intensity profile
flaval ligament
flawed image
flax-dresser's disease
Flechsig tract
Fleet bowel prep
Fleischer disease
Fleischmann bursa
Fleischner sign
fleur de lis pattern
Flexguard tip catheter
flexibility
flexible cardiac valve
flexible suction cannula
flexible surface coil
flexible surface-coil-type resonator (FSCR)
flexion deformity
flexion-distraction injury of spine
flexion maneuver on cervical spine x-ray
flexion-rotation injury of spine
flexor carpi ulnaris (FCU) muscle
flexor digitorum profundus (FDP) muscle
flexor digitorum superficialis (FDS) muscle
flexor hallucis longus (FHL) muscle
flexor pollicis longus (FPL) muscle
flexor tendon
FlexStrand cable
flexure
  caudal
  cephalic
  cerebral
  cervical
  colonic
  cranial

flexure *(cont.)*
   duodenojejunal
   hepatic
   left colic
   left colonic
   right colic
   right colonic
   sigmoid
   splenic
FlimFax teleradiology system
flip angle
flip-flop phenomenon
flipper hand
flips, value
Flo-Rester vessel occluder
floating leaflets
flocculation on barium enema
flocculent foci of calcification
flocculonodular lobe of cerebellum
flocculonodular tumors
flood section
floor
   bladder
   fibromuscular pelvic
   inguinal
   pelvic
   sellar
floppy aortic valve
floppy mitral valve
flotation catheter
flow
   antegrade
   antegrade bile
   antegrade blood
   antegrade diastolic
   aortic (AF)
   axoplasmic
   azygos
   azygos blood
   backward
   blood
   cerebral blood (CBF)

flow *(cont.)*
   cerebral brain
   cerebrospinal fluid (CSF)
   chronic reserve
   collateral
   collateral blood
   compromised
   coronary blood
   coronary reserve (CRF)
   dampened pulsatile
   decreased cerebral blood
   effective pulmonary blood (EPBF)
   effective pulmonic
   expiratory
   forward
   Ganz method for coronary sinus
   great cardiac vein (GCVF)
   hepatofugal
   hepatopetal
   high velocity
   inspiratory
   intercoronary collateral
   laminar
   left-to-right
   maximum midexpiratory
   midexpiratory tidal
   mitral valve
   myocardial blood (MBF)
   peak
   peak expiratory (PEF)
   peak tidal expiratory flow
   physiologic
   pulmonary blood (PBF)
   pulmonic output
   pulmonic versus systemic
   redistribution of pulmonary
      vascular
   regional cerebral blood (rCBF)
   regional myocardial blood
   regurgitant
   regurgitant systolic
   restoration of

**flow • fluid**

flow *(cont.)*
  retrograde
  retrograde systolic
  reversed vertebral blood (RVBF)
  sluggish
  systemic blood (SBF)
  systemic output
  time-averaged
  tissue
  total cerebral blood (TCBF)
  transmitral
  tricuspid valve
  turbulent blood
  turbulent intraluminal
flow arrest
flow-compensated gradient-echo sequence
flow-compromising lesion
flow cytometry
flow cytometry DNA analysis
flow cytometry Tpot
flow-dependent obstruction
flow-directed balloon catheter
flow-directed microcatheter
flow effect artifact
flow-guided Inoue balloon
flow images
flow-induced artifact
flowing spin
FloWire Doppler ultrasound
flow-limited expiration
flow mapping technique
flow quantification
flow redistribution
flow-related enhancement effects
flow scan, radionuclide
flow signal
flow study
flow-time curve
flow velocity profile
flow velocity signals
flow velocity waveforms
flow void
flow volume
flow-volume curve
flow-volume loop (in spirometry reports)
flowmeter
flowmetry
  blood
  Doppler
  laser-Doppler (LDF)
  Narcomatic
  Parks 800 bidirectional Doppler
  pulsed Doppler
  Statham electromagnetic
Fluckiger syndrome
fluctuant mass
fluffy infiltrate
fluffy rarefaction of Paget's disease
fluid
  amniotic
  articular
  ascitic
  bursal
  cavitary
  cerebrospinal (CSF)
  cystic
  extravascular
  free
  free abdominal
  high signal (on MRI) intratendinous collection of
  interstitial
  joint
  leakage of cerebrospinal
  loculated
  pelvic
  pericardial
  pericholecystic
  peritoneal
  pleural
  prostatic
  serosanguineous

fluid *(cont.)*
  spinal
  subgaleal cerebrospinal
  synovial
fluid accumulation in tissues
fluid-attenuated inversion recovery
  (FLAIR) imaging
fluid collection, loculated
fluid density
fluid enzymes
fluid expansion, rapid
fluid extravasation
fluid-filled bronchograms
fluid-filled mass in uterus
fluid flow between capillaries and
  interstitial tissue
fluid-fluid level
fluidification
fluid level
fluid mass
fluid overload
fluid resorption
fluid retention
fluid volume
fluid wave
fluke
  liver
  lung
fluorescein angiography
fluorescein uptake
fluorescence spectroscopy
fluorine (F)
  $^{18}$F (fluorine-18, F-18)
  $^{18}$FDG (fluorine-18 2-deoxy-D-
    glucose) PET scan
  $^{18}$F estradiol (FES)
  $^{18}$F fluoro-DOPA
  $^{18}$F fluorodeoxyglucose
  $^{18}$F fluorodeoxyglucose PET scan
  $^{18}$F fluorotamoxifen
  $^{18}$F labeled derivatives of
    m-tyrosine

fluorine *(cont.)*
  $^{18}$F labeled HFA-134a
  $^{18}$F labeled polyfluorinated ethyl
  $^{18}$F N-methylspiperone
  $^{18}$F spiperone
  $^{18}$F 2-deoxyglucose ($^{18}$FDG)
    uptake on PET scan
  $^{18}$F uptake
fluorocarbon-based ultrasound contrast
  agent
fluorodeoxyglucose (FDG) radioactive
  tracer
fluorography, spot-film
fluoroimmunoassay
fluorometer
fluorometry
  image intensification
  portable C-arm intensifier
  two-plane
FluoroPlus angiography
FluoroPlus Roadmapper digital
  fluoroscopy system
FluoroScan mini C-arm imaging
  system
fluoroscope (see *fluoroscopy*)
fluoroscopic assistance
fluoroscopic control, advanced under
fluoroscopic diskectomy
fluoroscopic guidance
fluoroscopic localization
fluoroscopic road-mapping technique
  in angioplastic vascular procedures
fluoroscopic view
fluoroscopy
  airway
  biplane
  C-arm
  C-arm digital
  chest
  digital
  electric joint
  FluoroPlus Roadmapper digital

fluoroscopy *(cont.)*
   mobile
   Orca C-arm
   real-time CT
   region-of-interest
FluoroPlus angiography
FluoroPlus Roadmapper digital
   fluoroscopy system
fluoroscopy-guided condylar lift-off
fluoroscopy-guided subarachnoid
   phenol block (SAPB)
Fluoro Tip cannula
flush aortogram
flush aortography
flushed
flushing of catheter
flutamide-associated liver toxicity
fluttering of valvular leaflet
fluximetry
fluxionary hyperemia
fly-through viewing, PVR
FMA cephalometric measurement
FMAP (feeding mean arterial pressure)
FMD (fibromuscular dysplasia)
FMH (first metatarsal head)
FMPIR (fast SE and fast IR) imaging
FMPSPGR (fast multiplanar spoiled
   gradient-recalled) imaging
FMPSPGR sequence
FMR (functional MR) imaging
fMRI or FMRI (functional magnetic
   resonance imaging)
fMRI signal change
FMS (fatty meal sonogram)
FNH (focal nodular hyperplasia)
FNTC (fine-needle transhepatic
   cholangiogram)
foam cell
foam embolus
foamy exudate in air spaces
focal abnormality
focal area of hemorrhage
focal area of hypometabolism
focal calcification
focal changes
focal damage
focal deficit
focal degenerative change
focal dilatations of air spaces
focal distortion
focal eccentric stenosis
focal edema
focal endocardial hemorrhage
focal hepatic hot spot
focal hyperinflation
focal inflammation in febrile
   granulocytopenia
focal interstitial infiltrate
focal intimal thickening
focal lesion
focal mass
focal nodular hyperplasia (FNH)
focal perivascular infiltrate
focal plaque-like defect
focal pooling of tracer
focal stenosis
focal uptake
focal wall motion abnormality
focal white matter signal abnormalities
foci of calcification
foci of tumor
focus (pl. foci)
   Assmann
   atrial
   ectopic
   epileptogenic
   hemorrhagic
   hypermetabolic activity
   junctional
   mesial frontal
   midline parasagittal
   multiple
   occipital
   radiolucent
   Simon

Fogarty adherent clot catheter
Fogarty arterial embolectomy catheter
Fogarty balloon biliary catheter
Fogarty-Chin extrusion balloon catheter
fog (or fogging) effect on CT
Foix-Alajouanine syndrome
fold
  adipose
  alar
  amniotic
  aryepiglottic
  caval
  cecal
  cholecystoduodenocolic
  circular
  circulator
  custocolic
  Douglas
  duodenojejunal
  duodenomesocolic
  epigastric
  esophageal
  falcif
  flattened duodenal
  gastric
  gastropancreatic
  genital
  giant gastric
  glossopalatine
  gluteal
  Guérin
  haustral
  Hensing
  hepatopancreatic
  ileocecal
  ileocolic
  Kerckring
  Kohlrausch
  mucosal
  Nélaton
  palatopharyngeal
fold *(cont.)*
  paraduodenal
  peritoneal
  prepyloric
  rectal
  rectouterine
  rugal
  sacrogenital
  semilunar
  sentinel
  sigmoid
  spiral
  superior duodenal
  superior transverse rectal
  thickened
  vestigial
folded fundus of gallbladder
folded step ramp
folding-potential analysis
Foley catheter
folinic acid, low-dose
follicle (pl. follicles)
  aggregated
  aggregated lymphatic
  anovular ovarian
  atretic ovarian
  gastric
  gastric lymphatic
  graafian
  intestinal
  malpighian
  nabothian
  ovarian
  primordial
  ruptured
  thyroid
  unruptured
follow-through, small-bowel
follow-up or followup (n., adj.)
  examination
follow up (v.)
Fonar Stand-Up MRI scanner

Fontan anastomosis of atrial
  appendage to pulmonary artery
fontanel (fontanelle)
fontanelle
  anterior
  anterolateral
  bregmatic
  bulging
  closed
  cranial
  frontal
  fused
  Gerdy
  mastoid
  occipital
  open
  overriding sutures of
  posterior
  posterolateral
  sagittal
  sphenoid
  tense
  triangular
foot (pl. feet)
  arch of
  arcuate artery of
  articulations of
  calcaneocavus
  Charcot
  digital artery of
  flail
  Friedreich
  Madura
  perforating artery of
  phalanges of
  rockerbottom
football finger
footballer's ankle
footling presentation
foramen (pl. foramina)
  alveolar
  anterior condyloid

foramen (cont.)
  aortic
  apical
  arachnoidal
  blind
  Bochdalek
  Botallo
  carotid
  cecal
  conjugate
  costotransverse
  cranial
  emissary sphenoidal
  epiploic
  ethmoidal
  Froesch
  frontal
  greater palatine
  great sacrosciatic
  greater sciatic
  intertransverse
  interventricular
  intervertebral
  Luschka
  Magendie
  Monro
  Morgagni
  sacrosciatic
  spinous
  stylomastoid
  superior maxillary
  vertebral
  Winslow
foramen magnum of skull
foramen ovale, patent
foramina (pl. of foramen)
foraminal encroachment
foraminal space
force (pl. forces)
Force balloon dilatation catheter
forcefully wedged
forearm

forefoot
  mid- and
  narrowing of
foreign body (FB)
  metallic
  retained
  tracheobronchial
foreign body aspiration
foreign body in respiratory passages
foreign body reaction
foreign body upper airway obstruction
foreign material artifact
Forestier disease
forking of sylvian aqueduct
form, wave
format
  cylindrical
  hemodynamic
  slice
  three-dimensional
  two-dimensional
formation
  bat-wing
  brain stem reticular
  bunion
  callosal
  callus
  Chiari
  eddy
  exuberant atheroma
  fistulous
  Gothic arch
  gray reticular
  hippocampal
  honeycomb
  lateral reticular
  marginal osteophyte
  mesencephalic reticular
  midbrain reticular (MRF)
  new bone
  osteophyte
  palisade

formation *(cont.)*
  paramedian pontine reticular
  periosteal bone
  pontine parareticular (PPRF)
  reticular
  rouleaux
  saccular
  spur
  thrombus
forme fruste (pl. formes frustes)
forme tardive
formication
formidable risk
formula
  Bayesian
  fan-beam
Forney syndrome
forniceal rupture
fornix (pl. fornices), flattening of
fornix cerebri
Forrester syndrome
forward failure
forward flow
forward flow of velocity
forward heart failure
forward subluxation
forward transport
forward triangle method
forward velocity (on Doppler)
fossa (pl. fossae)
  acetabular
  adipose
  amygdaloid
  anconeal (also anconal)
  antecubital
  anterior recess of ischiorectal
  articular
  axillary
  bony
  condylar
  coronoid
  cranial

fossa *(cont.)*
  crural
  cubital
  digastric
  digital
  duodenal
  duodenojejunal
  epigastric
  femoral
  floccular
  gallbladder
  glenoid
  Gruber
  hyaloid
  iliac
  infraspinous
  infrasternal
  infratemporal
  intercondylar
  intercondyloid
  interpeduncular
  ischiorectal
  Jobert
  navicular
  olecranon
  ovarian
  pararectal
  paravesical
  patellar
  pituitary
  popliteal
  posterior
  pterygopalatine
  radial
  retroappendiceal
  rhomboid
  Rosenmuller
  sphenoidal
  Sylvius
  temporal
  Treitz
  valve of navicular
  Waldeyer

fossa ovalis
fossa ovalis cordis
Foster-Kennedy syndrome
4-azido-2-([$^{14}$C]-methylamino)trifluorobenzonitrile imaging agent
four-chamber apical view
four-chamber plane on echocardiography
four-dimensional (4D) image
four-head camera
Fourier analysis of electrocardiogram
Fourier coefficients
Fourier domain
Fourier-encoded
Fourier transform (or transformation) imaging
Fourier transform infrared spectroscopy
Fourier transform Raman spectroscopy
Fourier transformation zeugmatography
Fourier two-dimensional (2D) imaging
Fourier two-dimensional (2D) projection reconstruction
four-part fracture
fourth branchial cleft pouch
fourth compartment
fourth cranial nerve (trochlear nerve)
fourth intercostal space
fourth left interspace
fourth ventricle tumor
four-vessel cerebral angiography
four-view chest x-ray:
  PA, lateral, both oblique
FOV (field of view) imaging
fovea
fovea centralis
fovea inferior
foveal fat pad
foveated chest
foveola, gastric

Fowler position
FP (frontopolar) artery
FPB (flexor pollicis brevis) muscle
FPL (flexor pollicis longus) muscle
F point of cardiac apex pulse
FR4 guiding catheter
fractal analysis
fractal-based method
fraction
  blood flow extraction
  ejection (EF)
  S-phase
  Teichholz ejection
  unattached
  ventricular ejection
fractional area
fractional moving blood volume estimation
fractional myocardial shortening
fractional shortening of left ventricle
fractionated radiation therapy
fractionated stereotaxic radiation therapy
fractionation
fraction dose
fracture
  abduction
  acute
  acute avulsion
  adduction
  agenetic
  Aitken classification of epiphyseal
  alveolar bone
  anatomic
  angulated
  ankle mortise
  annular
  AO classification of ankle
  apophyseal
  articular
  artificial
  Atkin epiphyseal

fracture *(cont.)*
  atrophic
  avulsion
  avulsion chip
  axial compression
  backfire
  Barton
  basal neck
  basal skull
  baseball finger
  basilar femoral neck
  basilar skull
  basocervical
  bending
  Bennett
  Berndt-Harty classification of transchondral
  bicondylar
  bimalleolar ankle
  bipartite
  birth
  blow-in
  blow-out
  boot-top
  Bosworth
  both-bone
  boxer's
  Boyd type II
  bucket-handle
  buckle
  bumper
  bunk bed
  burst (compression) (of atlas)
  bursting
  butterfly
  buttonhole
  Canale-Kelly talar neck
  capillary
  carpal navicular
  carpal scaphoid bone
  cartwheel
  Cedell (of talus)

**fracture**

fracture *(cont.)*
- cemental
- cementum
- cervical
- cervicotrochanteric
- Chance spinal
- chauffeur's
- chevron (V-shaped)
- chip
- chisel
- circumferential
- clay shoveler's
- cleavage
- closed
- closed break
- Colles
- collicular
- comminuted
- comminuted bursting
- comminuted intra-articular
- comminuted teardrop
- complete
- complex
- complicated
- composite
- compound
- compound skull
- compression (burst) (of atlas)
- condylar
- condylar compression
- condylar split
- congenital
- contrecoup
- cortical
- Cotton ankle
- cough (of a rib)
- crack
- craniofacial dysjunction
- crush
- cuboid
- cuneiform
- dancer's

fracture *(cont.)*
- Danis-Weber classification of ankle
- Darrach-Hughston-Milch
- dashboard
- decompression of
- Denis (A,B,C,D, or E) spinal
- dens
- dentate
- depressed
- depressed and compound skull
- depressed skull
- DeQuervain
- derby hat
- diacondylar
- diaphyseal
- diastatic
- direct
- dishpan
- dislocation
- displaced
- dogleg
- dome
- dorsal wing
- double
- Dupuytren
- Duverney
- dye punch
- dyscrasic
- endocrine
- epicondylar
- epiphyseal slip
- Essex-Lopresti calcaneal
- extra-articular
- extracapsular
- facial
- fatigue
- femoral neck
- fender
- fighter's
- finger
- fissure
- flake (of the hamate)

**fracture**

fracture *(cont.)*
flexion-burst
flexion-compression
flexion distraction
floating arch
four-part
Freiberg
Frykman radial
fulcrum
Galeazzi (of radius)
Garden femoral neck
Gosselin
greenstick
grenade-thrower's
gross
growth plate
Guérin
gutter
Hahn-Steinthal capitellum
hairline
hamate tail
hangman's (C2)
Hansen
Hawkins talar neck
healed
heat
hemicondylar
Herbert scaphoid bone
Hermodsson
hockey-stick
horizontal
horizontal maxillary
humeral head-splitting
hyperextension teardrop
hyperflexion
hyperflexion teardrop
idiopathic
impacted
impacted subcapital
impacted valgus
incomplete
indented (of skull)

fracture *(cont.)*
indirect
inflammatory
infraction
insufficiency
intercondylar
internally fixed
interperiosteal
intertrochanteric
intra-articular
intracapsular
intraperiosteal
intrauterine (of fetus)
irreducible
ischioacetabular
Jefferson burst
joint
joint depression
Jones
juvenile Tillaux
juxta-articular
Kocher
Kocher-Lorenz classification of
 capitellum
laryngeal
lateral column calcaneal
lateral wedge (of vertebral body)
laterally displaced
Lauge-Hansen classification of
 ankle
Le Fort I, II, and III
lead-pipe
linear
linear and depressed skull
Lisfranc
local compression
local decompression
long bone
longitudinal
loose
lorry driver's
low T humerus

fracture *(cont.)*
   lunate
   Maisonneuve fibular
   malar
   Malgaigne pelvic
   mallet
   malunited
   mandibular
   march
   maxillary
   medial column calcaneal
   medial epicondyle
   medial malleolar
   midfacial
   midshaft
   minimally displaced
   monomalleolar ankle
   Monteggia
   Monteggia fracture-dislocation
   Montercaux
   Moore
   Mueller classification of humerus
   multangular ridge
   multipartite
   multiple
   nasal
   navicular
   navicular body
   naviculocapitate
   neck
   Neer classification of shoulder
   neoplastic
   neurogenic
   neuropathic
   neurotrophic
   nightstick
   nonarticular radial head
   nondisplaced
   oblique
   occipital
   occult
   odontoid

fracture *(cont.)*
   Ogden classification of epiphyseal
   old
   olecranon
   olecranon tip
   one-part
   open
   open-break
   osteochondral
   Pais
   panfacial
   paratrooper
   parry
   patellar
   pathologic
   Pauwel
   pedicle
   pelvic rim
   pelvic ring
   perforating
   periarticular
   peripheral
   peritrochanteric
   phalangeal
   physeal plate
   Piedmont
   pillion
   pillow
   ping-pong
   plafond
   plaque
   plateau
   pond
   posterior element
   postmortem
   Pott ankle
   pressure
   puncture
   pyramidal
   Quervain (deQuervain)
   radial head
   radial styloid process

**fracture**

fracture *(cont.)*
  resecting
  retrodisplaced
  reverse Barton
  reverse Colles
  rib
  ring
  Rolando
  rotation burst
  Ruedi-Allgower tibial plafond
  sacral insufficiency
  Salter
  Salter-Harris (1 through 5)
  Salter-Harris-Rang classification of epiphyseal
  sandbagging (of long bones)
  scaphoid
  seat belt
  secondary
  segmental
  Segond
  senile subcapital
  SER-IV (supination, external rotation-type IV)
  shaft
  shear
  Shepherd
  sideswipe elbow
  silver-fork (Colles)
  simple
  simple skull
  skier's
  Skillern
  sleeve
  slice
  Smith
  Sneppen talar
  spiral
  splintered
  split compression
  spontaneous
  sprain

fracture *(cont.)*
  sprinter's
  stable
  stairstep
  Steinert classification of epiphyseal
  stellate
  stellate skull
  stellate undepressed
  step-off of
  Stieda
  straddle
  strain
  stress
  stress-type
  subcapital
  subcutaneous
  subperiosteal
  subtrochanteric
  supination (see *SER-IV*)
  supination-adduction
  supination-eversion
  supracondylar
  supracondylar femoral
  surgical neck
  T
  talar osteochondral
  T condylar
  T-shaped
  teardrop
  teardrop-shaped flexion-compression
  temporal bone
  thalamic (of calcaneal)
  three-part
  through-and-through
  tibial plafond
  tibial plateau
  tibiofibular
  Tillaux
  Tillaux-Kleiger
  tongue-type
  torsion

fracture *(cont.)*
  torus
  total condylar depression
  transcapitate
  transcervical femoral
  transchondral talar
  transcondylar
  transepiphyseal
  transhamate
  transscaphoid
  transtriquetral
  transverse
  trimalleolar ankle
  triplane
  triquetral
  trophic
  tuft
  two-part
  ulnar styloid
  undisplaced
  unilateral
  unstable
  ununited
  V-shaped (chevron)
  vertebra plana
  vertebral wedge compression
  vertical
  vertical shear
  wagon wheel
  Wagstaffe
  Watson-Jones navicular
  Watson-Jones spinal
  Weber C
  wedge
  wedge-compression
  wedged
  wedge flexion-compression
  willow
  Y
  Y-T
  Zickel
  zygomatic-malar complex (ZMC)
fracture classification
fracture deformity
fracture-dislocation, perilunate
  (PLFD)
fracture en rave
fracture fragment
fracture in close apposition
fracture line
fracture nonunion
fracture threshold
fracture zone
fragility, hereditary (of bone)
fragment
  alignment of fracture
  articular
  avulsed fracture
  avulsion
  bone
  bony
  butterfly fracture
  capital
  chondral
  cortical
  disk
  displaced
  displacement of fracture
  Fab (fragment antigen binding)
  fracture
  free
  free-floating cartilaginous
  loose
  major fracture
  osteochondral
  overriding of fracture
  retrolisthesed
  retropulsed bony
  smear
fragmentation myocarditis
fragmentation of apophysis
fragmentation therapy
frame
  robotics-controlled stereotactic
  stereotactic head

frameless stereotaxic DSA
frameless stereotaxic guidance tools
frank dislocation
frank hemorrhage
frank pulmonary edema
frank pus
Frank sign
Frank vectorcardiogram (VCG)
Frankel classification of spinal cord injury (Fraenkel)
Frankel white line
Frankfort horizontal plane
Frankfort mandibular incisor angle
fraught with error
fray
fraying of edges
fraying of meniscus
FRC (functional residual capacity)
free air
free air in body cavity
free air in diaphragm
free air passage
free air under diaphragm
free body in peritoneal cavity
free flap of cartilage
free-floating cartilaginous fragment
free fluid
free fragment
free hepatic venography
free induction decay (FID)
free induction delay curve
free induction signal
free intraperitoneal air
free intraperitoneal gas
free pericardial space
free pleural effusion
free radical
free-radical dosimeter
free wall, ventricular
free wall tract
freehand interventional sonography
freehand ultrasound

freely movable mass
Freiberg disease
Freiberg-Kohler disease
French 5 angiographic catheter
French MBIH catheter
French pigtail catheter
French scale for caliber of catheter
French shaft balloon
French T-tube
frequency analysis of Doppler signal
frequency domain imaging (FDI) in ultrasound
frequency
  halftone
  Larmor
  precisional
  raster
  vibration
frequency offset
frequency-related peak
friability
friable lesion
friable mass
friable mucosa
friable tumor
friable vegetation
friable wall
friction-reducing polymer
Friedel Pick syndrome
Friedreich foot
Frimodt-Moller syndrome
fringe field
fringe skeleton extraction
fringe, synovial
fringe thinning algorithms
frogleg view
frog-like appearance
Frohse ligamentous arcade
frond-like appearance
frontal bone
frontal defect

frontal foramina
frontal gyrus
frontal horn of lateral ventricle
frontal lobe
frontal lobe contusion
frontal lobe dysfunction
frontal lobe lesion
frontal lobe tumor
frontal plane
frontal plane loop
frontal pole
frontal sinus
frontal suture
frontal view
frontocentral convexity
frontocentral head region
frontoethmoidal encephalocele
fronto-orbital advancement
frontoparietal
frontoparietal suture
frontopolar region
frontosphenoid suture
frontosphenoidal encephalocele
frontotemporal (FT)
frontotemporal atrophy
frontotemporal muscle
frontotemporal region
frontozygomatic region
frothy colonic mucosa
Frykman classification of hand and wrist
FS (full scan) method/projection
FS-BURST MR imaging
FSCR, flexible surface-coil-type
FSE (fast SE) imaging
FSV (forward stroke volume)
FTA (femorotibial angle)
FTC (fibulotalocalacaneal) ligament
FTP (file transfer protocol)
F-1200 (and F-2000) Fluorescence Spectrophotometer
FUdR (5-fluorouracil deoxyribonucleoside)
Fuji AC2 storage phosphor computed radiology system
Fuji FCR9000 computed radiology system
Fukuyama congenital muscular dystrophy
fulcrum fracture
full-bladder ultrasound technique
full body echo planar system imager
full-blown cardiac tamponade
full-column barium enema
full energy peak efficiency
full-field digital mammography system
full-scan (FS) method/projection
full-scan with interpolation (FI) method/projection
full-thickness button of aortic wall
full-thickness Carrel button
full-thickness infarction of ventricular septum
full-volume loop spirometry
full width at half maximum (FWHM)
fulminant cerebral lymphoma (in AIDS)
fulminant course of disease
fulminant hepatic failure (FHF)
fulminant hydrocephalus
fulminant pulmonary edema
fulminant tuberculosis
fulminating ulcerative colitis
function
  atrial phasic volumetric
  commissural
  compromised ventricular
  depressed right ventricular contractile
  excitation
  exercise LV
  global ventricular

function *(cont.)*
  leaflet
  left atrial (LA)
  left ventricular (LV)
  left ventricular systolic/diastolic
  myocardial contractile
  point spread
  regional left ventricular
  regional ventricular
  reserve cardiac
  rest LV (left ventricular)
  rest RV (right ventricular)
  right and left atrial phasic volumetric
  right atrial (RA)
  right ventricular (RV)
  right ventricular systolic/diastolic
  sinusoid reference
  swallowing
  ventricular contractility (VCF)
  volumetric
functional abnormality
functional aerobic impairment (FAI)
functional bladder capacity
functional brain imaging
functional classification of congestive heart failure
functional correlation
functional cyst
functional disorder
functional disturbance
functional evaluation
functional impairment
functional magnetic resonance imaging (FMRI)
functional MRI (fMRI)
functional reentry
functional refractory period (FRP)
functional residual capacity (FRC)
functional ureteral obstruction
fundal
fundoplication
fundus
  aneurysmal
  bladder
  bald gastric
  eye
  gallbladder
  gastric
  stomach
  urinary bladder
  uterine
  vaginal
fundus of aneurysm
fundus uteri
fungal plaque
fungating
fungoides, mycosis
fungus ball
funic souffle
funicular souffle
funiculus (pl. funiculi)
funiculus cuneatus
funiculus dorsalis
funiculus gracilis
funiculus medullae spinalis
funiculus ventralis
funnel chest
funnel deformity
funnel pelvis
FUO (fever of undetermined origin)
Fürbringer sign (Fuerbringer)
furrier's lung
fused ankle
fused commissures
fused papillary muscle
fused physis
fusiform aneurysm
fusiform bronchiectasis
fusiform dilatation
fusiform narrowing of arteries
fusiform shadow

fusiform swelling
fusiform widening of duct
fusion
  ankle
  atlanto-occipital
  bone (bony)
  calcaneotibial
  carpal-metacarpal (CMC) (also carpometacarpal)
  cervical
  cervical interbody
  chevron
  diaphyseal-epiphyseal
  extra-articular hip
  facet
  interbody
  interphalangeal
  interspinous process
  intra-articular knee
  joint
  metatarsocuneiform joint

fusion *(cont.)*
  metatarsophalangeal joint
  multilevel
  occipitocervical
  pantalar
  spinal
  talar body
  talocrural
  tibiocalcaneal
  tibiotalar
  transfibular
  two-stage
fusion defect
fusion of two or more vertebral segments
fuzzy echo
fuzzy logic contrast correction
fuzzy rules
fuzzy set theory
FWHM (full width at half maximum)
fx (fracture)

# G, g

Ga (gallium)
GABA-BN complex
gadobenate dimeglumine imaging agent
gadodiamide imaging agent
gadolinium (Gd)
   Gd-BOPTA/Dimeg imaging agent
   Gd-DOTA contrast medium
   Gd-DOTA-enhanced subtraction dynamic study
   Gd-DTPA/Dimeg imaging agent
   Gd-DTPA-enhanced turbo FLASH MRI
   Gd-DTPA imaging agent
   Gd-DTPA-labeled albumin
   Gd-DTPA-labeled dextran
   Gd-DPTA PGTM imaging agent
   Gd-DTPA radioisotope
   Gd-DTPA with mannitol contrast
   Gd-enhanced imaging agent
   Gd-EOB-DTPA imaging agent
   Gd-FMPSPGR imaging
   Gd-HIDA chelate
   Gd-Hp-DO3A imaging agent
   Gd-labeled graft copolymer
   Gd-153 imaging agent
   Gd oxide contrast medium
gadolinium complex
gadolinium-enhanced MR imaging
gadopentetate dimeglumine imaging agent
gadoteridol contrast
Gaeltec catheter-tip pressure transducer
Gage sign
Gairdner disease
Gaisböck syndrome
galactography
galea aponeurotica
galeal extension of tumor
Galeazzi fracture-dislocation
Galeazzi fracture of radius
Galeazzi sign
Galen, great cerebral vein of
Galen Scan scanner
Galen teleradiology system
Gallannaugh bone plate
Gallavardin phenomenon
gallbladder
   bilobed
   body of
   chronically inflamed
   contracted
   Courvoisier

gallbladder *(cont.)*
  dilated
  distended
  double
  edematous
  fetal
  fish-scale
  floating
  folded fundus
  fundal portion of
  fundus of
  hourglass
  mobile
  multiseptate
  neck of
  nonvisualization of
  stasis
  thick-walled
  thin-walled
  wandering
gallbladder bed
gallbladder calculus
gallbladder ejection fraction
gallbladder hydrops
gallbladder lift
gallbladder polyp
gallbladder stasis
gallbladder study (oral cholecystogram)
gallbladder ultrasound
Gallie H-graft
gallium (Ga)
  $^{67}$Ga bone scan
  $^{67}$Ga citrate radioactive imaging
  $^{67}$Ga exam
  $^{68}$Ga GABA uptake carrier
  $^{67}$Ga imaging agent
gallium scan (scanning)
gallium scintigraphy
gallstone (see also *stone*)
  asymptomatic
  dissolution of

gallstone *(cont.)*
  faceted
  floating
  innocent
  radiolucent
  retained
  silent
  symptomatic
gallstone migration
GALT (gut-associated lymphoid tissue)
gamekeeper's thumb
gamma camera (see *camera*)
gamma counter
gamma irradiation
gamma probe
gamma ray attenuation
gamma spectrometric analysis
gamma unit
gamma knife for radiosurgery
Gammex RMI DAP (dose area product) meter
Gammex RMI scanner
Gamna-Gandy nodule
Gandy-Nanta disease
ganglia (pl. of ganglion)
ganglioglioma
gangliolysis, radiofrequency
ganglion (pl. ganglia)
  aberrent
  acousticofacial
  aorticorenal
  Acrel
  auditory
  auricular
  basal
  calcification of basal
  cardiac
  carotid
  celiac
  cervical
  cervicothoracic

ganglion *(cont.)*
  ciliary
  coccygeal
  diffuse
  dorsal root (DRG)
  ganglia
  gasserian
  geniculate
  intraosseous
  otic
  palmar
  paravertebral
  prevertebral
  petrosal
  posterior root
  radiocapitellar joint
  Scarpa
  sensory
  sphenopalatine
  submandibular
  spinal
  superior mesenteric
  sympathetic
  trigeminal
  uterine cervical
  vestibular
  Wrisberg
ganglioneuroma
ganglionic cyst in synovial tendon sheath
gangliosidosis, GM1 and GM2
gangrenous cholecystitis
Ganser diverticulum
gantry angulation in CT-guided percutaneous biopsy
gantry of CT scanner
gantry of lithotripsy machine
gantry room
gantry tilt
Ganz-Edwards coronary infusion catheter
Ganz formula for coronary sinus flow

gap
  Bochdalek
  intersection
  interslice
gap calculation
Garcin syndrome
Garden angle
Garden femoral neck fracture
Gardner-Diamond syndrome
Garland triangle
Garré disease
Garren-Edwards gastric (GEG) bubble
Garren gastric bubble
Gartland classification of supracondylar fracture
Gärtner (Gaertner) duct
gas
  abdominal
  aneurysmal wall
  bowel
  coursing of
  free subphrenic
  natural neon
  overlying bowel
  pulmonary
  small-bowel
  soft tissue
  subcutaneous tissue
  superimposed bowel
gas accumulation under serous tunic of intestine
gas-bloat syndrome
gas CT cisternography
gas cupula
gas density line
gaseous distention
gaseous drainage
gaseous oxygen artifact
gas-fluid level
gas nitrogen embolism
gas pattern
gasserian ganglion tumor

gassy
gas target
gastric air bubble
gastric antrum
gastric balloon (see *balloon*)
gastric bubble
gastric capacity
gastric catarrh
gastric channel
gastric contents
gastric distention
gastric fistula
gastric foveola
gastric fundus
gastric impression on liver
gastric mucosa imaging
gastric mucosal pattern
gastric outline
gastric partition
gastric pits
gastric pool
gastric pull-through segment
gastric reflux of bile
gastric remnant
gastric secretion
gastric ulcer
gastric window
gastrinoma, duodenal
gastritis
  acute
  antral
  atrophic
  chronic
  cirrhotic
  hemorrhagic
  hypertrophic
  necrotizing
  pseudomembranous radiation
gastroc (gastrocnemius muscle)
gastrocardiac syndrome
gastrocnemius muscle
gastrocnemius-soleus complex

gastrocnemius-soleus muscle group
gastrocolic ligament
gastrocolic omentum
gastroduodenal artery complex
gastroduodenitis
gastroduodenoscopy
gastroenteritis
gastroenterocolitis
gastroenteroptosis
gastroepiploic arcade
gastroepiploic artery
gastroepiploic vessel
gastroesophageal incompetence
gastroesophageal junction
gastroesophageal reflux (GER)
gastroesophageal reflux disease (GERD)
Gastrografin (meglumine diatrizoate) contrast medium
Gastrografin enema
gastrohepatic bare area
gastrohepatic omentum
gastrointestinal (GI)
  GI endoscopic ultrasound
  GI tract
gastrojejunocolic fistula
gastrolienal ligament
GastroMARK oral contrast medium
gastroparesis
Gastroport
gastroptosis
gastrosphincteric pressure gradient
Gastrovist contrast medium
gas ventilation study
gas volumes
gate arrays
gated blood (pool) cardiac wall motion study
gated blood pool ventriculogram
gated cardiac blood pool imaging
gated equilibrium blood pool scanning

gated exercise examination
gated imaging studies
gated inflow technique
gated magnetic resonance imaging
gated planar studies
gated radionuclide ventriculography
gated SPECT (GSPECT)
gated view (in MUGA, multiple gated acquisition scan)
gating (timing of images)
  cardiac
  diastolic
  ECG
  echocardiographic
  electrocardiogram
  heartbeat
  respiratory
  systolic
Gaucher disease
gauge
gauss
gaussian curve
gaussian dose-volume histogram
gaussian distribution
gaussian line saturation
gaussian mode profile laser beam
Gaynor-Hart position
GBM (glioblastoma multiforme)
GBP (gastric bypass)
GBS (Guillain-Barré syndrome)
GCSF, granulocyte colony stimulating factor
GCT (germ-cell tumor)
GCTSPS (germ-cell tumor with synchronous lesions in pineal and suprasellar regions)
GCVF (great cardiac vein flow)
Gd (gadolinium)
GE (gastroesophageal)
  GE junction
  GE reflux
GE (General Electric)
GE CT Advantage scanner
GE Advance PET scanner
GE CT Hi-Speed Advantage system
GE CT 8800 scanner
GE CT Max scanner
GE CT Pace scanner
GE detector
GE gamma camera
GE GN300 7.05T/89 mm bore multinuclear spectrometer
GE GN 500 MHz
GE HiSpeed Advantage helical CT scanner
GE HiSpeed CT scanner
GE Medical Systems
GE 9800 high-resolution CT scanner
GE MR Max scanner
GE MR Signa scanner
GE MR Vectra scanner
GE NMR spectrometer
GE Omega 500 MHz
GE QE 300 MHz GE PET scanner
GE scanner
GE Signa 5.4 Genesis MR imager
GE Signa 5.5 Horizon EchoSpeed MR imager
GE Signa MR system
GE Signa 1.5 tesla scanner
GE Signa 1.5 T magnet
GE Signa 4.7 MRI scanner
GE Signa 5.2 scanner
GE Signa 5.2 scanner with SR-230 3-axis EPI gradient upgrade
GE single axis SR-230 echo-planar system
GE single-detector SPECT-capable camera
GE SPECT (single-photon emission computerized tomography)

GE (General Electric) (cont.)
   GE Spiral CT scanner
   GE Starcam single-crystal tomographic scintillation camera
Gee-Herter disease
GEG (Garren-Edwards gastric) bubble
Geiger counter
gelatinous debris
gelatinous hematoma
Gelfoam powder embolization
gemellary pregnancy
gemellus (pl. gemelli) muscle
gene delivery imaging
general pattern matching
General Electric (see *GE*)
generalized
generator
   carbon dioxide
   $^{166}$Dy (dysprosium)
   extraction
   $^{166}$Ho (holmium in vivo)
   172Hf-172Lu
   molybdenum-99
   Van de Graaff
generator-produced $^{188}$Re (rhenium)
genial tubercle of mandible
geniculate body
geniculate ganglion
geniculocalcarine region
geniculocalvarium
geniculum
genitourinary tuberculosis
Gennari
   band of
   line of
   stripe of (in brain)
Gensini catheter
Gentle-Flo suction catheter
genu valgum (knock-knee) deformity
genu varum (bowleg) deformity
geographic lesion
geometric distortion
geometry, coronary vessel
geometry factor
geophagia artifact
GER (gastroesophageal reflux)
GERD (gastroesophageal reflux disease)
Gerdy ligament
Gerdy tubercle in knee
Gerhardt sign
Gerhardt triangle
geriatric features on chest x-ray
germ-cell tumor (GCT), intracranial
germinal matrix
germinoma, primary central nervous system
Gertzbein classification of seat belt injury
gestation
   extrauterine
   intrauterine
gestational age
gestational sac diameter (GS)
gestational trophoblastic disease
gestational trophoblastic neoplasia (GTN)
GF cassette
GFR (glomerular filtration rate)
Ghon complex
Ghon primary lesion
Ghon-Sachs complex
Ghon tubercle
ghosting artifact
GI (gastrointestinal)
giant aneurysm
giant bullous emphysema
giant cell carcinoma
giant cell interstitial pneumonia (GIP)
giant gastric folds
Gianturco-Roehm bird's nest vena caval filter
Gianturco-Rösch Z-stent esophageal stent

Gianturco-Roubin flexible coil stent
Gianturco-Wallace venous stent
Gianturco wool-tufted wire coil stent
giardiasis
gibbous deformity
Gibbs artifact
Gibbs random field
gibbus (n.)
GIF (graphics interchange format)
gigantism, cerebral
GIP (giant cell interstitial pneumonia)
girdle
   limb
   pelvic
   shoulder
girth, abdominal
gland
   absorbent
   accessory
   admaxillary
   adrenal
   Albarran
   alveolar
   anteprostatic
   aortic
   apical
   aporic
   arterial
   arteriococcygeal
   axillary sweat
   Bartholin
   bulbocavernous
   bulbourethral
   calcification of pineal
   carotid
   coccygeal
   Cowper
   Duverney
   endocrine
   globate
   glomiform
   haversian

gland *(cont.)*
   hilar
   interscapular
   lacrimal
   lymph
   mammary
   ovaries
   pancreas
   parathyroid
   parotid
   pineal
   pituitary
   salivary
   Skene
   sublingual
   submandibular
   suprarenal
   testes
   urethral
   thymus
   thyroid
gland volume
glandular proliferation
glandular tissue
Glasgow sign
glass blower's emphysema
glass eye artifact
glass track detector
Gleason grade
Glénard disease
glenohumeral joint
glenohumeral ligament
glenoid cavity
glenoid fossa
glenoid process
GLF lymphography method
glial disease
glial nodule
glial scarring
glial tumor
Glidewire
   long taper/stiff shaft
   Radiofocus

glioblast
glioblastoma
glioblastoma multiforme (GBM)
glioma
  anaplastic cerebral
  brain stem
  butterfly-type
  cerebral
  high-grade
  intracranial
  low-grade
  malignant
  non-anaplastic
  optic nerve
  pontine
  rolandoparietal
  supratentorial
glioma tumor
gliomatosis cerebri
glioneural hamartoma
gliosarcoma
gliosis
  astrocytic
  progressive subcortical
  reactive
gliosis of sylvian aqueduct
Glisson capsule
global cardiac disease
global cerebral hypoperfusion
global cerebral ischemia
global cortical defect
global ejection fraction
global hypokinesis
global hypometabolism
global left ventricular dysfunction
global systolic left ventricular dysfunction
global tissue loss
global ventricular dysfunction
global wall motion abnormality
globally depressed ejection fraction
globe, optic

globe-orbit relationship
globoid heart
globular chest
globular sputum
globus hystericus
globus pallidus
glomeriform arteriovenous anastomosis
glomeriform arteriovenular anastomosis
glomerular basement membrane
glomerular filtration agent
glomerular filtration rate (GFR)
glomeruloid formation
glomerulonephritis
  acute
  membranous
  necrotizing
  proliferative
  segmental necrotizing
glomus (subungual) tumor
glomus-type arteriovenous malformation (AVM)
glossopharyngeal nerve (ninth cranial nerve)
glottic larynx
glottis
glove phenomenon (artifact)
gloves, radiation-attenuating surgical
glow curve
GLP7 film
glucagon
Glucarate $^{99m}$Tc hot spot imaging agent
glucose metabolism within the myocardium
glue, percutaneous fibrin
glutamate spectroscopy
glutathione
gluteal bonnet
gluteal lines
gluteus maximus muscle

gluteus medius muscle
gluteus minimus muscle
gm (gram)
goiter
  Basedow
  colloid
  cystic
  diffuse
  diving
  exophthalmic
  familial
  fibrous
  intrathoracic
  iodide
  iodine deficiency
  lingual
  multinodular
  nodular
  parenchymous
  retrovascular
  simple
  substernal
  suffocative
  thyroid
  toxic
  toxic nodular
  vascular
  wandering
Golay coil
gold radioactive source
gold standard of diagnosis
gold-195m radionuclide
Goldblatt phenomenon
Goldenhar syndrome
golfer's elbow
GoLytely bowel prep
gonial angle (of mandible)
gonion-gnathion plane
Goodale-Lubin cardiac catheter
Goodpasture syndrome
gooseneck concept
gooseneck deformity of outflow tract
gooseneck shape of ventricular outflow
Gore-Tex catheter
gorge
gorging
Gorham disease
Gorlin catheter
Gorlin formula for aortic valve area
Gorlin hydraulic formula for mitral valve area
Gorlin method for cardiac output
Gorlin syndrome
Gosling pulsatility index
Gosselin fracture
Gosset, spiral band of
Gothic arch formation
Gottschalk staging
Gould PentaCath 5-lumen thermodilution catheter
Gould Statham pressure transducer
Gouley syndrome
gout, tophaceous
gouty tophus
Gowers bundle
Gowers column
Gowers fasciculus
Gowers syndrome
GP (gastroplasty)
graafian follicle
graafian vesicle
Grace method of ratio of metatarsal length
grade 1 tear
grade 2 tear
grade 3 tear
grade
  Gleason
  Hyams
  osteoarthritis
  placental
graded compression sonography
graded infusion

**gradient**

gradient
  aortic outflow
  aortic valve (AVG)
  aortic valve peak instantaneous
  arteriovenous pressure
  atrioventricular
  biliary-duodenal pressure
  brain-core
  conjugate
  coronary perfusion
  dephasing
  diastolic
  duodenobiliary pressure
  elevated
  encoding
  end-diastolic aortic–left ventricular pressure
  Ficoll
  gastrosphincteric pressure
  hepatic venous pressure
  holosystolic
  instantaneous
  left ventricular outflow pressure
  maximal estimated
  mean mitral valve
  mean systolic
  mitral valve
  negligible pressure
  outflow tract
  peak diastolic
  peak instantaneous
  peak pressure
  peak right ventricular–right atrial systolic
  peak systolic (PSG)
  peak-to-peak pressure
  perfusion
  pressure
  pressure-flow
  pulmonary artery diastolic and wedge pressure (PADP-PAWP)

gradient *(cont.)*
  pulmonary artery to right ventricle diastolic
  pulmonary outflow
  pulmonic valve
  rephasing
  residual
  right ventricular to main pulmonary artery pressure
  stenotic
  subvalvular
  systolic
  transaortic systolic
  translesional
  transmitral diastolic
  transpulmonic
  transstenotic pressure
  transtricuspid valve diastolic
  transvalvar
  transvalvular pressure
  tricuspid valve
  ventricular
gradient across valve
gradient amplifier
gradient coil
gradient drive current
gradient echo cine technique
gradient echo image
gradient echo imaging sequence
gradient echo MR with magnetization transfer
gradient echo pulse sequence
gradient echo sequence
gradient echo phase image
gradient echo pulse sequence
gradient echo sequence imaging
gradient magnetic field
gradient-recalled acquisition in a steady state (GRASS)
gradient-recalled echo (GRE)
gradient sheet coils
gradient waveforms

grading, histologic
graft
   coronary artery bypass (CABG)
   Dacron-covered stent
   endovascular aortic
graft copolymer
grafting
graft patency
graft-versus-host disease (GVHD)
Graham-Burford-Mayer syndrome
Graham-Cole cholecystography
grain-handler's lung
gram (gm)
Grancher sign
Grancher triad
grand mal seizure
Granger view
Grantham classification of femur
   fracture
granularity
granulated
granulation stenosis
granulation tissue
granulocyte colony stimulating factor
   (GCSF)
granulocytic leukemia
granuloma (pl. granulomata)
   amebic
   apical
   beryllium
   calcified
   cholesterol
   coccidioidal
   coli
   eosinophilic
   epithelioid
   extravascular
   fishtank
   foreign body
   frontoethmoidal giant cell
      reparative
   Hodgkin

granuloma *(cont.)*
   inguinal
   laryngeal
   lethal midline
   lipoid
   Majocchi
   malarial
   midline
   Mignon
   miliary
   noncaseating
   paracoccidioidal
   periapical
   pseudopyogenic
   reticulohistiocytic
   rheumatic
   silicotic
   stellate
   swimming pool
   thorium dioxide
   tricophytic
   tuberculous
   umbilical
   xanthomatous
granulomatosis
   allergic
   Wegener
granulomatous enterocolitis
granulomatous gastritis
granulomatous inflammation of
   bronchi
granulosa-theca cell tumor
granulovacuolar degeneration
graphics interchange format (GIF)
graphite fibrosis of lung
Graser diverticulum
GRASS (gradient-recalled acquisition
   in a steady state)
   GRASS MR imaging
   GRASS pulse sequence
Gratiolet convolutions
Graupner method

grave prognosis
Graves disease
gravid uterus
gravida
gravis, myasthenia
gravitational edema
gravity drainage
gray (Gy)
gray commissure (of spinal cord)
gray horns in spinal canal
gray matter
gray radiation absorbed dose (Gy rad)
gray-scale Doppler
gray-scale images (imaging)
gray-scale range
gray-scale ultrasound
gray to white matter activity ratio
gray to white matter utilization ratio
gray-white differentiation on CT scan
gray-white matter contrast ratio
gray-white matter junction
Grayson ligament in hand
GRE (gradient-recalled echo)
    GRE breath-hold hepatic imaging
    GRE-in images
    GRE-out images
    GRE magnetic resonance imaging
greater curvature of stomach
greater multangular bone
greater saphenous vein
greater sciatic notch
greater superficial petrosal nerve
greater trochanter
greater tuberosity
great vessels, transposition of
Greene sign
Greenfield IVC (inferior vena cava) filter
greenstick fracture
Greer EZ Access drainage pouch
grenade thrower's fracture
grenz ray

Greulich and Pyle, bone age according to
grey (see *gray*)
grid, megavoltage
grid therapy
Griesinger sign
Grollman pigtail catheter
groove
    alveolingual
    alveolobuccal
    alveololabial
    anal intersphincteric
    anterolateral
    anteromedian
    arterial
    atrioventricular (AV)
    auriculoventricular
    basilar
    bicipital
    bronchial
    buccal
    carotid
    carpal
    cavernous
    central
    coronary
    costal
    dental
    developmental
    digastric
    esophageal
    ethmoidal
    gastric
    genital
    gingivobuccal
    gingivolabial
    Harrison
    infraorbital
    interatrial
    intertubercular
    interventricular
    labial
    lacrimal

groove *(cont.)*
   Liebermeister
   neural
   paravertebral
   radial
   radial neck
   sagittal
   Sibson
   spindle colonic
   ulnar
   urethral
   venous
   Verga lacrimal
   vertebral
Groshong double-lumen catheter
Groshong tunneled catheter
Grossman scale for regurgitation
Grossman sign
ground-glass appearance of lungs
ground-glass attenuation
ground-glass density
ground-glass infiltrates in lungs
ground-glass opacity
ground plate
ground state
group viewing
growth arrest line
growth center of bone
growth plate arrest
growth plate fracture
growth plate injury
growth plate widening
Gruber fossa
Gruentzig (Grüntzig)
grumous debris
grumous tissue
Grüntzig (Gruentzig)
Grüntzig balloon catheter angioplasty
Grüntzig Dilaca catheter
Grüntzig technique for PTCA
GS (gestational sac)
GSA imaging agent for liver
   scintigraphy

Gsell-Erdheim syndrome
GSPECT (gated SPECT)
GSW (gunshot wound)
GSWH (gunshot wound to head)
GTN (gestational trophoblastic
   neoplasia)
guanylate cyclase (enzyme)
Guérin fracture
Guglielmi detachable coil (GDC)
guidance
   active biplanar MR imaging
   fluoroscopic
   radiologic
   under fluoroscopic
guide wire entrapment
Guidezilla guiding catheter
guiding catheter
guiding shots
guilt screen
Gull disease
gumma (pl. gummas or gummata)
gummas of rib
gun stock deformity
Gunn crossing sign
gunshot wound (GSW)
gunshot wound to head (GSWH)
Gustilo-Anderson classification of
   tibial plafond fracture
Gustilo classification of tibial fractures
gut (intestine)
   blind
   large
   mid-
   small
gutter
   lateral
   left
   paracolic
   parapelvic
   peritoneal
   right
   sacral

**gutter • gyrus**

gutter fracture
Guyon canal
Gy (gray) radiation absorbed dose
gymnast's wrist
gynecoid pelvis
gyral crest
gyration
gyri cerebri
gyriform calcification
gyromagnetic ratio
Gyroscan, Philips
Gyroscan S15 scanner
gyrus (pl. gyri)
  angular (AG)
  annectant
  ascending parietal
  Broca
  callosal
  central
  cingulate
  contiguous supramarginal
  dentate
  fasciolar
  first temporal
  flattening of
  frontal
  fusiform
  Heschl transverse
  hippocampal
  inferior frontal
  inferior temporal
  infracalcarine
  insular
  lamination of
  lateral occipitotemporal
  lingual
  marginal

gyrus *(cont.)*
  medial occipitotemporal
  middle frontal
  middle temporal
  occipital
  occipitotemporal
  olfactory
  orbital
  paracentral
  parahippocampal
  paraterminal
  parietal
  postcentral
  posterior central
  precentral
  preinsular
  quadrate
  short insular
  subcallosal
  subcollateral
  superior frontal
  superior parietal lobule
  superior temporal
  supracallosal
  supramarginal
  temporal
  transverse temporal
  Turner marginal
  uncal
  uncinate
gyrus cerebelli
gyrus cingulatus
gyrus cinguli
gyrus fornicatus
gyrus hippocampi
gyrus isthmus fornicatus
gyrus rectus

# H, h

H1 (halistatin-1) imaging agent
H1 spectroscopy
$H_2$ $^{15}O$ (water O-15) radioactive
  diagnostic agent
$H_2$ $^{15}O$ PET (positron emission
  tomography)
habenula
habitus
  body
  gracile
  large
Haglund deformity
Hagner disease
Hahn-Steinthal classification of
  capitellum fracture
Haifa camera
Haines-McDougall medial sesamoid
  ligament
hairline crack in bone cortex
hairline fracture
Hale syndrome
half-Fourier acquisition single-shot
  turbo spin-echo (HASTE)
half-Fourier imaging (HFI)
half-Fourier three-dimensional
  technique
half-life
  antibody
  biological
  effective
  radioactive
  short
half-moon artifact
half-moon shape
half-scan (HS) method/projection
half-scan with extrapolation (HE)
  method/projection
half-scan with interpolation (HI)
  method/projection
half-time, clearance
halftone banding
halftone frequency
half-wedged field technique
halistatin-1 (H1) imaging agent
Hallberg biliointestinal bypass
Hallermann-Streiff-François syndrome
hallucal pronation
hallux abductovalgus
hallux elevatus
hallux extensus
hallux flexus deformity
hallux interphalangeal joint

hallux interphalangeus angle
hallux limitus (HL)
hallux malleus deformity
hallux migration
hallux rigidus deformity
hallux valgus (HV)
  bilateral
  unilateral
hallux valgus angle (HVA)
hallux valgus deformity
hallux valgus interphalangeus angle
hallux valgus-metatarsus primus varus complex
hallux varus deformity
halo cast
halo effect
halo ring
halo sign
halogenated thymidine analogue (radiosensitizer)
HAMA (human anti-murine antibodies) response
hamartoma
  cardiac
  cartilaginous
  chondromatous
  duodenal wall
  glioneural
  pancreatic
  pulmonary
  subependymal
  vascular
  ventromedial hypothalamic
hamartomatous lesion
hamartomatous polyp
hamate bone
hamate tail fracture
Hamilton-Stewart formula for measuring cardiac output
Hamman pneumopericardium sign

Hamman-Rich syndrome (idiopathic pulmonary fibrosis)
hammer-marked skull secondary to thinning
hammer toe (or hammertoe)
  dynamic
  fixed
hammock mitral valve
hammock valve
hammocking of mitral valve leaflet
Hampton hump
Hampton line
hamstring muscle
Hanafee catheter
hand
  articulations of
  digital artery of
  phalanges of
hand grip exercise
hand-held probe
hand injection of contrast medium
Hand-Schüller-Christian disease
hangman's fracture
HAPE (high-altitude pulmonary edema)
Hara classification of gallbladder inflammation
Harbitz-Mueller syndrome
HARC-C wavelet compression technique
hard disk herniation
hard metal disease
hardening of arteries
hardware optimized trapezoid (HOT) pulse
Hardy-Clapham sesamoid classification
Harkavy syndrome
harmonic imaging
Harrison sulcus
Hartmann closure of rectum
Hartmann point

Hartmann pouch
Hartnup disease
Hartzler ACX-II or RX-014 balloon
  catheter
Hartzler angioplasty balloon
Hartzler LPS dilatation catheter
Hartzler Micro XT dilatation catheter
harvester lung
harvesting
  bone
  graft
  vein
Hashimoto thyroiditis
HASTE (half-Fourier acquisition
  single-shot turbo spin-echo) MR
  cholangiography
HAT-transformed images
Hatcher-Smith cervical fusion
hatchet-head deformity
Hatle method to calculate mitral valve
  area
Hausdorff error
Hausdorff metric measure
haustral blunting
haustral fold
haustral indentation
haustral markings
haustral pattern
haustral pouch
haustrations
haustrum (pl. haustra)
haversian canal
haversian gland
Hawkins breast localization needle
  with FlexStrand cable
Hawkins classification of talar neck
  fractures
Hawkins II talar neck fracture
Hawkins impingement sign
Hawkins line
Hayem-Widal syndrome

Haygarth node
hazy density
hazy infiltrate
HBCT (helical biphasic contrast CT)
H-benzapine imaging agent
HC (head circumference)
HC/AC ratio (head circumference to
  abdominal circumference)
HCTH (helical CT holography)
HDI (HDTV-interlaced)
HDI (high-definition imaging) 3000
  ultrasound system
HDIC (hepatodiaphragmatic
  interposition of the colon)
HDM bronchial provocation test
HDM challenge
HDR (high dose rate)
HE (half-scan with extrapolation)
  method/projection
head
  cartilaginous cap of phalangeal
  clavicular head of sternocleido-
    mastoid
  femoral
  first metatarsal (FMH)
  forward positioning of
  humeral
  long
  metatarsal
  pancreas
  radial
  short
  terminal
  transillumination of
  ulnar
head and neck, femoral
head circumference (HC)
headhunter catheter
head of barium column
healing infarct
health physics

**heart**

heart
  abdominal
  air-driven artificial
  alcoholic
  ALVAD (intra-abdominal left ventricular assist device)
  artificial
  angiosarcoma of
  aortic opening of
  apex of
  armored
  artificial
  athlete's
  athletic
  axis of
  balloon-shaped
  Baylor total artificial
  beer
  beriberi
  boat-shaped
  bony
  booster
  boot-shaped
  bovine
  bread-and-butter
  bulb of
  cardiogenic shock
  cervical
  chaotic
  conical
  coronary artery of
  crisscross
  degeneration of
  diaphragmatic surface of
  dome-shaped
  donor
  drop
  dynamite
  enlargement of
  elongated
  empty
  encased

heart *(cont.)*
  enlarged
  failing
  fat
  fatty
  fibroid
  fibroma of
  flabby
  flask-shaped
  globoid
  hairy
  hanging (suspended)
  holiday
  horizontal
  hyperdynamic
  hyperkinetic
  hyperthyroid
  hypertrophied
  hypoplastic
  hypothermic
  inferior border of
  inflammation of
  intermediate
  irritable
  ischemic
  left (atrium and ventricle)
  left border of
  left ventricle of
  luxus
  lymphosarcoma of
  malposition of
  massively enlarged
  mildly enlarged
  movable
  myxedema of
  myxoma of
  one-ventricle
  ovoid
  ox
  paracorporeal
  parchment
  pear-shaped

heart *(cont.)*
  pectoral
  pendulous
  pulmonary
  Quain fatty
  resting
  rhabdomyoma of
  right (atrium and ventricle)
  right border of
  right ventricle of
  round
  sabot
  semihorizontal
  semivertical
  single-outlet
  snowman
  soldier's
  spastic
  sternocostal surface of
  stone
  superior border of
  superoinferior
  suspended
  systemic
  teardrop
  three-chambered
  thrush breast
  tiger
  tiger lily
  tobacco
  total artificial (TAH)
  transplanted
  transverse
  Traube
  triatrial
  trilocular
  univentricular
  University of Akron artificial
  upstairs-downstairs
  Utah artificial
  Utah TAH (total artificial heart)
  venous

heart *(cont.)*
  venting of
  vertical
  wandering
  water-bottle
  wooden shoe
heart and great vessels
heart and lung transplantation
heart apex
heart attack (myocardial infarction)
heart border
heart catheterization (also cardiac)
  femoral
  retrograde
  transseptal
  transvenous
heart in sinus rhythm
heart overload
heart decortication
heart disease, atherosclerotic
heart failure
  acute
  backward
  chronic
  compensated congestive
  congestive
  decompensated congestive
  diastolic
  fetal
  forward
  high-output
  left-sided
  low-output
  refractory
  right-sided
  systolic
heart-lung transplant (transplantation)
heart power failure
heart prosthesis
heart sac
heart tamponade
heart remnant

heart-to-background ratio
heart-to-lung ratio (HLR)
heat-damaged Tc-RBCs
heat-expandable stent
heat fracture
heat-generating source
Heath-Edwards classification of
 pulmonary vascular disease
heave and lift
heaving precordial motion
heavy-particle irradiation
Heberden disease
Heberden nodes
Heberden sign
Heckathorn disease
Hector, tendon of
heel bone
heel, Sorbol
heel tendon
Heerfordt syndrome
Hegglin syndrome
Heim-Kreysig sign
Helbing sign
helical biphasic contrast-enhanced CT
 (HBCT)
helical coil stent
helical computed tomography (CT)
helical CT holography (HCTH)
helical pattern
helical thin-section CT scan
helical-tip Halo catheter
Helios diagnostic imaging system
helium-filled balloon catheter
Helix camera
Helmholtz coil
Helmholtz configuration
heloma (pl. helomata)
heloma durum
heloma molle
hemal arch
hemangioblastoma tumor
hemangioendothelioma

hemangioma
 cavernous
 verrucous
hemangiomatosis
hemangiopericytoma
hematemesis
hematochezia
hematocystic spot (HCS)
hematogenous dissemination
hematogenous spread of metastases
hematologic parameters
hematoma
 aneurysmal
 balancing subdural
 carotid plaque
 chronic subdural (CSDH)
 corpus luteum
 dissecting aortic
 dural
 encapsulated subdural
 epidural (EDH)
 evolving
 extracerebral
 extradural
 gelatinous
 hemispheral
 intracerebral
 intracranial
 intramural
 intraparenchymal
 intrarenal
 intraventricular
 mural
 nasal septum
 organized
 perianal
 pericardial
 perirenal
 posterior fossa
 primary intracerebral
 rectus sheath
 retromembranous

hematoma *(cont.)*
   retroperitoneal
   scalp
   spinal epidural
   spontaneous spinal epidural
   subcapsular
   subdural
   subgaleal
hematoma cap
   azygos
   left pleural apical
hematoma formation on bowel wall
hematomediastinum (hemomediastinum)
hematopericardium (hemopericardium)
hematuria
hemiagenesis
hemiarch
hemiatrophy
hemiaxial view
hemiazygos vein
hemibody irradiation
hemic calculus
hemicardium
hemicolon
hemicranium
hemidiaphragm
   attenuation by
   tenting of
hemidiaphragm depression
hemidiaphragmatic
hemifacial microsomia
hemihypertrophy
hemipelvis
hemisection of spinal cord
hemispheral mass effect
hemisphere
   cerebellar
   cerebral
   dominant
   left
   mesial
   right

hemisphere atrophy
hemisphere damage
hemisphere lesion
hemisphere stroke
hemithorax (pl. hemithoraces)
hemivertebra
   balanced
   unbalanced
hemodynamic alterations
hemodynamic assessment
hemodynamically significant findings
hemodynamically weighted echo planar MR imaging
hemodynamic impotence
hemodynamic penumbra
hemodynamic reserve impairment
hemodynamic response
hemodynamic support
hemodynamics, cardiovascular
hemomediastinum (hematomediastinum)
hemoperfusion
hemopericardium
hemoperitoneum
hemopleuropneumonia syndrome
hemopneumothorax
hemoptysis
hemorrhage
   anastomotic
   aneurysmal
   arterial
   brain stem
   capillary
   central nervous system
   cerebellar
   chronic parenchymal
   concealed
   delayed traumatic intracerebral (DTICH)
   diffuse subarachnoid
   Duret
   eight-ball

hemorrhage *(cont.)*
  epidural
  exsanguinating (into pleural space)
  external
  extradural
  extrapleural
  focal endocardial
  frank
  hypothalamic
  internal
  interstitial
  intertrabecular
  intra-abdominal
  intracerebral (ICH)
  intracranial
  intramural arterial
  intraparenchymal
  intraplaque (IPH)
  intrapleural
  intrapulmonary
  intraventricular (IVH)
  life-threatening
  lobar intracerebral
  massive exsanguinating
  meningeal
  neonatal intracranial
  nondominant putaminal
  nontraumatic epidural
  old
  parenchymal
  parenchymatous
  periaqueductal
  peribronchiolar
  perirenal
  pontine
  postoperative mediastinal
  pulmonary
  putaminal
  retrobulbar
  salmon-patch
  sentinel transoral
  slit

hemorrhage *(cont.)*
  spinal epidural (SEH)
  spinal subarachnoid
  spinal subdural (SSH)
  splinter
  striate
  subacute
  subarachnoid (SAH)
  subchorionic
  subdural (SDH)
  subependymal
  submucosal
  subserosal
  thalamic
  traumatic meningeal
  variceal
  venous
hemorrhagic consolidation
hemorrhagic corpus luteum cyst
hemorrhagic cyst
hemorrhagic duodenitis
hemorrhagic gastritis
hemorrhagic infarct
hemorrhagic necrosis
hemorrhagic pericarditis
hemorrhagic pleurisy
hemorrhagic stroke
hemorrhagic zone, pyramidal
hemostatic puncture closure device (HPCD)
hemothorax (pl. hemothoraces)
hemotympanum
Henderson-Jones chondromatosis
Henderson-Jones disease
Henke trigone
Henle
  jejunal interposition of
  ligament of
Henle loop
Henle sheath
Henry
  master knot of
  vertebral artery of

Henry and Wrisberg, ligaments of
Hensing fold
heparin
heparinization
heparinized blood
hepatic angiography (angiogram)
hepatic angiomyolipoma
hepatic arterial phase (HAP)
hepatic arteriovenous fistula
hepatic artery thrombosis
hepatic bed
hepatic cirrhosis
hepatic congestion
hepatic cord
hepatic cyst
hepatic diverticulum
hepatic duct bifurcation
hepatic flexure of colon
hepatic insufficiency
hepatic necrosis
hepatic vein thrombosis
hepatic venography with hemodynamic evaluation
hepatic veno-occlusive disease
hepatic venous outflow
hepatic venous web disease
hepatic web dilation
hepatitis, fulminant
hepatization
hepatobiliary disease
hepatobiliary ductal system imaging with quantitative measurement of gallbladder function
hepatobiliary ductal system imaging with pharmacologic intervention
hepatobiliary imaging
hepatobiliary scintigraphy
hepatobiliary tree
hepatocarcinoma
hepatocellular carcinoma
hepatocellular dysfunction
hepatoclavicular view

hepatodiaphragmatic interposition of colon (HDIC)
hepatoduodenal-peritoneal reflection
hepatofugal flow
hepatojugular reflux
hepatolithiasis
hepatoma
hepatomalacia
hepatomegaly
hepatopetal flow
hepatopleural fistula
hepatoptosis
hepatorenal bypass graft
hepatorenal saphenous vein bypass graft
hepatorenal syndrome (HRS)
hepatosplenomegaly
hepatotoxicity
herald bleed
Herbert-Fisher fracture classification system
Hering canal
Hermodsson fracture
hernia (pl. hernias)
   abdominal wall
   axial hiatal
   Bochdalek
   cecal
   congenital
   diaphragmatic
   direct inguinal
   epigastric
   esophageal
   femoral
   funicular inguinal
   hiatal
   hiatus
   incarcerated
   incisional
   incomplete
   indirect inguinal
   inguinal

**hernia • heterotopia**

hernia *(cont.)*
    inguinofemoral
    interstitial
    intrapericardial diaphragmatic
    mediastinal
    obturator
    ovarian
    pantaloon
    paraesophageal hiatal
    paraileostomal
    parastomal
    peritoneal
    properitoneal
    rolling hiatal
    scrotal
    sliding hiatal
    sliding-type hiatal
    spigelian
    strangulated
    umbilical
    ventral
hernia defect
hernia pouch
hernia sac
herniated abdominal contents
herniated cerebellar tonsil
herniated cervical disk
herniated disk
herniated intervertebral disk (HID)
herniated nucleus pulposus (HNP)
herniated preperitoneal fat
herniation
    brain
    brain tissue
    central
    cerebellar
    cerebral
    cingulate
    concentric
    disk
    fatal
    foramen magnum

herniation *(cont.)*
    frank disk
    hard disk
    hippocampal
    impending
    internal disk
    intraspongy nuclear disk
    lumbosacral intervertebral disk
    phalangeal
    soft disk
    subfalcine (subfalcial)
    subligamentous disk
    supraligamentous disk
    temporal lobe
    tentorial notch
    thoracic intervertebral disk
    tonsillar
    transtentorial
    uncal
herniation of brain tissue
herniation of nucleus pulposus into adjacent vertebral body
HER-2 neu oncoprotein expression
Heschl convolution
Heschl transverse gyrus
Hesselbach ligament
Hesselbach triangle
heterocyclic free radicals
heterogeneous appearance
heterogeneous hyperattenuation
heterogeneous isodense enhancement
heterogeneous microdistribution
heterogeneous perfusion pattern
heterogeneous system disease
heterogeneous uptake
heterologous graft
heterotaxy
    abdominal
    visceral
heterotaxy syndrome
heterotopia
    gastric
    gray matter

heterotopic bone formation
heterotopic gray matter
heterotopic ossification
heterotopic pancreas
heterotopic pregnancy
Hetzel forward triangle method for cardiac output
Heubner, recurrent artery of
Hewlett-Packard color flow imager
Hewlett-Packard phased-array imaging system
Hewlett-Packard scanner
Hewlett-Packard ultrasound unit
Hexabrix contrast medium
hexadactyly
hexamethylpropyleneamine oxime
Hey amputation
HFD (high frequency Doppler) ultrasound
HFLA duration
HI (half-scan with interpolation) method/projection
hiatal hernia
hiatus
   adductor
   diaphragmatic
   esophageal
   popliteal
hiatus hernia
Hibbs metatarsocalcaneal angle
hibernating myocardium
hibernation, myocardial
hibernoma
Hickman indwelling right atrial catheterf
Hickman tunneled catheter
hickory-stick fracture
HID (herniated intervertebral disk)
HIDA (hepatoiminodiacetic acid) scan
Hidalgo catheter
hierarchical information
hierarchical scanning pattern

Hieshima coaxial catheter
HIFU (high-intensity focused ultrasound)
high altitude pulmonary edema (HAPE)
high amplitude impulse
high attenuation
high contrast film
high defect in atrial septum
high definition imaging (HDI) 3000 ultrasound system
high definition television (HDTV)
high density barium
high density linear array
high dose film dosimeter
high dose rate (HDR)
high dose rate remote afterloading
high energy imaging
high energy protons
high energy trauma
high field open MRI scanner
high field strength MR imaging
high field strength scanner
high field system
high filling pressure
high flow, low resistance pattern
high frequency Doppler ultrasound
high frequency miniature probe
high frequency therapeutic ultrasound
high frequency ultrasound imaging
high grade stenosis
high grade tumor
high impedance circulation
high interstitial pressure
high lateral wall myocardial infarction
high left main diagonal artery
high minute ventilation
Highmore, antrum cardiacum of
high order curve recognition
high osmolar media (HOM)
high output circulatory failure
high output heart failure

high-pitched signal
high pontine lesion
high power field
high power, thin section quantitative MT
high rate detect interval
high rate pacing
high rate ventricular response, atrial fibrillation with
high reflectivity
high resolution B-mode imaging
high resolution computed tomography (HRCT) scan
high resolution coronal cuts on CT scan
high resolution CT mammography
high resolution diffraction
high resolution EEG
high resolution infrared (HRI) imaging
high resolution, low-speed radiography
high resolution magnification
high resolution storage phosphor imaging
high-riding patella (patella alta)
high right atrium
high sensitivity measurement
high signal mass
high spatial frequency reconstruction algorithm
high spatial resolution cine CT (HSR-CCT)
high spatial resolution mode (volumetric imaging)
high speed rotation dynamic angioplasty catheter
high take-off of left coronary artery
high temperature diffraction
high temporal resolution cine CT (HTRCCT)
high temporal resolution mode (multi-time point imaging)
high torque (see *Hi-Torque*)

high velocity gunshot wound
high velocity jet
hilar area
hilar artery
hilar dance
hilar gland enlargement
hilar haze
hilar lymph node enlargement
hilar mass
hilar plate
hilar prominence
hilar reaction
hilar shadows
hilar structures
hilar vessels
Hilight Advantage System CT scanner
Hill sign
Hill-Sachs deformity
Hill-Sachs shoulder lesion
Hillock arch
Hilton law
hilum (formerly hilus) (pl. hila)
  hepatic
  kidney
  lips of
  lung
  renal
  splenic
hilus (pl. hili) tuberculosis
hindbrain deformity
hindfoot excursion
hindfoot instability
hindfoot joint complex
hindfoot valgus
hinged implant
hip
  congenital dislocation of (CDH)
  congenital dysplasia of (CDH)
  developmental dysplasia (DDH) of
  dislocated
  hanging
hip bone (os coxae)

hip bump
hip dislocation
Hippel-Lindau syndrome
hip prosthesis
hip replacement
hippocampal formation
hippocampal gyrus
hippocampal herniation
hippocampal infarction
hippocampal MR volumetry
hippocampal region
hippocampal sclerosis
hippocampal volume
hippocampus
Hippuran contrast medium
Hirschsprung-associated enterocolitis (HAEC)
His
  angle of
  atrioventricular node of
  atrioventricular opening of
  bundle of
His band
His bundle
His spindle
His-Haas muscle transfer
Hislop-Reid syndrome
Hispeed CT scanner
histamine
histiocytic origin
histiocytoma
  angiomatoid
  benign fibrous
  fibrous
  low-grade malignant
  malignant fibrous
Hi-Star midfield MRI system
histiocytosis, sinus
histiocytosis X
histogram
  dose-volume
  gaussian dose-volume
  multisectional dose-volume

histogram equalization algorithms
histologic grading
histology
histopathological subtype
histopathologic comparison
histopathologic-CT correlation
histoplasmoma
histoplasmosis
Hitachi CT scanner
Hitachi MR scanner
Hitachi Open MRI System
Hitachi ultrasound
Hi-Torque Floppy (HTF) guide wire
HIV-related metabolic abnormality
HIV-seronegative
HIV-seropositive
HJB (high jugular bulb)
HL (hallux limitus)
HLA (horizontal-long axial) images
HLHS (hypoplastic left heart syndrome)
HLR (heart-to-lung ratio)
H-mode echocardiography
HMPAO (hexamethyl propylene amine oxime) for SPECT scan
HNA (hypothalamoneurohypophyseal axis)
HNP (herniated nucleus pulposus)
Ho:YAG (holmium yttrium aluminum garnet) laser
Hobb view
HOC or HOCM (hypertrophic obstructive cardiomyopathy)
hockey-stick appearance of catheter tip
hockey-stick deformity of tricuspid valve
Hodgkin disease
Hodgkin lymphoma
Hodgkin tumor
Hodgson aneurysmal dilatation of the aorta
Hodgson disease

Hoffa disease
Hoffmann atrophy
Hofmeister anastomosis
Hohl tibia condylar fracture classification
Holdsworth classification of spinal injury
hole burning, selective
hole pattern
holiday heart syndrome
hollow chest syndrome
hollow foot
hollow-point bullet
Holmes cortical cerebellar degeneration
Holmes heart
Holmes syndrome
holmium (Ho)
holmium-166 imaging agent
holmium:YAG (yttrium aluminum garnet) laser for angioplasty
holocrania
Hologic QDR 1000W dual-energy x-ray absorptiometry scanner
Hologic 2000 scanner
hologram
holography
    MEVH
    multiple-exposure volumetric (MEVH)
    3-D
    volumetric multiplexed transmission
    Voxgram multiple exposure
holosystolic mitral valve prolapse
Holt-Oram syndrome
Holthouse hernia
Holzknecht space
Holzknecht stomach
HOM (high osmolar media)
homoartery
homogeneity
homogeneous appearance

homogeneous echo pattern
homogeneous opacity
homogeneous perfusion
homogeneous soft tissue density
homogeneous thallium distribution
homology mapping
homonuclear spin systems
homotransplantation
Honda sign appearance
H-1-H (headhunter) catheter
H-1 CSI scan
H-1 MR spectroscopic imaging
H1 spectroscopy
$H_2$ $^{15}O$ positron emission tomography
honeycomb formation
honeycomb lung
honeycomb pattern
honeycombing, fibrotic
hooklike osteophyte formation
hook-shaped ureter
hook wire localization, CT-directed
hoop-shaped loops of bowel
Hoover sign
Hope sign
horizontal fissure
horizontal fissure of lung
horizontal fracture
horizontal gaze
horizontal lie
horizontal long axis SPECT image
horizontal-long axial images (HLA)
horizontal plane
horizontal plane loop
horizontal striping
hormone, immunoreactive parathyroid (iPTH)
horn
    Ammon
    anterior
    central
    dorsal spinal cord
    enlarged frontal

horn *(cont.)*
   frontal
   lateral
   meniscal
   occipital
   posterior
   posterior gray (of spinal cord)
   projectile
   spinal cord
   spinal dorsal
   splaying of frontal
   temporal
   uterine
   ventral
   ventricular
Horner syndrome
horseshoe appearance
horseshoe configuration on thallium imaging
horseshoe kidney
horseshoe shape
Horsley anastomosis
Horton disease
hose-pipe appearance of terminal ileum
host, immunocompromised
hot area
"hot" contrast
hot-cross-bun skull
hot nodule
hot nose sign
hot spot artifact
hot spot imaging agent
hot spot on scan
hot-tip laser
Hough transform (HT)
Hounsfield calcium density measurement unit (on CT scan)
Hounsfield unit (HU) (on CT scan)
hourglass bladder
hourglass constriction of gallbladder
hourglass deformity on myelogram
hourglass-shaped lesion
hourglass stomach
House grading system
housemaid's knee
Howtek Scanmaster DX scanner
HPCD (hemostatic puncture closure device)
hpf (high-power field)
HPGe detector
HRA (high right atrium)
HRCT (high resolution computed tomography) image
HRI (high resolution infrared) imaging
HRS (hepatorenal syndrome)
HS (half-scan) method/projection
H/S or HSG (hysterosalpingography) catheter
HSS ligament rating scale
HSSG (hysterosalpingosonography)
HT (Hough transform)
HTML (hypertext markup language)
HTTP (also http) (hypertext transfer protocol)
HU (Hounsfield unit)
Huchard disease
Hughes-Stovin syndrome
Hughston Clinic classification of injury
Hughston view
human anti-murine antibodies (HAMA)
human serum-albumin imaging agent
human visual sensitivity weighting
humeral bone
humeral head-splitting fracture
humeroradial articulation
humeroulnar articulation
humerus
humidifier lung

hump
  buffalo
  hip
    dowager's
  Hampton
humpback
Hunter canal
Hunter syndrome
Hunter-Sessions inferior vena cava balloon occluder
hunterian ligation of aneurysm
Hunt-Hess aneurysm grading system
Hunt-Hess subarachnoid hemorrhage scale
Hunt-Kosnik classification of aneurysm
Huppert disease
Hurler syndrome
Huschke ligament
Hutchinson-type neuroblastoma
Hutinel-Pick syndrome
HV (hallux valgus)
HVA (hallux valgus angle)
Hx (history)
hyaline-cartilage endplate of the intervertebral disk
hyaline membrane disease
hyaloid fossa
hybrid MRI imaging agent
hybrid-RARE imaging
hydatid
  alveolar
  sessile
  Virchow
hydatid cyst
hydatidiform mole (molar pregnancy)
HydraCross TLC PTCA catheter
Hydradjust IV table
hydramnios
hydranencephaly
hydrocephalus
hydrated proteoglycan gel of annulus fibrosus

hydration
hydrencephalomeningocele
hydrencephaly
hydrocele
hydrocephalic
hydrocephalocele
hydrocephalus
  acquired
  acute
  asymptomatic
  bilateral
  chronic
  communicating
  congenital
  delayed
  idiopathic
  infantile
  noncommunicating
  normal-pressure (NPH)
  normotensive
  obstructive
  occult
  posthemorrhagic
  postinfectious
  post-traumatic
  primary
  progressive
  secondary
  symptomatic
  unilateral
  unshunted
hydrocephalus ex vacuo
hydrodynamic potential of disk
hydroencephalocele
hydroencephaly
hydrogen proton imaging
Hydrolyser microcatheter for thrombectomy systems
hydroma (see *hygroma*)
hydronephrosis
hydronephrotic kidney
hydropericardium

hydroperitoneum
hydrophilic-coated catheter
hydrophone, needle
hydropic changes
hydropic degeneration
hydropneumothorax
hydrops
  endolymphatic
  gallbladder
  labyrinthine
  semicircular canal
hydrosalpinx
hydrostatic pressure of blood
hydrosyringomyelia
hydrothorax
hydroureter
hydroureteronephrosis
hygroma
  cystic
  subdural
hyoid bone
hyoscine butylbromide imaging agent
Hypaque contrast medium
Hypaque-Cysto contrast medium
Hypaque-M contrast medium
Hypaque Meglumine contrast medium
Hypaque myelography
Hypaque-76 contrast media
Hypaque Sodium contrast medium
Hypaque swallow
hyparterial bronchi
hyperabduction maneuver
hyperacute renal transplant rejection
hyperacute stroke
hyperaeration
hyperaldosteronism
hyperattenuation, heterogeneous
hypercalcemia-supravalvular aortic stenosis
hyperconcentration of contrast medium
hyperdense middle cerebral artery sign

hyperdynamic abductor hallucis
hyperdynamic AV fistulae
hyperechoic area
hyperechoic region
hyperechoicity
hyperemia
  active
  arterial
  collateral
  diffuse
  fluxionary (active)
  mucous membrane
  passive
  reactive
  venous
hyperemic flow
hyperexpanded lobe
hyperexpansion, compensatory lobe
hyperextensibility of joints
hyperextension injury
hyperextension of neck
hyperextension teardrop fracture
hyperfixation
Hyperflex steerable wire
hyperflexion/hyperextension cervical injury
hyperflexion injury
hyperflexion teardrop fracture
hyperfractionated radiation therapy
hyperinflation
  dynamic pulmonary
  pulmonary
hyperintense marrow space
hyperintense mass
hyperintense ring sign
hyperintense signal
hyperintensity
  cortical
  white matter signal
hyperkinetic segmental wall motion
hyperlordosis, functional
hyperlucency

hyperlucent lung
hypermetabolic nodule
hypermetabolic region
hypermotility
hypermyelination
hypernephroma
hyperosmotic solution
hyperostosis
  ankylosing spinal
  Caffey
  diffuse idiopathic sclerosis (DISH)
  diffuse idiopathic skeletal (DISH)
  idiopathic cortical (ICH)
  infantile cortical
  senile ankylosing (of spine)
  skull
hyperostosis associated with venous malformation
hyperostosis frontalis interna
HyperPACS system
hyperperistalsis
hyperplasia
  adaptive
  adenomatous
  adrenal
  adrenocortical
  angiofollicular lymph node
  angiolymphoid
  benign prostatic
  compensatory
  congenital adrenal (CAH)
  cortical nodular
  ductal
  endometrial
  epiphyseal
  fibrous tissue
  focal nodular (FNH)
  follicular
  giant follicular
  hematopoietic bone marrow
  intravascular papillary endothelial
  lipoid adrenal

hyperplasia *(cont.)*
  lung lymphoid
  lymphoid
  mucosal
  myointimal
  neoplastic
  nodular adrenal
  nodular lymphoid
  nodular regenerative
  parathyroid
  pituitary
  prostatic
  pseudoangiomatous stromal
  reactive
  sinus
  smooth
  splenic
  Swiss-cheese
  thymus
  thyroid
hyperplastic adenomatous polyp
hyperplastic lesion
hyperpolarized He-3 imaging agent
hyperpolarized helium
hyperpolarized $^{129}$Xe (xenon-129) gas
hyperprolactinemia
hyperrugosity
hypersplenism
hypertelorism
hypertension (HTN, Htn)
  benign intracranial (BIH)
  intracranial
  primary pulmonary (PPH)
  pulmonary artery
  renovascular
  striate hemorrhage in intracranial
hypertension injury
hypertensive cardiomegaly
hypertensive cardiopathy
hypertensive contrast concentration
hypertensive crisis
hypertensive diathesis

hypertensive heart disease
hypertensive hemorrhage
hypertensive ischemic ulcer
hypertensive left ventricular
   hypertrophy
hypertensive renal disease
hypertensive stroke
hypertensive vascular degeneration
hypertensive vascular disease
hypertext markup language (HTML)
hypertext transfer protocol (HTTP,
   http)
hyperthermia
   capacitive
   loco-regional
   radiotherapy with
   radiotherapy without
   volumetric interstitial
   whole body
hyperthermia probe
hyperthermia treatment
   deep
   external
   interstitial
   intracavitary
   low energy radiofrequency
      conduction
   microwave
   superficial
   ultrasound
hypertonic airways
hypertonicity
hypertransradiancy
hypertrophic cardiomyopathy (HC)
hypertrophic marginal spurring
hypertrophic nonunion
hypertrophic obstructive cardiomyopathy (HOC or HOCM)
hypertrophic pyloric stenosis
hypertrophic spurring
hypertrophic subaortic stenosis

hypertrophy
   adaptive
   asymmetric septal (ASH)
   biatrial
   biventricular
   bladder
   bone
   cardiac
   compensatory
   complementary
   concentric left ventricular
   eccentric left ventricular
   epiphyseal
   four-chamber
   functional
   left atrial
   left ventricular (LVH)
   ligamentous-muscular
   lipomatous (of the interatrial
      septum)
   muscular
   myocardial
   myocardial cellular
   olivary
   panchamber
   physiologic
   pyloric
   right atrial
   right ventricular (RVH)
   scalenus anticus muscle
   smooth-muscle
   trigonal
   type A (B or C) right ventricular
   unilateral
   ventricular
   villous
   Wigle scale for ventricular
hypervascular arterialization
hypervolemia
hypervolemic pulmonary edema
hypoaeration
hypoattenuating (CT scan)

hypoattenuation
hypocycloidal ankle tomography
hypodense area
hypodense lesion
hypoechogenic
hypoechoic area on ultrasound
hypoechoic band
hypoechoic fluid collection
hypoechoic halo
hypoechoic layer
hypoechoic mantle
hypoechoic rim
hypofractionated radiation therapy
hypofrontality
hypoganglionosis of colon
hypogastric artery
hypogastric region
hypogastrium
hypogenetic lung syndrome
hypoglossal canal
hypoglossal nerve (twelfth cranial nerve)
hypointense signal
hypokinesia
  apical
  cardiac
  diffuse
  diffuse ventricular
  global
  inferior wall
  regional
  septal
hypokinetic left ventricle
hypokinetic segmental wall motion
hypolucency of lung
hypometabolic area
hypometabolism, global
hypoparathyroidism
hypoperfused state
hypoperfusion
  acute alveolar
  apical

hypoperfusion *(cont.)*
  global cerebral
  peripheral
  pulmonary
  resting regional myocardial
  septal
  systemic
hypoperistalsis
hypopharyngeal diverticulum
hypopharynx
hypophyseal (or hypophysial)
hypophysial (or hypophyseal)
hypophysial Rathke duct
hypophysis, infundibulum
hypoplasia
hypoplastic aorta syndrome
hypoplastic aortic arch
hypoplastic emphysema
hypoplastic heart
hypoplastic heart ventricle
hypoplastic horizontal ribs
hypoplastic left (or left-sided) heart syndrome (HLHS)
hypoplastic left heart syndrome
hypoplastic left ventricle syndrome
hypoplastic lung
hypoplastic right heart
hypoplastic subpulmonic outflow
hypoplastic tricuspid orifice
hyposensitive carotid sinus syndrome
hyposensitization
hypospadias
hypostatic bronchopneumonia
hypostatic congestion
hypostatic pneumonia
hypostatic pulmonary insufficiency
hypotension, cerebral
hypotensive challenge
hypothalamic lesion
hypothalamus tumor
hypothenar eminence
hypothenar muscle groups of hand

hypothermia
hypotonic duodenography
hypotonic patient
hypovolemia
hypovolemic shock
hypoxic brain damage
hypoxic cell sensitizer
hypoxic injury
hypoxic ischemic encephalopathy
hypoxic ischemic insults
hypoxic pulmonary hypertension
hypoxic pulmonary vasoconstriction
hypoxic vasoconstriction
hysterogram
hysterography
hysterosalpingogram
hysterosalpingography
hysterosalpingosonography (HSSG)
hysterosonography
hysterotubogram
Hz (hertz or cycles per second)

# I, i

I (iodine)
IAB (intra-aortic balloon) catheter
IABP (intra-aortic balloon pump)
IADSA (intra-arterial digital subtraction angiography)
IAM (internal auditory meatus)
IAS (interatrial septum)
iatrogenic carotid-cavernous fistula
iatrogenic dural tear
iatrogenic injury
IBD (inflammatory bowel disease)
IBM field-cycling research relaxometer
IBM NMR spectrometer
IBM Speech Server clinical reporting system
I-B1 radiolabeled antibody
IBS (irritable bowel syndrome)
IBZP (chloro-hydroxy-iodophenyl-methyl-tetrahydro-H-benzapine) imaging agent
ICA (internal carotid artery)
ICAM-1 (intercellular adhesive molecule)
ICE (intracardiac echocardiography)
ICEDP (intracranial epidural pressure)
ICEUS (intracaval endovascular ultrasonography)
ice-pick view on M-mode echocardiogram
ICH (intracerebral hemorrhage)
ICP (intracranial pressure)
ICRU 50 radiotherapy
ICS (improved Chen-Smith) coder
ICS (intercostal space)
ictal hyperperfusion
ictal phase study
ictal SPECT
ictal technetium Tc-99m HMPAO brain SPECT
ictus site
ICU (intensive care unit)
ICUS (intracoronary ultrasound)
ICV (internal cerebral vein)
IDD (intraluminal duodenal diverticulum)
identification
    particle
    peak
    phase
    topographic
idiopathic calcium pyrophosphate dihydrate (iCPPD) deposition disease

idiopathic cardiomegaly
idiopathic disease
idiopathic fibrosis, pulmonary interstitial
idiopathic fracture
idiopathic hypertrophic subaortic stenosis (IHSS)
idiopathic inflammatory bowel disease (IBD)
idiopathic intestinal pseudo-obstruction
idiopathic megacolon
idiopathic mural endomyocardial disease
idiopathic pleural calcification
idiopathic pulmonary arteriosclerosis (IPA)
idiopathic pulmonary fibrosis
idiopathic scoliosis
idiopathic unilobar emphysema
idiopathic varicocele
IDIS (intraoperative digital subtraction) angiography system
IDK (internal derangement of knee)
IDSA (intraoperative digital subtraction angiography)
IDSI (Imaging Diagnostic Systems Inc.) scanner
IEA (inferior epigastric artery) graft
IgG autoantibodies
Ig2b kappa monoclonal antibody
IHSS (idiopathic hypertrophic subaortic stenosis)
IJV (internal jugular vein)
ileal conduit
ileal motility
ileal neo-bladder
ileal pouch-anal anastomosis
   H-shaped
   J-shaped
   S-shaped
   W-shaped
ileal reservoir
ileitis
   backwash
   Crohn
   distal
   granulomatous
   obstructive dysfunctional
   prestomal
   regional
   terminal
ileoanal endorectal pull-through
ileocecal fat pad
ileocecal junction
ileocecal region
ileocecal valve
   competent
   incompetent
ileococcygeus muscle
ileocolic disease
ileocolic fold
ileocolic vessel
ileocolitis
ileoconduit
ileogram
ileostogram (loopogram)
ileostomate
ileostomist
ileotransverse colon anastomosis
ileum, terminal
ileus
   adhesive
   adynamic
   adynamic/paralytic
   dynamic
   dynamic/spastic
   gallbladder
   gallstone
   mechanical
   meconium
   occlusive
   paralytic
   postoperative
   spastic

Ilfeld-Holder deformity
iliac artery angioplasty
iliac artery disease
iliac artery stent
iliac atherosclerotic occlusive disease
iliac bone
iliac crest
iliac dowel
iliac fossa
iliac lesion
iliac-renal bypass graft
iliac spine
iliac stenosis
iliac tuberosity
iliac vessel
iliac wing
iliocaval compression syndrome
iliocaval junction
iliocaval thrombolysis
iliocaval tree
iliofemoral bypass
iliofemoral vein thrombosis
iliofemoral venous stenosis
ilioinguinal ring
ilioinguinal syndrome
iliopectineal eminence
iliopectineal line
iliopopliteal bypass
ilioprofunda bypass graft
iliopsoas muscle
iliopsoas ring
iliotibial band friction syndrome
ilium
Ilizarov ring
ill-defined consolidation
ill-defined mass
Illumen-8 guiding catheter
ILP (interstitial laser photocoagulation)
IM (intermetatarsal) joint
IM (intramedullary) rod (rodding)
IMA (inferior mesenteric artery)
IMA (intermetatarsal angle)
IMA (internal mammary artery)
image (see *imaging*)
   artifact
   attenuated
   stereotactic CT scan
image acquisition gated examination
image acquisition time
image analysis system
image coder, Chen-Smith
image control
imaged (verb)
image edge profile acutance
image fusion
image-guided radiosurgery
image intensification
image intensifier
image matrix
image noise
Imagent GI imaging agent
image post-processing errors artifact
image quality degradation
imager (see *scanner*)
image reconstruction
image restoration algorithm
image volume
imaging (also *image*; *scan*; *scanner*)
   Adenoscan
   adenosine echocardiography
   adrenal
   aerosol ventilation scan
   A-FAIR (arrhythmia-insensitive
      flow-sensitive alternating
      inversion recovery)
   air contrast
   air enema fluoroscopic
   airway fluoroscopy
   Aloka
   Aloka color Doppler real-time 2D
      blood flow imaging with Cine
      Memory
   amplitude

**imaging**

imaging *(cont.)*
  AMT-25-enhanced MR angiography
  angiography for controlling GI bleeding
  angiotensin II, AT$_1$ receptor
  anisotropic 3D
  annotated
  anterior planar
  anthropometric
  antifibrin antibody
  antegrade
  antegrade pyelography
  aortography
  aperiodic functional MR
  arrhythmia-insensitive flow-sensitive alternating inversion recovery (A-FAIR)
  arterial flow phase
  arteriovenous shunt
  arthrography
  Artoscan MRI
  A-scan
  ascending contrast phlebography
  Aspire continuous (CI)
  ATL real-time Neurosector scan
  attenuation
  Aurora MR breast
  axial
  axial grade echo
  axial transabdominal
  balloon expulsion
  balloon test occlusion
  barium enema
  barium swallow
  Biad SPECT
  bile duct scan
  biliary tract
  biliary tract CT scan
  binary
  "black blood" T2-weighted inversion recovery MR

imaging *(cont.)*
  blood flow
  blood pool
  blood pool phase
  BMIPP SPECT scan
  B-mode
  body coil
  body section radiography
  BOLD
  bolus challenge
  bone age
  bone density
  bone length
  bone mineral content
  bone phase
  bone scintiscan
  brain scan
  breath-hold, contrast-enhanced 3D MR angiography scan
  breath-hold T1-weighted MP-GRE MR
  breath-hold ungated
  breath-hold velocity-encoded cine MR
  bronchial provocation
  bronchography
  B-scan
  bull's eye
  Captopril-stimulated renal
  cardiac
  cardiac blood pool
  cardiac catheterization
  cardiac MRI for function
  cardiac MRI for morphology
  cardiac MRI for velocity flow mapping
  cardiac positron emission tomography (PET)
  cardiac radiography
  CAT (computerized axial tomography)
  cardiac wall motion

**imaging**

imaging *(cont.)*
   cardiokymography (CKG)
   cardiovascular radioisotope scan and function
   Cardiolite scan
   CardioTek (Cardiotec) scan
   cardiotocography
   carotid duplex
   carotid sinus
   CathTrack catheter locator system
   CDI (color Doppler imaging)
   celiac and mesenteric arteriography
   cephalogram
   cerebral perfusion SPECT
   chemical-selective fat saturation
   chemical shift
   cholangiography
   cine
   cine CT (computed tomography)
   cine gradient-echo
   cine PC (phase contrast)
   cineradiography
   cine view in MUGA scan
   cisternography
   cold spot myocardial imaging
   collimation
   colloid shift on liver-spleen scan
   color amplitude
   color-coded pulmonary blood flow
   color Dopper (CDI)
   color flow
   color-flow duplex
   column mode sinogram
   combined leukocyte-marrow
   combined multisection diffuse-weighted and hemodynamically weighted echo planar MR
   combined thallium-Tc-HMPAO
   Compuscan Hittman computerized
   computed axial tomography (CAT)

imaging *(cont.)*
   computed tomography (CT)
   computed transmission tomography
   chondroitin sulfate iron colloid (CSIS)-enhanced MR
   cone-beam
   contiguous
   contrast-enhanced magnetization transfer saturation
   contrast material enhanced
   conventional planar (CPI)
   convergent color Doppler
   coronary artery scan (CAS)
   corpus cavernosonography
   correlative diagnostic
   cross-sectional
   CSF-suppressed T2-weighted 3D MP-RAGE MR
   CT (computed tomography)
   CTAT (computerized transverse axial tomography)
   CT guidance for cyst aspiration
   CT guidance for needle biopsy
   CT guidance for placement of radiation therapy fields
   cystography
   cystourethroscopy
   dacryocystography
   delayed
   delayed bone
   DentaScan
   DEXA (dual energy x-ray absorptiometry) bone density scan
   dexamethasone suppression test for Cushing syndrome
   diagnostic
   diffusion and perfusion magnetic resonance
   diffusion magnetic resonance
   diffusion-weighted MR

**imaging**

imaging *(cont.)*
  digitally fused CT and
    radiolabeled
  digital radiography
  digital vascular (DVI)
  dipyridamole echocardiography
  dipyridamole handgrip
  dipyridamole infusion
  dipyridamole thallium stress
  dipyridamole thallium-201
  displacement field-fitting MR
  diuretic renal
  Doppler
  Doppler color flow
  Doppler tissue
  Doppler ultrasonography
  Doppler venous
  double contrast
  double-dose gadolinium
  double-helical CT
  double-phase technetium Tc 99m
    sestamibi
  DSC (dynamic susceptibility
    contrast) MR
  dual-echo DIET fast SE (spin
    echo)
  dual energy x-ray absorptiometry
    (DEXA)
  dual isotope
  dual-phase
  duodenography
  duplex
  duplex carotid
  duplex Doppler
  dynamic contrast-enhanced
    subtraction MR
  dynamic scintigraphy
  dynamic susceptibility contrast
    (DSC) MR
  echocardiography (ECG)
    ECG-gated multislice MR
    ECG-gated spin-echo MR

imaging *(cont.)*
  echo-planar (EPI)
  echo-planar FLAIR (fluid attenu-
    ated inversion-recovery)
  echo-planar MRA
  ED (end-diastolic)
  electric joint fluoroscopy
  electrocardiogram-gated MRI
  electrocardiography-gated echo-
    planar
  electrodiagnostic
  electronic portal
  electron radiography
  electromagnetic blood flow
  endoanal MR
  endorectal coil MR
  endoscopic catheterization of
    biliary ductal system
  endoscopic catheterization of
    pancreatic ductal system
  EPI (echo-planar imaging)
  epididymography
  EPR spatial
  equilibrium MUGA
  ERCP (endoscopic retrograde
    cholangiopancreatography)
  esophageal function
  esophagography
  ETL 3D FSE
  excitation-spoiled fat-suppressed
    T1-weighted ST
  excretory urography
  exercise
  exercise thallium-201 stress
  ex vivo MR
  fast cardiac phase contrast cine
  fast Fourier transform (FFT)
  fast low-angle shot (FLASH)
  fast multiplanar spoiled gradient-
    recalled (FMPSPGR)
  fast SE
  fast SE and fast IR (FMPIR)

**imaging**

imaging *(cont.)*
fast spin-echo MR
fast spoiled gradient-recalled MR
fat-suppressed three-dimensional spoiled gradient-(FDG)
FDG myocardial
FDG PET
ferumoxides-enhanced MR
filmless
511-keV high-energy
50 msec low resolution
first-pass myocardial perfusion
FLAIR (fluid-attenuated inversion-recovery)
FLAIR-FLASH
FLASH (fast low-angle shot)
flawed
flow
fluid-attenuated inversion-recovery (FLAIR)
FluoroPlus angiography
FluoroPlus Roadmapper digital fluoroscopy
fluoroscopic
fluoroscopic localization for transbronchial biopsy or brushing
fluoroscopy-guided condylar lift-off
flush aortogram
FMPIR
FMPSPGR
Fonar Stand-Up MRI
four-dimensional (4D)
four-hour delayed thallium
frequency domain (FDI) in ultrasound
FS-BURST MR
fSE (functional SE)
functional MR (FMR)
gadolinium (Gd) (see *imaging agent*)
gallbladder

imaging *(cont.)*
gallium (Ga) (see *imaging agent*)
gastric emptying
gastric mucosa
gastrointestinal motility
gas ventilation
gated MR
gated cardiac blood pool
gene delivery
gradient-echo
gradient-echo phase
gradient-echo sequence
gradient-recalled-echo (GRE) MR
GRASS MR (gradient-recalled acquisition in steady state)
gray-scale
GRE (gradient-recalled echo)
GRE breath-hold hepatic
GRE gadolinium-chelate enhanced
GRE-in
GRE-out
H-1 MR spectroscopic
half-Fourier, three-dimensional technique
harmonic
HAT-transformed
HBCT (helical biphasic computed tomography)
HCTH (helical CT holography)
Helios diagnostic
hemodynamically weighted echo planar MR
hepatobiliary scan
Hewlett-Packard phased-array
HIDA (hepatoiminodiacetic acid)
high-definition (HDI)
high-energy
high-field-strength MR
high frequency Doppler ultrasound
high frequency ultrasound
high resolution B-mode
high resolution storage phosphor

**imaging**

imaging *(cont.)*
  HLA (horizontal long axial)
    SPECT scan
  Hologic QDR 1000W dual-energy
    x-ray absorptiometry
  holography
  H-1 CSI (halostatin-1 CSI)
  horizontal long axis (HLA)
    SPECT scan
  hot spot imaging
  hot spot myocardial imaging
  HRCT (high-resolution CT)
  hybrid-RARE
  hydrogen proton
  hypotonic duodenography
  hysterosalpingography
  image acquisition gated scan
  immunoglobulin (Ig), monoclonal
  infarct avid
  infrared
  initial
  in-phase
  in-phase GRE
  intermediate
  interventional
  intracoronary
  intracranial
  intraoperative
  intraperitoneal technetium sulfur
    colloid
  intravenous fluorescein
    angiography (IVFA)
  in vivo
  in vivo He-3 MR
  iodine (see *imaging agent*)
  iodomethylnorcholesterol ($^{59}$NP)
    scintigraphy
  irreversible compression of MR
  Isocam scintillation
  isotope
  isotope-labeled fibrinogen
  isotope shunt

imaging *(cont.)*
  isotropic 3D
  Judkins coronary arteriography
  kidney function
  kidneys, ureters, bladder (KUB)
  kinematic MR
  kinestatic charge detector (KCD)
  laser-polarized helium MR
  limited
  line
  linear scan
  lipid-polarized helium MR
  lipid-sensitive MR
  liver-spleen
  localizing
  loopogram
  lower extremity
  lower limb venography
  low-field MR
  low-field-strength
  low resolution
  lymphangiography
  macromolecular contrast-enhanced
    MR
  magic-angle spinning
  Magnes 2500 WH (whole head)
  magnetic resonance (MR)
  magnetic resonance angiography
    (MRA)
  magnetic resonance cholangiog-
    raphy with HASTE sequence
  magnetization transfer
  magnetoacoustic
  mammary ductogram
  mammary galactogram
  marker transit
  mass
  Matrix LR3300 laser
  maximum intensity projection
  Meckel $^{99m}$Tc pertechnetate
    gastric-mucosa scan
  microwave

imaging *(cont.)*
   middle-field-strength MR
   midsagittal MR
   miniature
   minimum intensity projection
   mirror
   misleading
   M-mode echocardiogram
   monoclonal antibody
   MRA (magnetic resonance angiography)
   MRI (magnetic resonance imaging)
   MUGA (multiple gated acquisition) cardiac blood pool
   multi-echo
   multi-echo coronal
   multimodality
   multiorgan
   multiplanar MR
   multiplanar reformatted radiographic and digitally reconstructed radiographic
   multiple gated acquisition (MUGA) cardiac blood pool
   multipulse
   multisection diffuse-weighted
   multisection MR
   multislice first-pass myocardial perfusion
   multitime point
   multitracer
   MUSTPAC ultrasound
   myelography
   myocardial perfusion
   Myoscint
   native
   navigated spin-echo diffusion-weighted MR
   needle biopsy of intrathoracic lesion with follow-up films
   nephrostogram

imaging *(cont.)*
   nephrotomography
   neurodiagnostic
   neuroradiologic
   noninvasive
   nonsubtraction
   $^{59}$NP (iodomethylnorcholesterol) scintigraphy
   nuclear bone
   nuclear gated blood pool
   nuclear perfusion
   oblique axial MR
   off-resonance saturation pulse
   one-dimensional chemical shift (1D-CSI)
   100 msec high resolution
   on-line portal
   opposed GRE
   opposed-phase GRE
   opposed-phase MR
   optical
   oral cholecystogram (OCG)
   Orca fluoroscopic C-arm
   orthopantogram
   orthoroentgenogram
   out-of-phase GRE
   overlapping
   oxygenation-sensitive functional MR
   pancreas ultrasonography
   pancreatography
   panoramic
   parallel hole
   parallel-tag MR
   parathyroid ultrasonography
   PASTA (polarity-altered spectral-selective acquisition)
   PC (phase contrast)
   PDI
   pelvimetry with placental localization
   pelvimetry without placental localization

imaging *(cont.)*
 percutaneous drainage of abscess
 percutaneous intracoronary angioscopy
 percutaneous placement of enteroclysis tube
 percutaneous placement of gastrostomy tube
 percutaneous transhepatic cholangiography
 percutaneous transhepatic dilatation of biliary duct stricture with stent placement perfusion
 perfusion and ventilation lung
 perfusion MR
 perfusion-weighted
 perineogram
 peritoneogram
 periorbital Doppler
 peripheral vascular
 Persantine-thallium
 PET (positron emission tomography)
 PET metabolic
 PET myocardial fatty acid
 PET perfusion
 PET perfusion metabolism
 PETT (positron emission transaxial tomography)
 phase
 phase contrast (PC)
 phased-array surface coil MR
 phase encode time reduced acquisition sequence
 phase velocity
 pinhole
 PIPIDA hepatobiliary
 plain films
 planar (2D)
 planar spin
 planar thallium
 point

imaging *(cont.)*
 polarity-altered spectral-selective acquisition (PASTA)
 positron
 postcontrast MR
 postdrainage
 postexercise
 post-injection
 postmetrizamide CT
 postoperative
 postoperative biliary duct stone removal
 postoperative cholangiography
 post-stress
 power Doppler (PDI)
 pre-contrast
 preoperative
 pressure perfusion
 pretherapy
 protodensity MR
 proton density
 proton density-weighted
 pseudodynamic MR
 pullback
 pulmonary perfusion
 pulmonary ventilation
 pulsed electron paramagnetic
 pulsed magnetization transfer MR
 pyelography
 pyelostogram
 PYP (pyrophosphate) technetium myocardial
 pyrophosphate (PYP)
 QCT (quantitative computed tomography) (for bone loss)
 quantitative
 quantitative fluorescence
 quantitative spirometrically controlled CT
 radioactive fibrinogen
 radioactive iodine uptake (RAIU)
 radiographically normal

imaging *(cont.)*
   radioisotope
   radioisotope cisternography
   radioisotope gallium
   radioisotope indium-labeled white blood cell scan
   radioisotope lung scan
   radioisotope technetium
   radioisotope uptake in bone
   radioisotope uptake in vascular brain tumor
   radioisotope voiding cystography
   radionuclide
   radionuclide gated blood pool
   radionuclide milk
   radionuclide renal
   radionuclide renography
   radionuclide thyroid
   rapid axial MR
   rapid-sequence
   RARE MR
   real-time
   real-time echocardiogram
   real-time 2D blood flow
   reconstructed radiographic
   rectilinear bone scan
   redistributed thallium
   redistribution
   redistribution myocardial
   redistribution thallium-201
   regional ejection fraction (REFI)
   registration and alignment of 3D
   renal angiography
   renal computed tomography (CT)
   renal cyst
   renal duplex
   renal ultrasonography
   renal venography
   renogram
   rest (resting)
   rest myocardial perfusion
   rest-redistribution

imaging *(cont.)*
   rest thallium-201 myocardial
   resting MUGA
   retrograde
   retrograde cystography
   retrograde ureteropyelography
   ring-type
   rose bengal sodium $^{131}$I biliary
   row mode sinogram
   R-to-R
   sagittal
   sagittal gradient echo
   sagittal oblique
   sagittal T1
   sagittal transabdominal
   saline-enhanced MR
   scanogram
   scintigraphic scan
   scintillation
   scout
   scrambled
   SE (spin echo)
   sector scan echocardiography
   segmented k-space turbo gradient echo breath-hold sequence
   segmenting dual echo MR
   selective
   selenium ($^{75}$Se)-labeled bile acid
   sequential
   sequential plane
   sequential point
   sequential quantitative MR
   serial
   serial contrast MR
   serial static
   serial duplex
   serialography
   sestamibi stress scan
   shaded surface display (SSD)
   shuntogram
   sialography
   SieScape ultrasound

**imaging**

imaging *(cont.)*
  silhouette
  simultaneous volume
  single-dose gadolinium
  single-voxel proton brain
    spectroscopy (PROBE)
  sinus tract
  sliding-thin-slab maximum
    intensity projection CT
  slip-ring
  small field-of-view (FOV)
  SmartSpot high resolution digital
  Sones coronary arteriography
  source
  SPECT (single photon emission
    CT) thallium
  spine CT with contrast
  spine CT without contrast
  spin-echo (SE)
  spin-echo cardiac
  spin-echo MR
  spin-lock
  spin-lock induced T1rho weighted
  SPIO (superparamagnetic iron
    oxide)
  spirometrically controlled CT
  splanchnic vascular
  spleen ultrasonography
  splenoportography (transsplenic
    portography)
  split-brain
  spot
  spot-film
  SSD (shaded surface display)
  stacked scans
  static
  static 3D FLASH (fast low-angle
    shot)
  stent placement
  stereotactic localization for breast
    biopsy
  STIR (short T1 inversion
    recovery)

imaging *(cont.)*
  stop action
  strain-rate MR
  stress
  stress-redistribution
  stress thallium-201 myocardial
  stroke volume
  subtraction
  superparamagnetic iron oxide-
    enhanced
  SureStart
  survey-view
  susceptibility-weighted MR
  tagging cine MR
  TechneScan MAG3
  technetium (see *imaging agent*)
  thallium (Tl)
    $^{201}$Tl exercise
    $^{201}$Tl myocardial
    $^{201}$Tl SPECT brain
  thallium myocardial perfusion
  thallium rest-redistribution
  thallium scintigraphy
  thallium stress
  thick-slice
  thin-collimation
  thin-slice
  three-dimensional (3D)
    3D Fourier transform (3DFT)
    3DFT GRASS MR
    3DFT SPGR MR
    3D H-1 MR spectroscopic
    3D reformations of MR
    3D turbo SE (spin echo)
  three-phase
  ThromboScan
  thyroid
  thyroid ultrasonography
  time of flight (TOF)
  timed
  TIPS (transjugular intrahepatic
    protosystemic shunt)

**imaging** *(cont.)*
tissue Doppler
TOF (time of flight)
tomographic
total body scan
T1 weighted
T1 weighted coronal
T1 weighted sagittal
Toshiba Aspire continuous
transabdominal
transaxial
transcervical catheterization of fallopian tube
transesophageal Doppler color flow
transluminal atherectomy
transluminal balloon angioplasty
triple-dose gadolinium
triple-phase bone scan
TSPP (technetium stannous pyrophosphate) rectilinear bone
T2-QMRI (T2-quantitative magnetic resonance imaging)
T2 weighted
T2 weighted coronal
turboFLAIR (fluid-attenuated inversion recovery)
turboFLASH (fast low-angle shot)
two-dimensional (2D)
2D Fourier transform
2D gradient-recalled echo
two-phase CT
ultrafast
ultrafast CT
ultrasonic tomographic
ultrasound backscatter microscopy (UBM)
ultrasonography
unenhanced MR
unsuppressed
upper GI and small bowel series

**imaging** *(cont.)*
ureteral reflux
urethrocystography
urography
vaginogram
variance
vascular flow
vectorcardiography
velocity-encoded MR
venography
venous
ventilation
ventilation-perfusion (V/Q)
vertical-long axial (VLA)
vesiculography
videofluoroscopic
video radiography
virtual reality
Vitrea 3D
VLA (vertical-long axial)
voiding cystourethrography
volume-rendered
volumetric
V/Q (ventilation-perfusion)
wall motion
water selective SE (spin echo)
white blood cell
whole body scan
whole body thallium
wide-beam scan
xenon-133 ($^{133}$Xe) SPECT
xeroradiography
Xillix LIFE-GI fluorescence endoscopy
x-ray sensitive vidicon
**imaging agent** (including contrast media, radioactive drugs, radioisotopes, and technetium)
ABGd
Adenoscan
aerosolized technetium Tc DTPA

**imaging agent** *(cont.)*
   aggregated albumin with technetium
   aggregated iodinated $^{131}$I serum
      albumin
   air
   Albunex ultrasound heart
   AMI 121 and 227
   aminopolycarboxylic acid
   Amipaque
   Angio-Conray
   Angiocontrast
   Angiografin
   Angiovist 282, 292, 370
   antifibrin antibody
   antifibrin-MoAb antibody
   antimony
   antimyosin monoclonal (with Fab)
      antibody
   B-19036 chelate
   baby formula with ferrous sulfate
   Baricon
   barium sulfate
   Baro-CAT
   Baroflave
   Barosperse 110
   benzamide
   Biligrafin
   Biliscopin
   Bilivist
   Bilopaque
   Biloptin
   Bis-Gd-mesoporphyrin (Bis-Gd-MP)
   bromospirone (Br)
      $^{76}$Br
   bromodeoxyuridine
   bromophenol blue
   bunamiodyl (also buniodyl)
   C (carbon)
   CA15-3 antigen radioimmunoassay
   calcium (Ca)
      $^{45}$Ca
      $^{47}$Ca

**imaging agent** *(cont.)*
   carbogen radiosensitizer
   carbon (C)
      $^{11}$C acetate
      $^{11}$C butanol
      $^{11}$C carbon monoxide
      $^{11}$C carfentanil
      $^{11}$C deoxyglucose
      $^{11}$C flumazenil
      $^{11}$C-labeled cocaine
      $^{11}$C-labeled fatty acids
      $^{11}$C L-159
      $^{11}$C L-884
      $^{11}$C lumazenil
      $^{11}$C L-methylmethionine
      $^{11}$C methionine
      $^{11}$C methoxystaurosporine
      $^{11}$C N-methylspiperone
      $^{11}$C N-methylspiroperidol (NMS)
      $^{11}$C nomifensine
      $^{11}$C palmitate
      $^{11}$C palmitic acid radioactive
      $^{11}$C raclopride
      $^{11}$C thymidine
   carbonated saline solution
   carcinoma-specific monoclonal
      antibody
   Cardiografin sodium
   Cardio-Green (indocyanine green)
   Cardiolite
   CardioTec (or Cardiotec)
   CEAker
   CentoRx
   Ceretec radioisotope
   cerium silicate
   cesium chloride ($^{137}$Cs)
   Cholebrine
   Cholografin
   Cholografin Meglumine
   chromated $^{51}$Cr serum albumin

imaging agent *(cont.)*
  chromium (Cr)
  Cr-HIDA
  Cr-HIDA chelate
  chromium-labeled red blood cells
  $CO_2$ negative
  Conray
  Conray 30; 43; 60; 280; 325; 400
  copper (Cu)
  $^{62}$Cu PTSM
  $^{67}$Cu (copper-67)
  Cu/Zn-SOD (copper-zinc superoxide dismutase)
  corn oil and ferric ammonium citrate
  Cr (chromium)
  Cs (cesium)
  Cu (copper)
  cyanocobalamin
  Cysto-Conray
  Cysto-Conray II
  Cystografin
  Cystokon
  d,1-HMPAO
  DDFP (dodecafluoropentane)
  degassed tap water
  denatured technetium Tc RBCs
  deuterium
  dextrose 5% in water
  diatrizoate meglumine
  diatrizoate sodium
  Diatrizoate-60
  diazepam
  diethylenetriaminepentaacetic acid (DTPA)
  dihydroxyphenylalanine [DOPA]
  Diodrast
  Dionosil
  diprotrizoate
  dodecafluoropentane (DDFP)
  DOPA (dihydroxyphenylalanine)
  DTPA (diethylenetriaminepentaacetic acid)

imaging agent *(cont.)*
  Duografin
  Dy-DTPA-BMA
  dysprosium HP-DO3A
  Echogen or EchoGen ultrasound
  Echovist
  EDTMP
  etanidazole
  Ethiodol
  Ethodian (iophendylate)
  Evans blue
  exametazime
  F (fluorine)
  FCR 9501HQ
  Fe TPPS4
  Fe-EHPG chelate
  Feridex
  ferric ammonium citrate
  ferric ammonium citrate-cellulose paste
  ferric chloride
  ferrioxamine methanesulfonate
  Ferrixan
  ferromagnetic
  ferumoxsil
  5-chlorodeoxycytidine
  5-iodoacetamidofluorescein
  5-iodo-2-deoxyuridine
  fludeoxyglucose ($^{18}$F)
  fluorine (F)
  $^{18}$F estradiol (FES)
  $^{18}$F fludeoxyglucose ($^{18}$FDG)
  $^{18}$F fluoro-DOPA (6FD)
  $^{18}$F fluorodeoxyglucose (FDG)
  $^{18}$F fluoroisonidazole
  $^{18}$F fluorotamoxifen
  $^{18}$F-labeled HFA-134a
  $^{18}$F-labeled polyfluorinated ethyl
  $^{18}$F L-DOPA
  $^{18}$F N-methylspiperone
  $^{18}$F spiperone

imaging agent *(cont.)*
   fluorocarbon-based ultrasound
   fluorodeoxyglucose (FDG)
   4-azido-2([$^{14}$C]-methylamino)
      trifluorobenzonitrile
   furosemide
   Ga (gallium)
   gadobenate dimeglumine
   gadobenic acid
   gadobutrol
   gadodiamide
   gadolinium (Gd)
      $^{153}$Gd (gadolinium-153)
      Gd-BOPT (benzyloxypropionic-
         tetraacetate)
      Gd-BOPTA/Dimeg
      Gd-DOTA
      Gd-DTPA (diethylenetriamine-
         pentaacetic acid)
      Gd-DTPA/Dimeg
      Gd-DTPA-labeled albumin
      Gd-DTPA-labeled dextran
      Gd-DPTA PGTM
      Gd-DTPA with mannitol
      Gd-EOB-DTPA
      Gd-gadopentetate dimeglumine
      Gd-HIDA chelate
      Gd-Hp-DO3A
   gadolinium oxide contrast medium
   gadoteridol
   gadoversetamide
   gallium (Ga)
      $^{67}$Ga bone scan
      $^{67}$Ga citrate scan
      $^{68}$Ga-EDTA
   Gastrografin (meglumine
      diatrizoate)
   GastroMark oral
   Gastrovist
   Gd (gadolinium)

imaging agent *(cont.)*
   glucagon
   Glucarate $^{99m}$Tc hot spot
   gold-195m
   H$_2$ $^{15}$O (water O-15) radioactive
   halistatin-1 (H-1)
   hand-agitated
   H-benzapine
   Hedspa
   Hexabrix
   high-density barium
   high osmolar
   Hippuran
   Hipputope
   holmium (Ho)
   holmium-1-66-labeled tetraazacy-
      clododecane tetramethylene
      hybrid
   H-1 (halistatin-1)
   hot spot
   human serum-ABGd
   human serum-albumin
   hydrogen peroxide
   hyoscine butylbromide
   hybrid MRI
   hyoscine butylbromide
   Hypaque
   Hypaque-Cysto
   Hypaque-50
   Hypaque-M
   Hypaque Meglumine
   Hypaque-76
   Hypaque Sodium
   hyperpolarized He-3
   hyperpolarized $^{129}$Xe
   I (iodine)
   IBZP (chloro-hydroxy-iodophenyl-
      methyl-tetrahydro-H-benzapine)
   Ig2b kappa monoclonal antibody
   Imagent GI
   Imagopaque

**imaging agent**

imaging agent *(cont.)*
  imidoacetic acid
  immunoglobuin G ($^{111}$I-IgG)
  ImmuRAID (CEA Tc99m) antibody
  Immurait (IgG 2A monoclonal
    antibody)
  In (indium)
  Indiclor
  indium (In)
    $^{111}$In altumomab pentetate
      monoclonal antibody
    $^{111}$In antimyosin antibody
    $^{111}$In DTPA (diethylenetriamine
      pentaacetic acid)
    $^{111}$In-Fab-DTPA
    $^{111}$In-IgG
    $^{111}$In imciromab pentetate
    $^{111}$In-labeled antimyosin anti-
      body
    $^{111}$In-labeled human nonspecific
      immunoglobulin G
    $^{111}$In-labeled leukocyte bone
    $^{111}$In-labeled white blood cell
    $^{111}$In murine anti-CEA mono-
      clonal antibody type ZCE 025
    $^{111}$In murine monoclonal anti-
      body Fab to myosin
    $^{111}$In pentetreotide (OctreoScan)
    $^{111}$In satumomab pendetide
    $^{111}$In scintigraphy
    $^{111}$In white blood cell imaging
  indocyanine green
  Intropaque
  iobenzamic acid
  iobitridol
  iocarmic acid
  iocetamic acid
  iodamine meglumine
  iodinated
  iodinated $^{131}$I human serum albumin
  iodinated $^{125}$I radioactive

imaging agent *(cont.)*
  iodine (I)
    $^{123}$I ABZM
    $^{125}$I brachytherapy
    $^{123}$I BMIPP SPECT
    $^{125}$I fibrinogen scan
    $^{123}$I heptadecanoic acid
    $^{131}$I-Hippuran
    $^{123}$I IBZM
    $^{123}$I IBZP
    $^{192}$I high-dose-rate remote
      afterloader
    $^{123}$I IMP (iodomethamphetam-
      mine)
    $^{125}$I interstitial radiation
      implant
    $^{131}$I iodocholesterol
    $^{125}$I iodopyracet
    $^{131}$I iodopyracet
    $^{131}$I iofendylate
    $^{123}$I iofetamine HCl
    $^{123}$I IPPA (pentylpentadecanoic
      acid)
    $^{131}$I-labeled anti-CEA MoAb
      (CC49) and IFN-alpha
    $^{131}$I-labeled human MoAb
    $^{131}$I labeled monoclonal Fab
      fragment directed against a
      tumor antigen
    $^{131}$I-MIBG
  iodipamide meglumine
  iodized oil
  Iodo-gen
  iodohippurate sodium
  iodomethamate sodium
  iodo-phenylated chelates
  iodophthalein sodium
  Iodotope
  iodoxamate meglumine
  iodoxamic acid
  iohexol
  ionic

**imaging agent**

imaging agent *(cont.)*
ionic paramagnetic
iopamidol
Iopamiron 310; 370
iopanoic acid
iopentol
iopentol nonionic
iophendylate
iopydol
iopydone
iosefamic acid
iotetric acid
iothalamate
iothalamate meglumine
iothalamate sodium
iothalmic acid
iotrol
iotroxic acid
ioversol
ioxaglate meglumine
ioxaglate sodium
ioxilan with iohexol
ipodate
ipodate calcium
ipodate sodium
Ir (iridium)
Iriditope radioactive
iridium (Ir)
$^{192}$Ir (iridium-192)
isoflurane
Isopaque
Isovue nonionic
Isovue-128; 200; 300; 370
Isovue-M 200; 300
K (potassium)
K4-81
kinase C antiglioma monoclonal antibody
Kinevac
Kontrast U
krypton-81m ($^{81m}$Kr) radioactive
LeukaScan

imaging agent *(cont.)*
Levovist
Lipiodol
Lipiodol myelographic
lipophilic
Liquipake
L-methyl $^{11}$C-methionine
L-[1-$^{11}$C] tyrosine
long-scale
low osmolality
low-osmolar
lymphangiographic
L-tyrosine ($^{11}$C)
Lymphazurin (isosulfan blue)
MAA (macroaggregated albumin)
macromolecular
Macrotec
magnetite albumin
Magnevist
Mallinckrodt
mangafodipir trisodium
manganese (Mn)
    MnCl (manganese chloride)
    Mn DPDP (dipyridoxal diphosphate) chelate
    MnPcS4
    Mn-SOD
    Mn TPPS4
mannitol and saline 1:1 solution
MD-50; MD-60; MD-76
MD-Gastroview
MDP
meglumine
meglumine diatrizoate
meglumine iodipamide
meglumine iotroxate
meso-HMPAO
metabolic 8-hydroxyquinolyl-glucuronide
metaiodobenzylguanidine (MIBG)
Metastron
methiodal sodium

**imaging agent**

imaging agent *(cont.)*
methoxy-poly (ethylene glycol)-poly-L-lysine-DTPA
methyl methacrylate
metrizamide
metrizoate
metrizoate sodium
metrizoic acid
MIBG (metaiodobenzylguanidine)
MIBI
microbubble contrast
mineral oil
MMCM (macromolecular)
Mn (manganese)
monoclonal (MOAB, MoAb) antibody
monoclonal antibody 7E3
monoclonal antibody B72.3 labeled with indium
MS-325
myelographic
Myoscint
Myoview
N (nitrogen)
$^{13}$N (nitrogen-13 ammonia)
$^{59}$NP (nifurpipone-59)
N-butyl cyanoacrylate
naloxone
nanoparticulate
NCL-Arp monoclonal antibody
NCL-ER-LHZ monoclonal antibody
negative contrast
nephrotropic MR imaging contrast
Neurolite
neurotropic
nicotinamide
nimodipine
Niopam
nitrogen-13 ammonia ($^{13}$N)
nitrous oxide

imaging agent *(cont.)*
no-carrier-added $^{18}$F
nonionic
nonionic contrast
nonionic paramagnetic contrast
nonsteroidal antiphlogistics
normal human serum albumin
Novopaque
$^{59}$NP (iodomethylnorcholesterol)
Nycomed
O (oxygen)
OctreoScan
Octreotide
oil emulsion
OKT3 monoclonal antibody
olsalazine
Omnipaque
Omnipaque (nonionic)
Omniscan
OncoScint
OncoScint breast
OncoScint CR/OV
OncoScint CR103
OncoScint CR372
OncoScint OV103
OncoScint PR356
OncoScint-NSC
OncoSpect
OncoTrac
Optiray
Optiray 320
Optiray nonionic
Orabilix sodium
Oragrafin
Oragrafin Calcium
Oragrafin Sodium
oral
oral contrast
Oralex ultrasound
Oxilan (ioxilan)

**imaging agent**

imaging agent *(cont.)*
  oxygen (O)
    inhaled (MR contrast)
    $^{15}$O (oxygen-15)
    $^{15}$O carbon dioxide (inhaled)
    $^{15}$O carbon monoxide
    $^{15}$O oxygen
    $^{15}$O labeled water
    $^{17}$O NMR spectroscopy
  P (phosphorus)
  palladium (Pd)
    $^{103}$Pd radioactive
  Pantopaque
  paramagnetic
  paramagnetic Cr-labeled red blood cells
  $^{212}$Pb-labeled monoclonal antibody
  pentagastrin
  pentavalent DMSA
  pentetreotide $^{111}$I
  Pentreotide
  peppermint oil (with barium enema)
  peptide
  Perchloracap
  perflubron
  perfluoro-1H,-1H-neopentyl
  perfluorocarbon
  perfluorocarbon $^{19}$F
  perfluoroctylbromide (PFOB)
  perfluoro-1H,-1H-neopentyl
  pertechnetate sodium
  phenobarbital
  Phentetiothalein
  phosphoric acid
  phosphorus (P)
    $^{32}$P chromic phosphate
    $^{32}$P sodium phosphate
  PMT (pyridoxyl-5-methyl tryptophan)
  polygelin colloid

imaging agent *(cont.)*
  potassium (K)
    $^{43}$K (potassium-43)
    $^{81}$Kr-m (krypton-81m) radioactive
  Priodax
  ProHance (gadoteridol) nonionic gadolinium
  propyliodone
  Prostascint diagnostic
  Prostascint monoclonal antibody
  P623-Gd (gadolinium)
  pSV-b-Gal plasmid
  QW 3600
  Racobalamin-57 radioactive agent
  radioactive iodinated serum albumin (RISA)
  radioactive isotope
  radiolabeled MoAb
  radiolabeled peptide alpha-M2
  radiopaque
  Rb (rubidium)
    $^{82}$Rb-based cardiac
  Re (rhenium)
  Reno-M-Dip
  Reno-M-30
  Reno-M-60
  Renografin
  Renografin-60
  Renografin-76 microbubbles
  Reno-M
  Reno-M-Dip
  Renotec
  Renovist
  Renovist II
  Renovue-Dip
  Renovue-65
  residual
  reticuloendothelial
  rhenium (Re)
    $^{186}$Re hydroxyethylidene diphosphate (HEDP)

imaging agent *(cont.)*
RIGScan CR49
Robengatope radioactive agent
rose bengal sodium $^{131}I$ radioactive biliary agent
rubidium chloride ($^{82}Rb$)
$^{82}Rb$ (rubidium-82)
$^{86}Rb$ (rubidium-86)
$^{86}Rb$-35S-33P
Rubratope-57 radioactive agent
Salpix
samarium (Sm)
$^{153}Sm$ ethylene diamine tetramethylene phosphoric acid
satumomab pendetide (OncaScint CR/OV)
selenium (Se)
$^{75}Se$ (selenium-75)
sestamibi
Sethotope radioactive
7E3 monoclonal antiplatelet antibody
7-methoxy $^{11}C$ methoxystaurosporine
SHU 454 (Echovist)
SHU 508A (Levovist)
Sinografin
Skiodan
Sm (samarium)
SmartPrep
sodium bicarbonate solution
sodium chloride 0.9%
sodium diatrizoate
sodium diatrizoate with Menoquinon
sodium iodide
sodium iodide ring
sodium iodipamide
sodium iodohippurate
sodium iodomethamate
sodium iothalamate

imaging agent *(cont.)*
sodium ipodate
sodium methiodal
sodium pertechnetate Tc99m
sodium thorium tartrate
sodium tyropanoate
Solu-Biloptin
Somatostatin
sonicated
sonicated meglumine sodium
sonicated Renografin-76
sorbitol 70%
SPIO (superparamagnetic iron oxide)
spontaneous echo
SPP (superparamagnetic particle)
sprodiamide
Sr (strontium)
Sterling
strontium (Sr)
$^{82}Sr$ (strontium-82)
$^{85}Sr$ (strontium-85)
$^{89}Sr$ (strontium-89)
sucrose polyester
sulfobromophthalein (BSP)
sulfur colloid labeled with Tc 99m
superparamagnetic iron oxide (SPIO)
suppo-cire C
tantalum (Ta)
$^{183}Ta$
Tc (technetium)
TcHIDA (technetium HIDA)
Tc $O_4$
teboroxime
Techneplex
TechneScan MAG3 ($^{99m}Tc$ mertiatide) renal diagnostic
TechneScan Q-12
technetated aggregated human albumin

**imaging agent**

imaging agent *(cont.)*
   technetium (Tc, $^{99m}$Tc)
      $^{99m}$Tc albumin
      $^{99m}$Tc albumin aggregated
      $^{99m}$Tc albumin colloid
      $^{99m}$Tc albumin microaggregated
      $^{99m}$Tc albumin microspheres
      $^{99m}$Tc anti-granulocyte monoclonal murine antibody Fab fragments
      $^{99m}$Tc antimelanoma murine monoclonal antibody
      $^{99m}$Tc antimony-trisulfide colloid
      $^{99m}$Tc biciromab
      $^{99m}$Tc bicisate (Neurolite)
      $^{99m}$Tc BIDA
      $^{99m}$Tc colloid
      $^{99m}$Tc DIEDA
      $^{99m}$Tc dimercaptosuccinic acid
      $^{99m}$Tc DISIDA
      $^{99m}$Tc disofenin
      $^{99m}$Tc DMSA
      $^{99m}$Tc DTPA
      $^{99m}$Tc DTPA aerosol
      $^{99m}$Tc DTPA-galactosyl-human serum-albumin
      $^{99m}$Tc ECD
      $^{99m}$Tc etidronate
      $^{99m}$Tc exametazine
      $^{99m}$Tc Fab fragment of anti-CEA antibody IMMU-4
      $^{99m}$Tc ferpentetate
      $^{99m}$Tc furifosmin
      $^{99m}$Tc GH (glucoheptonate)
      $^{99m}$Tc GHP
      $^{99m}$Tc Glucarate hot spot
      $^{99m}$Tc gluceptate
      $^{99m}$Tc GSA
      $^{99m}$Tc HDP
      $^{99m}$Tc HIDA
      $^{99m}$Tc HMPAO (hexamethylpropylamine oxime)

imaging agent *(cont.)*
   technetium *(cont.)*
      $^{99m}$Tc human serum albumin
      $^{99m}$Tc IDA (iminodiacetic acid)
      $^{99m}$Tc IMMU-4 monoclonal antibody
      $^{99m}$Tc iron-ascobate-DTPA
      $^{99m}$Tc labeled A.C. (albumin colloid)
      $^{99m}$Tc labeled anti-alpha-fetoprotein
      $^{99m}$Tc labeled anti-CEA MoAb
      $^{99m}$Tc labeled antifibrin DD-3B6/22 Fab monoclonal antibody fragments
      $^{99m}$Tc labeled antigranulocyte antibodies
      $^{99m}$Tc labeled fibrinogen
      $^{99m}$Tc labeled red blood cells
      $^{99m}$Tc labeled stannous methylene diphosphonate
      $^{99m}$Tc lidofenin
      $^{99m}$Tc MAA (macroaggregated albumin)
      $^{99m}$Tc MAG3 (mercaptoacetyltriglycerine)
      $^{99m}$Tc MDP
      $^{99m}$Tc mebrofenin
      $^{99m}$Tc medronate
      $^{99m}$Tc medronate disodium
      $^{99m}$Tc mertiatide
      $^{99m}$Tc MIBI uptake
      $^{99m}$Tc MISO
      $^{99m}$Tc murine monoclonal antibody IgG2a to B cell
      $^{99m}$Tc murine monoclonal antibody to human alpha-fetoprotein
      $^{99m}$Tc murine monoclonal antibody to human chorionic gonadotropin
      $^{99m}$Tc oxidronate

imaging agent *(cont.)*
  technetium
    $^{99m}$Tc pentetate sodium
    $^{99m}$Tc pentetate calcium trisodium
    $^{99m}$Tc pentetic acid
    $^{99m}$Tc PIPIDA
    $^{99m}$Tc PMT
    $^{99m}$Tc polyphosphate
    $^{99m}$Tc PYP (pyrophosphate)
    $^{99m}$Tc RBC (red blood cells)
    $^{99m}$Tc SC (sulfur colloid)
    $^{99m}$Tc sestamibi
    $^{99m}$Tc siboroxime
    $^{99m}$Tc sodium
    $^{99m}$Tc sodium gluceptate
    $^{99m}$Tc sodium pertechnetate
    $^{99m}$Tc SPP (stannous pyrophosphate)
    $^{99m}$Tc succimer
    $^{99m}$Tc sulfur colloid
    $^{99m}$Tc sulfur microcolloid
    $^{99m}$Tc teboroxime
    $^{99m}$Tc tetrofosmin
    $^{99m}$Tc tin-pyrophosphate
    $^{99m}$Tc triisocyanide
    $^{99m}$Tc trimetaphosphates
  technetium antimony trisulfide colloid
  technetium bound to DTPA
  technetium bound to serum albumin
  technetium bound to sulfur colloid
  technetium ethylene cysteine diethylester
  technetium pertechnetate sodium
  technetium-tagged RBCs
  Telepaque
  Tesuloid
  thallium (Tl)
    $^{201}$Tl (thallium-201)
  thallous chloride

imaging agent *(cont.)*
  TheraSeed (palladium 103) active isotope in titanium capsule
  Thixokon
  thorium dioxide
  Thorotrast
  ThromboScan
  tissue
  Tl (thallium)
  TmDOTP-5
  Tomocat
  triisocyanide $^{99m}$Tc
  triiodinated
  Tru-Scint AD
  TSPP (technetium stannous pyrophosphate)
  tyropanoate
  tyropanoate sodium
  Tyropaque
  U (uranium)
    $^{235}$U (uranium-235)
  ultrasmall particle superparamagnetic iron oxide
  Ultravist (iopromide)
  uniphasic
  Urografin
  Urografin-76
  Urografin 290
  urokinase
  Urovist Cysto
  Urovist Meglumine
  Urovist Sodium
  USPIO (ultrasmall superparamagnetic iron oxide)
  Vascoray
  visualization of
  water-soluble
  water-soluble iodinated
  water-soluble nonionic positive
  whole blood monoclonal antibody
  Xe (xenon)

imaging agent *(cont.)*
  xenon (Xe)
    $^{127}$Xe (xenon-127)
    $^{133}$Xe (xenon-133)
  xylenol orange
  ZK44012
imaging anatomic correlation
imaging-based stereotaxis in tumor neurosurgery
imaging-directed 3D volumetric information on intracranial lesion
imaging pathologic correlation
imaging plane
imaging renogram
imaging system (see *scanner*)
imaging workstation
Imagopaque contrast media
Imatron C-100 ultrafast CT scanner
Imatron C-100 scanner
Imatron C-100XL CT Scanner
Imatron C-150L EBCT scanner
Imatron Fastrac C-100 cine x-ray CT scanner
Imatron Ultrafast CT scanner
imbalance of phase or gain artifact
imbricate
imbrication
  capsular
  facetal
IMED intravenous infusion device
IMI (inferior myocardial infarction)
imidoacetic acid radioactive agent
immediate intervention
immediate post-ictal period
immersion B-scan ultrasound
imminent death
imminent demise
immobilization
immobilized
immune electron microscopy
immuno-lymphoscintigraphy
immunoblastic

immunocompetency
immunocompromised patient
immunoelectrophoresis
Immunomedics system
immunoreactive parathyroid hormone (iPTH)
immunoscintigraphy
immunoscintimetry
ImmuRAID (CEA-Tc 99m) antibody imaging agent
Immurait (IgG 2A monoclonal antibody)
IMPA cephalometric measurement
IMP SPECT scan
impacted fracture
impacted subcapital fracture
impacted urethral stones
impacted valgus fracture
impaction
  fecal
  stone
impaired renal function
impaired venous return
impaired ventilation-perfusion
impairment
  circulatory
  functional
  inspiratory muscle function
  motor
  renal function
  sensory
ImpaxPACS system
impedance phlebography
impedance plethysmography (IPG)
impede filling
impediment
impending myocardial infarction
imperfect regeneration
imperforate aneurysm
imperforate anus
impinge
impinged upon

impingement
  dural
  lateral
  ligamentous (ankle)
  nerve root
  talar
  talofibular
impingement exostosis
impingement syndrome
impinging
implant (also prosthesis)
  biodegradable
  cochlear
  double-lumen breast
  double-stem silicone
  double-stem silicone lesser MP
  epidural
  hinged
  hydroxyapatite
  interstitial
  iodine I-125 interstitial radiation
  iridium-192 endobronchial
  iridium-192 wire
  mammary
  methyl methacrylate beads
  open cord tendon
  otologic
  palladium ($^{103}$Pd) prostate
  permanent interstitial
  PMMA (poly-methyl methacrylate)
  synthetic bone
  prostate
  retropectoral mammary
  silicone
  silicone elastomer rubber ball
  silicone wrist
  single-lumen breast
  temporary interstitial
  total knee
  VDS (ventral derotating spinal)
implantable bone growth stimulator, Osteo Stim

implantation of radioactive sources
implanted imaging-opaque marker
implanted pacemaker
importance, prognostic
impression
  cardiac (on liver)
  colic
  digastric
  duodenal
  esophageal
  gastric
  liver
  renal
  suprarenal
improved Chen-Smith (ICS) coder
improvement, interval
impulse, apical
inactive mode
inadequate cardiac output
inadequate runoff
inadequate visualization
inanition
incarcerated hernia
incarceration
incarial bone
"incidentaloma" (on sonography)
incisional hernia
incisural sclerosis
inciting event
inciting factors
inclination of treadmill
inclinometer
incoherence, magnetic resonance spin
incompetence
  aortic
  aortic valve
  chronotropic
  communicating vein
  deep venous
  mitral valve
  postphlebitic
  pulmonary

incompetence *(cont.)*
  sphincter
  traumatic tricuspid
  tricuspid valve
  valve
  valvular
incompetent valve
incomplete closure
incomplete dislocation
incomplete fracture of bone
incomplete Kartagener syndrome
incomplete pulmonary fissure
incomplete stroke
incongruity, angle of
incontinence
incorporation of new-bone formation
increased activity, surrounding halo of
increased AP (anterior/posterior) diameter of chest
increased attenuation
increased basilar cisterns
increased central venous pressure
increased cerebral vascular resistance
increased density
increased echo signal on ultrasound
increased extracellular fluid volume
increased interstitial fluid
increased interstitial markings
increased intracranial pressure
increased intrapericardial pressure
increased left ventricular ejection time
increased markings
increased myocardial oxygen requirements
increased outflow resistance
increased peripheral resistance
increased prominence of pulmonary vessels
increased pulmonary arterial pressure
increased pulmonary obstruction
increased pulmonary vascular markings
increased pulmonary vascular resistance
increased tracer uptake
increased ventricular afterload
increases, incremental
increment of perfusion
incremental doses
incremental increases
incremental pacing
incremental risk factors
increments in luminal diameter
incus bone
indecisiveness
indentation of myelography dye with incomplete tumors
indented fracture of skull
indeterminate age
index (pl. indexes, indices)
  angiographic muscle mass
  ankle–arm
  ankle–brachial (ABI)
  apnea–hypopnea (AHI)
  arch
  arch length
  Ashman
  Benink tarsal
  body mass
  bromodeoxyuridine labeling
  cardiac (CI)
  cardiothoracic
  Chippaux-Smirak arch
  contractile work
  contractility
  coronary stenosis (CSI)
  coronary vascular resistance (CVRI)
  Detsky modified cardiac risk
  diastolic left ventricular
  diastolic pressure-time (DPTI)
  dye fluorescence (DFI)
  eccentricity
  effective pulmonic

index *(cont.)*
  ejection phase
  ellipticity
  end-diastolic volume (EDVI)
  end-systolic stress wall (ESWI)
  end-systolic volume (ESVI)
  exercise
  fetal-pelvic
  Fick cardiac
  Fourier pulsatility
  Fourmentin thoracic
  Gosling pulsatility
  hemodynamic
  ischemic
  left ventricular end-diastolic
    volume (LVEDI)
  left ventricular end-systolic
    volume (LVESVI)
  left ventricular fractional
    shortening
  left ventricular mass (LVMI)
  left ventricular stroke volume
  left ventricular stroke work
  maturation
  mean ankle-brachial systolic
    pressure
  mean wall motion score
  mitral flow velocity
  myocardial infarction recovery
    (MIRI)
  myocardial jeopardy
  myocardial $O_2$ demand
  Nakata
  $O_2$ consumption
  penile brachial pressure (PBPI)
  pipe stemming of ankle-brachial
  postexercise (PEI)
  poststress ankle/arm Doppler
  predicted cardiac
  profundal popliteal collateral
  pulmonary arterial resistance
  pulmonary blood volume (PBVI)

index *(cont.)*
  pulmonic output
  pulsatility
  QOL (quality of life)
  regurgitant
  resistive
  resting ankle/arm Doppler
  resting ankle-arm pressure
    (RAAPI)
  right and left ankle
  runoff resistance
  Singh osteoporosis
  stroke (SI)
  stroke volume (SVI)
  stroke work (SWI)
  systemic arteriolar resistance
  systemic output
  systolic pressure-time
  systolic toe/brachial
  talocalcaneal
  tension-time (TTI)
  thoracic
  truncated arch
  valgus
  venous distensibility (VDI)
  wall motion score
  water perfusable tissue
  Wood units
indicator dilution curve
indicator-dilution method for cardiac
  output measurement
indicator dilution therapy
indicator fractionation principle
indices (pl. of index)
Indiclor imaging agent
indigestion
indirect blood supply
indirect computed tomography
indirect fracture
indirect hernia
indirect MR arthrography

indium (In)
   $^{111}$In (indium-111, In-111)
   $^{111}$In antimyosin antibody
   $^{111}$In DTPA (diethylenetriamine pentaacetic acid)
   $^{111}$In-Fab-DTPA
   $^{111}$In-IgG
   $^{111}$In imciromab pentetate
   $^{111}$In-labeled antimyosin antibody
   $^{111}$In-labeled human nonspecific immunoglobulin G
   $^{111}$In-labeled leukocyte bone
   $^{111}$In-labeled white blood cell
   $^{111}$In murine monoclonal antibody Fab to myosin
   $^{111}$In pentetreotide (OctreoScan)
   $^{111}$In scintigraphy
   $^{111}$In white blood cell imaging
indocyanine dilution curve
indocyanine green angiography
indocyanine green dye for detection of intracardial shunt
indocyanine green dye method for cardiac output measurement
indolent radiation-induced rectal ulcer
indolent ulcer
induced thrombosis of aortic aneurysm
inducibility basal state
inducible
inductance
induction anesthesia
indurated mass
indurated tissue
induration
indurative pleurisy
indwelling catheter
indwelling Foley catheter
indwelling nonvascular shunt
indwelling stent
inelastic collision

inelastic pericardium
inequality, limb-length
inexorable progression
in extremis
Inf (infarction)
infant, profoundly obtunded
infantile hydrocephalus
infantile lobar emphysema
infantile-onset spinocerebellar ataxia
infantile pneumonia
infantile syndrome
infantile thoracic dystrophy
infarct (see *infarction*)
infarcted heart muscle
infarcted lung segment
infarct expansion
infarct size limitation
infarction (also infarct)
   acute myocardial (AMI)
   age indeterminate
   anemic
   anterior communicating artery distribution
   anterior myocardial (AMI)
   anterior-wall myocardial
   anteroinferior myocardial
   anterolateral myocardial
   anteroseptal myocardial
   apical myocardial
   arrhythmic myocardial
   atherothrombotic
   atherothrombotic brain
   atrial
   bicerebral
   bland
   bone
   brain stem
   capsular
   capsulocaudate
   capsuloputaminal
   capsuloputaminocaudate
   cardiac

**infarction**

infarction (cont.)
  cerebellar
  cerebral
  cerebral artery
  concomitant
  cortical
  diaphragmatic myocardial (DMI)
  dominant-hemisphere
  embolic
  evolving myocardial
  extensive anterior myocardial
  focal skin
  frontal lobe
  full-thickness
  gyral
  healing
  hemispheric
  hemorrhagic
  high lateral myocardial
  hippocampal
  hyperacute myocardial
  impending
  impending myocardial
  inferior myocardial (IMI)
  inferolateral myocardial
  inferoposterolateral myocardial
  intestinal
  intraoperative myocardial
  ischemic brain stem
  lacunar brain
  lateral myocardial
  livedo reticularis, digital
  medullary
  mesencephalic
  mesenteric
  multifocal
  multiple cortical
  myocardial (MI)
  nonarrhythmic myocardial
  nonembolic
  nonfatal myocardial

infarction (cont.)
  non-Q wave myocardial
  nonseptic embolic brain
  nontransmural myocardial
  occipital lobe
  old myocardial
  papillary muscle
  paramedian
  parenchymal
  pituitary
  pontine
  posterior cerebral territory
  posterior myocardial
  posteroinferior myocardial
  postmyocardial
  pulmonary
  Q wave myocardial
  red
  recent myocardial
  renal
  right ventricular
  segmental bowel
  septal myocardial
  septic pulmonary
  severe
  silent myocardial
  sinoatrial node
  spinal cord
  subacute myocardial
  subcortical
  subendocardial (SEI)
  subendocardial myocardial
  temporal lobe
  testicular
  thalamic
  thrombotic
  transmural myocardial
  uninfected
  ventral pontine
  watershed
  white matter

infarct avid imaging (hot spot scan, technetium pyrophosphate scan)
infarctoid cardiomyopathy
infected thrombosed graft
infectious disease
infective thrombosis (or thrombus)
inferior basal segment
inferior border
inferior cerebellar peduncle
inferior dorsal radioulnar ligament
inferior epigastric artery
inferior facet
inferior frontal gyrus
inferior ligaments
inferior lobe of lung
inferior margin of superior rib
inferior mediastinum
inferior mesenteric artery
inferior parietal lobule
inferior pubic ramus (pl. rami)
inferior pulmonary ligament
inferior pulmonary vein
inferior quadriceps retinaculum
inferior temporal gyrus
inferior temporal lobule
inferior thyroid vein
inferior tip of scapula
inferior vena cava (IVC) orifice
inferior vena cava syndrome
inferior vena caval filter
inferior wall akinesis
inferior wall hypokinesis
inferior wall MI (myocardial infarction)
inferiormost
inferoapical wall
inferobasal
inferolateral displacement of apical beat
inferolateral wall myocardial infarction
inferolaterally
inferomedial
inferomedially
inferoposterior wall myocardial infarction
inferoposterolateral
INFH (ischemic necrosis of femoral head)
infiltrate (also infiltration)
 active
 aggressive interstitial
 aggressive perivascular
 alveolar
 apical
 basilar
 basilar zone
 bilateral interstitial pulmonary
 bilateral upper lobe cavitary
 bronchocentric inflammatory
 butterfly pattern of
 calcareous
 calcium
 cavitary
 circumscribed
 confluent
 consolidated
 diffuse
 diffuse aggressive polymorphous
 diffuse alveolar interstitial
 diffuse bilateral alveolar
 diffuse interstitial
 diffuse perivascular
 diffuse reticulonodular
 eosinophilic
 epituberculous
 fatty
 fibronodular
 fluffy
 focal interstitial
 focal perivascular
 ground glass
 hazy

infiltrate • inflammation

infiltrate *(cont.)*
  interstitial
  interstitial nonlobar
  invasive angiomatous interstitial
  leukemia
  linear
  lung
  lung base
  lymphocytic
  massive
  meningeal
  micronodular
  migratory
  mononuclear
  multifocal aggressive
  mural
  parasitic
  patchy
  peribronchial
  perihilar
  peripheral
  perivascular
  plasmacytic
  pneumonic
  pulmonary
  pulmonary eosinophilic
  pulmonary parenchymal
  pulmonic
  punctate
  reticular
  reticulonodular
  retrocardiac
  strandy
  sulfasalazine-induced pulmonary
  transient
  tuberculous
infiltration (see *infiltrate*)
infiltration pattern
infinitesimal Z spectrum
Infiniti catheter from Cordis
inflamed edematous medium-sized
  bronchi
inflamed pleura
inflammation
  acute phase of
  adhesive
  alveolar septal
  atrophic
  bursal
  calcaneal bursa
  cardiac muscle
  cirrhotic
  diffuse
  disseminated
  fibrosing
  fibrinous
  focal
  granulomatous (of bronchi)
  hyperplastic
  hypertrophic
  interstitial
  meningeal
  metastatic
  mucosal
  necrotic
  obliterative
  parenchymatous
  polyarticular symmetric
    tophaceous joint
  proliferative
  pseudomembranous
  sclerosing
  spleen
  subacute
  suppurative
  thyroid gland
  vein
inflammation causes
  burning
  crushing
  cutting
  foreign body
  fungus
  parasite
  radiation

inflammatory adhesions
inflammatory bowel disease (IBD)
inflammatory disease
inflammatory fracture
inflammatory lesion
inflammatory polypoid mass
inflammatory process
inflammatory reaction
inflammatory response syndrome
inflammatory response, whole body
inflate
inflation
  air
  balloon
  sequential balloon
  simultaneous balloon
inflow
  aortic
  blood
inflow cuff
inflow disease progression
inflow tract of left ventricle
influenza
information, hierarchical
infra-apical
infra-auricular
infracardiac type total anomalous venous return
infraclavicular pocket
infracolic midline
infracristal ventricular septal defect
infradiaphragmatic vein
infragastric
infragenicular popliteal artery
infragenicular position
infrageniculate artery
infraglenoid tuberosity
infragluteal crease
infrahepatic vena cava
infrainguinal bypass stenosis
infrainguinal revascularization
infrainguinal vein bypass graft

inframammary crease
inframammary syndrome
inframyocardial
infrapatellar contracture syndrome (IPCS)
infrapatellar fat pad
infrapopliteal artery occlusion
infrapopliteal vessel
infrapulmonary position
infrared imaging
infrared light-emitting diode
infrarenal abdominal aortic aneurysm
infrarenal aorta
infrarenal stenosis
infrascapular
infraspinous fossa
infrasternal angle
infratemporal fossa
infratentorial approach
infratentorial compartment
infratentorial Lindau tumor
infraumbilical mound
infravesical obstruction
infundibular atresia
infundibular chamber
infundibular pulmonary stenosis
infundibular septum
infundibular stalk
infundibular subpulmonic stenosis
infundibuloventricular crest
infundibulum
  bile duct
  cerebral
  gallbladder
  hypophysis
  os
  right ventricular
  tumor of
Infuse-a-port catheter
infusion line, peripheral intravenous
infusion transcatheter therapy

Ingram-Bachynski classification of
　hip fracture
ingrowth, bone
inguinal bulge
inguinal crease
inguinal floor
inguinal fold
inguinal hernia
inguinal ligament syndrome
inguinal node
inguinal region
inguinal ring
inguinal trigone
inhalation by slow inspiration
inhalation of krypton-77 to measure
　cerebral blood flow on PET scan
inhalation of radioactive xenon gas
inhalation pneumonia
inhalation study
inhalation technique
inhalation tuberculosis
inhaled oxygen brain MR contrast
　agent
inhaled radionuclide
inherently unstable condition
inhomogeneity correction
inhomogeneity, off-axis dose
inhomogeneous distribution
inhomogeneous echo pattern
inhomogeneous image
inhomogeneous tracer distribution
inion bump
initial delay in appearance time of
　contrast material
initial shock
initial staging evaluation
initiation
injection
　air
　barium (through colostomy)
　bolus
　contrast medium

injection *(cont.)*
　double
　hand (done by hand)
　intra-amniotic
　intra-arterial
　intramuscular (I.M., IM)
　intramuscular fetal
　intraperitoneal fetal
　intrathecal
　intravascular
　intravenous (I.V., IV)
　intravenous bolus
　intravenous fetal
　machine (done by machine)
　manual
　Omnipaque (iohexol) intrathecal
　opacifying
　percutaneous ethanol
　power
　rest
　sclerosing
　selective arterial
　serial
　straight AP pelvic
　venous
injection port
injection test for pneumoperitoneum
injector
　auto
　Hercules power
　Medrad power angiographic
　power
　pressure
　PulseSpray
injury (pl. injuries)
　acute stretch
　axial compression (of spine)
　ballistic
　barked
　bilateral incomplete ureteral
　blunt
　brachial plexus

**injury**

injury *(cont.)*
  burst
  cervical spine
  closed head (CHI)
  cocking
  compression flexion
  compression-plus-torque theory of cervical
  compressive hyperextension
  concomitant tracheal
  crush
  crushing
  decelerative
  degloving
  discoligamentous
  distraction hyperflexion
  Erb (to brachial plexus)
  Erb-Duchenne-Klumpke
  extension (of spine)
  extensive head
  flexion-distraction
  flexion-rotation
  forced flexion
  growth plate
  head (HI)
  high-caliber, low-velocity handgun
  hyperextension
  hyperflexion
  hyperflexion/hyperextension cervical
  hypertension
  hypoxic
  hypoxic/ischemic
  iatrogenic ureteral
  immunologic
  intercostal nerve
  intraperitoneal
  inversion
  ischemic
  Klumpke (to brachial plexus)
  lateral bending (of spine)
  Lisfranc

injury *(cont.)*
  low back
  matrix
  meniscal
  mild head
  motor vehicle (MVI)
  nerve
  obstetrical
  penetrating lung
  perinatal
  peripheral nerve
  physeal
  plexus
  postnatal
  prenatal
  pronation-external rotation (P-ER)
  pulmonary parenchymal
  radial vascular thermal
  radiation-induced skin
  rapid deceleration
  repetitive strain (RSI)
  repetitive stress (RSI)
  seat belt
  severe head
  skier's
  soft tissue
  softball sliding
  spinal cord (SCI)
  straddle
  strain-sprain
  subendocardial
  supination-outward rotation
  three-column (spinal column)
  through-and-through
  throwing-arm
  transcutaneous crush
  traumatic
  traumatic brain (TBI)
  traumatic head
  two-column
  ultrasonic assessment of
  vesical

injury *(cont.)*
   weight-bearing rotational
   whiplash
   windup
Injury Scale, Abbreviated
Injury Severity Score (ISS)
injury to nerve roots
inlay graft
inlet
   esophageal
   pelvic
   thoracic
inner adrenal cortex
inner stripe of Baillinger (in brain)
inner table
innermost intercostal muscles
Innervision MR scanner
innocuous
innominate (*not* innominant)
innominate aneurysm
innominate angiography
innominate artery buckling
innominate artery kinking
innominate artery stenosis
innominate bone
innominate vein
Innovator Holter system
inoperable brain tumor
inoperable disease
Inoue balloon catheter
in-phase GRE imaging
in-phase image
in-phase sequence
in-plane vessels
Inrad HiLiter ultrasound-enhanced
   stylet
insertion
   anomalous
   Bosworth bone peg
   ligamentous
   percutaneous (via femoral vein)
   percutaneous pin
   tendinous

insidious onset
insidious progression
in situ
in situ bypass
in situ grafting
in situ pinning
insonation, Doppler
insonifying wave field
inspiration, inhalation by slow
inspiration phase
inspiratory effort
inspiratory flow
inspiratory flow rates
inspiratory flow-volume, tidal
inspiratory increase in venous
   pressure
inspiratory phase
inspiratory reserve volume (IRV)
inspiratory retraction
inspiratory spasm
inspired air
inspissated mucus
inspissation of feces
instability
   anterolateral rotary knee
   articular
   atlantoaxial
   chronic functional
   dorsal intercalary segment (DISI)
   first ray
   hindfoot
   inversion
   joint
   lateral rotatory ankle
   ligamentous
   osseous
   postlaminectomy
   rotary
   rotary ankle
   rotational
   rotatory
   shoulder joint

**instability • integration**

instability *(cont.)*
  spinal
  subtalar
  truncal
  varus-valgus
  volarflexed intercalated segment (VISI)
instantaneous enhancement rate
instantaneous gradient
InstaScan scanner
in-stent balloon redilation
instillation, subarachnoid
insufficiency
  acute cerebrovascular
  acute coronary
  aortic (AI)
  aortic valve
  arterial
  autonomic
  basilar
  basilar artery
  brachial-basilar
  cardiac
  cardiopulmonary
  cerebrovascular
  chronic venous
  congenital pulmonary valve
  coronary
  gastric
  hepatic
  hypostatic pulmonary
  ileocecal
  mitral (MI)
  muscular
  myocardial (MI)
  nonocclusive mesenteric arterial
  nonrheumatic aortic
  parathyroid
  postirradiation vascular
  post-traumatic pulmonary
  pulmonary (PI)
  pulmonary arterial flow

insufficiency *(cont.)*
  pulmonary valve
  pyloric
  renal
  respiratory
  Sternberg myocardial
  thyroid
  transient ischemic carotid
  tricuspid (TI)
  uterine
  valvular
  valvular aortic
  velopharyngeal
  venous
  vertebrobasilar arterial
insufficiency fracture
insufflation
  air
  $CO_2$
  gas
  tubal
insular gyrus
insular lobe
insula, roof of
insular region of brain
insulative development
insulinoma
insult
  aortic
  bihemispheral
  cerebrovascular
  infectious
  mechanical (to spine)
  myocardial
  occlusive cerebrovascular
  toxic
intact valve cusp
intact ventricular septum
integral, Choquet fuzzy
integral dose
integrated bipolar sensing
integration, telecom

Integris 3000 scanner
Integris V3000 imager
integrity, spinal
integrity and alignment
Intel PC Link2 board
Intel Plink Ethernet card
intensified radiographic imaging system (IRIS)
intensifier, image
intensifying screen artifact
intensity
   angina with recent increase in
   beam
   CIDNP signal
   decreased
   equal in
   fat-signal
   low signal
   maximal
   radiation
   signal (SI)
   variable
intensity-modulated photon beams
intensity windowing
intensive care unit (ICU)
intentional reversible thrombosis
interactive electronic scalpel
interactive MR-guided biopsy
interactive visual approach
interarticular disk
interarticularis, pars
interatrial baffle
interatrial communication
interatrial groove
interatrial septal defect
interatrial septum, lipomatous hypertrophy of the
interatrial transposition of venous return
interbody fusion
interbronchial mass
intercalary defect

intercarpal articulation
intercarpal coalition
intercarpal joints
intercaudate distance
intercaval band
intercavernous anastomosis
intercellular adhesive molecule (ICAM-1)
intercellular edema
intercellular space
interchondral joint
interchordal space fenestration
interclavicular notch
intercollicular groove
intercom, noise reduction
intercomparison measurement technique
intercondylar eminence
intercondylar fossa
intercondylar fracture
intercondylar groove
intercondylar notch
intercondyloid eminence
intercondyloid fossa
intercondyloid notch
intercoronary anastomosis
intercoronary collateral flow
intercoronary steal syndrome
intercostal artery
intercostal muscle
intercostal nerve injury
intercostal retraction on inspiration
intercostal space (ICS)
intercostal vein
intercostal vessels
intercostobrachial nerve
intercristal diameter
interdigital clavus
interdigital ligament
interdigital neoplasm
interdigital neuroma
interdigitating coil stent

interdigitation of vastus lateralis with
 fascia
interface
 acetabular-prosthetic
 acoustic
 air
 air-tissue
 bone-implant
 bony
 catheter-skin
 DICOM
 fat-water
 joint
 media-adventitia
 muscle-fat
 socket/residuum
 socket-stump
interface spacing, multiple-beam
interference dissociation
interferometry, phase shifting
interfibrosis
interfraction interval
interfragmental compression
interfragmentary plate
intergluteal cleft
interhemispheric cyst
interhemispheric fissure
interictal PET FDG study
interictal phase
interictal SPECT study
interictal spiking
interlaminar
interleaved axial slabs
interleaved GRE sequence
interleaved imaging passes
interleaved inversion-readout segment
interlobar empyema
interlobar fissure
interlobar pleurisy
interlobar septum (pl. septa)
interlobular emphysema
interlobular pleurisy

interlobular septa thickening
interlobular vasculature
interlobular vessels
interlocking detachable coils
interloop abscess
intermaxillary spine
intermediate artery
intermediate bursa
intermediate coronary syndrome
intermediate cuneiform fracture-
 dislocation
intermediate images
intermediate signal mass
intermediate slices
intermediolateral gray column
intermesenteric abscess
intermetacarpal articulation
intermetatarsal angle (IMA)
intermetatarsal angle-reducing
 procedure
intermetatarsal joint (IM)
intermetatarsal ligament
intermetatarsal space
intermetatarsophalangeal bursa
intermittent diffuse esophageal spasm
intermittent occlusion
intermittent venous claudication
intermuscular septum
internal auditory meatus
internal caliber
internal capsule and basal ganglia
 tumor
internal capsule intracerebral hemorrhage
internal carotid artery (ICA)
internal clot
internal conjugate diameter
internal cyclotron target
internal derangement of knee (IDK)
internal disk herniation
internal echogenicity
internal-external drainage catheter

internal femoral rotation
internal iliac artery
internal intercostal muscles
internal intermuscular septum
internal jugular approach for cardiac
  catheterization
internal jugular bulb
internal jugular triangle
internal jugular vein
internal jugular venous cannula
internal mammary artery (IMA)
internal pudendal artery
internal retention mechanism
internal rotation in extension (IRE)
internal rotation in flexion (IRF)
internal snapping hip syndrome
internal thoracic artery
internal thoracic vein
internal tibial torsion (ITT)
internal tibiofibular torsion
internuclear distance
interopercular distances
interorbital distance
interosseous ligament
interosseous membrane
interosseous muscle groups of hand
interosseous nerve
interosseous space
interosseous talocalcaneal ligament
interparietal bone
interpedicular distance
interpediculate
interpeduncular cistern
interpeduncular notch
interpeduncular space
interperiosteal fracture
interphalangeal (IP)
interphalangeal dislocation
interphalangeal fusion
interphalangeal joint
interpleural space
interpolate cues

interpolation
  color space
  cubic convolution
  linear
  nearest neighbor
  prism
  trilinear
interpolation algorithm
interpolation kernel
Interpore bone replacement material
interposed colon segment
interposition graft
interposition, soft tissue
interpretive criteria
interpretive variability
interpulse time
interrenal stenosis
interrogation
  color-duplex
  pulse Doppler
  radiation
  transtelephonic ICD
interruption, aortic arch
intersection gap
intersegmental aberration
interseptal region
intersesamoid ligament
intersigmoid recess
interslice distance
interslice gap
interspace
  ballooning of vertebral
    disk
  vertebral disk
  wedging of vertebral
intersperse
intersphincteric abscess
interspinal ligament
interspinous distance
interspinous ligament
interspinous process
interspinous widening

interstices, bone
interstitial boost
interstitial brachytherapy
interstitial changes
interstitial diffuse pulmonary fibrosis
interstitial edema
interstitial emphysema
interstitial fibrosis
interstitial fluid
interstitial heat generating source
interstitial hyperthermia treatment
interstitial implant
  permanent
  temporary
interstitial infiltrate
  diffuse alveolar
  invasive angiomatous
interstitial insertion of temperature sensors
interstitial laser photocoagulation (ILP)
interstitial lung disease (ILD)
interstitial markings, increased
interstitial meniscal tear
interstitial nonlobar infiltrates
interstitial pneumonia air leak
interstitial prematurity fibrosis
interstitial probe
interstitial prominence
interstitial pulmonary edema
interstitial pulmonary fibrosis
interstitial radioactive colloid therapy
interstitial radioelement application, ultrasonic guidance for
interstitial radiotherapy
interstitial scarring
interstitial shadowing
interstitial space
interstitial template irradiation
interstitial thermoradiotherapy
interstitial tissues
intertarsal

interthalamic bridge
intertrabecular hemorrhage
intertrabecular soft tissue
intertrochanteric plate
intertubercular diameter
interval
  acromiohumeral (AHI)
  atlantoaxial
  atlantodens (ADI)
  supracricoid
interval change
interval development
interval improvement
interval intra-atrial conduction
interval progression
interval resolution
intervention
  immediate
  surgical
  therapeutic
interventional limb salvage
interventional neuroradiology
interventional procedure
interventional radiography
interventional radiology
interventricular (IV)
interventricular foramen
interventricular groove
interventricular septal defect
interventricular septum
interventricular sulcus, posterior
interventricular vein, posterior
intervertebral disk narrowing
intervertebral disk space
intervertebral foramen
intervertebral joint
intervertebral ligament
interzone
intestinal atresia
intestinal diverticulum
intestinal emphysema
intestinal follicle

intestinal hypoperistalsis syndrome
intestinal infantilism
intestinal malrotation
intestinal ureter, construction of
intestinal villous architecture
intestinal web
intestine
 blind
 coils of
 kink in
 large
 malrotation of
 small
"in the magnet" (in magnetic resonance imaging)
intima
 arterial
 diffuse thickening of arterial
 friable thickened degenerated
 hypertrophied
 tunica
intimal attachment of diseased vessel
intimal atherosclerotic disease
intimal debris
intimal dissection
intimal flap
intimal irregularity
intimal proliferation
intimal remodeling
intimal tear
intimal thickening
intimal-medial dissection
intimomedial thickness
in toto
intra-abdominal arterial bypass graft
intra-abdominal fat
intra-acetabular
intra-acinar pulmonary arteries
intra-alveolar fibrosis
intra-aneurysmal thrombus
intra-aortic balloon assist

intra-aortic balloon counterpulsation
intra-aortic balloon double-lumen catheter
intra-aortic balloon pump(ing) (IABP)
intra-arterial chemotherapy
intra-arterial digital subtraction angiography (IADSA)
intra-arterial DSA
intra-arterial filling defects
intra-arterial injection of water-soluble iodinated contrast agent
intra-arterial intracerebral thrombolysis
intra-arterially
intra-arterial superselective nimodipine
intra-arterial thrombosis
intra-arterial thrombus
intra-articular adhesion
intra-articular body
intra-articular calcaneal fracture
intra-articular fracture
intra-articular ligament
intra-articular loose body
intra-articular radiopharmaceutical therapy
intra-atrial baffle
intra-atrial filling defect
intra-atrial reentry
intra-atrial thrombi
intra-axial brain tumor
intra-axial cyst
intra-axial varix
intra-orbital air
intra-pixel sequential processing (IPSP)
intracanalicular
intracapsular fracture
intracardiac baffle
intracardiac calcium
intracardiac echocardiography (ICE)
intracardiac mass

intracardiac pressure in Doppler
  echocardiogram
intracardiac right-to-left shunt
intracardiac shunt(ing)
intracardiac thrombus
Intracath catheter
intracatheter
intracaval endovascular ultrasonography (ICEUS)
intracavitary afterloading applicators
intracavitary brachytherapy
intracavitary clot formation
intracavitary extension of tumor
intracavitary filling defect
intracavitary hyperthermia treatment
intracavitary prostate ultrasonography
intracavitary radiation source
intracavitary radioactive colloid therapy
intracavitary radioelement application
intracavitary radiotherapy
intracellular DNA double-strand
intracerebral hematoma
intracerebral hemorrhage
  basilar
  bulbar
  cerebellar
  cerebral
  cerebromeningeal
  cortical
  internal capsule
  intrapontine
  pontine
  subcortical
  ventricular
intracerebral lesion
intracerebral lymphoma
intrachondrial bone
intracompartmental ischemia and edema
intracondyloid
intracoronary imaging
intracoronary stent placement
intracoronary stenting
intracoronary ultrasound (ICUS)
intracortical osteogenic sarcoma
intracranial air
intracranial aneurysm
  arteriosclerotic
  congenital
  dissecting
  mycotic
  traumatic
intracranial berry aneurysm
intracranial calcification
intracranial circulation
intracranial cyst
intracranial electroencephalography
intracranial fat proplase
intracranial glioma
intracranial hemorrhage
intracranial imaging
intracranial malformation
intracranial mass
intracranial neoplasm
intracranial sinus thrombosis
intracranial tuberculoma
intracranial tumor
intracranial vascular lesion
intracranial vascular occlusion
intracranial vessel
intractable bleeding disorder
intractable heart failure
intractable ulcer
intradermal injection of Tc-HSA
intradiaphragmatic aortic segment
intradiskal
intraductal mucin-producing tumor
intraductal pressure
intradural abscess
intradural anastomosis
intradural arteriovenous fistula
intradural extramedullary tumor of spinal cord

intradural nerve root
intradural retromedullary arteriovenous fistula
intradural vessels
intraesophageal stent
intraforaminal approach
intrahepatic atresia (IHA)
intrahepatic biliary drainage catheter
intrahepatic biliary duct dilatation
intrahepatic biliary radicles
intrahepatic biliary tract dilatation
intrahepatic biliary tree
intralabyrinthine
intralaminar thalamus
intralobular fibrosis
intraluminal air
intraluminal brachytherapy
intraluminal defect
intraluminal dilation
intraluminal dimension
intraluminal duodenal diverticulum (IDD)
intraluminal filling defect
intraluminal flow
intraluminal foreign bodies
intraluminal low dose rate brachytherapy
intraluminal mass
intraluminal membranes
intraluminal Silastic esophageal stent
intraluminal sutureless prosthesis
intraluminal thrombus, laminated
intramammary
intramedullary epidermoid cyst
intramedullary fixation
intramedullary rod (rodding)
intramedullary spinal cord tumor
intramedullary spinal lesion
intramural air in colon
intramural arterial hemorrhage
intramural clot
intramural colonic air

intramural coronary artery aneurysm
intramural diverticulum
intramural gas
intramural hematoma
intramural portion of the distal ureter
intramural thrombus
intramural tunnel
intramuscular aortic segment
intramuscular hemangioma
intramyocardially
intraneural ganglion cyst
intraneuronal neurofibrillary tangles
intranodal architecture
intranuclear diskogram
intraoperative arteriography
intraoperative digital subtraction angiography (IDSA)
intraoperative electrocortical stimulation (IOECS) mapping
intraoperative gamma probe
intraoperative high dose rate (IOHDR) brachytherapy
intraoperative imaging
intraoperative laser ablation
intraoperative laser photocoagulation of ventricular tachycardia
intraoperative myocardial infarction
intraoperative pancreatography
intraoperative radiation therapy (IORT)
intraoperative radiography
intraoperative radiolymphoscintigraphy
intraoperative radiotherapy (IORT)
intraoperative scanning technique
intraoperative ultrasound
intraoperative x-ray visualization of fixation devices
intraoral periapical radiograph
intraosseous ganglia
intraosseous vascular malformations
intraosseous venography

intraosseous wiring
intrapapillary terminus
intraparenchymal cyst
intrapedicular fixation
intrapericardial bleeding
intrapericardial pressure
intraperiosteal fracture
intraperitoneal air
intraperitoneal cavity
intraperitoneal exposure
intraperitoneal fluid
intraperitoneal injury
intraperitoneal rupture
intraperitoneal Tc-sulfur colloid scan
intrapleural hemorrhage
intrapleural pressure
intrapleurally
intrapontine intracerebral hemorrhage
intraportal endovascular ultrasonography (IPEUS)
intrapulmonary barotrauma
intrapulmonary disease
intrapulmonary hemorrhage
intrapulmonary pressure
intrapulmonary shunt(ing)
intrarenal collecting system
intrarenal hematoma
intrarenal pelvis
intrarenal reflux
intrasellar Rathke cleft cyst (RCC)
intrasellar tumor
intraspinal adenoma
intraspinal lesion
intraspinal tumor
intrastitial afterloading nylon tubes
intrastitial radiation source
intratendinous fluid collection
intratentorial lipoma
intrathecal imaging
intrathecal injection of metrizamide
intrathecal injection of radiopharmaceutical

intrathecal ionics
intrathecal roots
intrathecal space
intrathoracic airways obstruction
intrathoracic dimension
intrathoracic dislocation of shoulder
intrathoracic goiter
intrathoracic Kaposi sarcoma
intrathoracic pressure
intrathoracic stomach
intrathoracic thyroid
intrathoracic upper airway obstruction
intratracheal
intratumoral agent
intratumoral necrosis
intratumoral structure
intrauterine cardiac failure
intrauterine cytomegalic inclusion disease
intrauterine fetal transfusion, ultrasonic guidance for
intrauterine fracture (of fetus)
intrauterine growth retardation (IUGR)
intrauterine heart failure
intrauterine pregnancy
intrauterine sac
intravascular clotting process
intravascular coagulation of blood (ICD), disseminated
intravascular contents, secondary extravasation of
intravascular filling defect
intravascular guide wire
intravascular mass
intravascular prosthesis
intravascular radiopharmaceutical therapy
intravascular sickling, lung
intravascular space
intravascular stenting

intravascular thrombosis
intravascular tumor thrombus
intravascular ultrasound (IVUS)
intravascular ultrasound catheter
intravascular volume depletion
intravascular volume status
intravenous (I.V. or IV)
intravenous bolus injection of contrast medium
intravenous cholangiography (IVC)
intravenous coronary thrombolysis
intravenous DSA (digital subtraction angiography)
intravenous fetal injection
intravenous fluorescein angiography (IVFA)
intravenous infusion line, peripheral
intravenous injection of isotope as bolus
intravenous line
intravenous pyelogram (IVP)
intravenous pyelography
   excretory
   rapid-sequence
intravenous urogram (IVU)
intravenous urography
intravenously enhanced CT scan
intraventricular aberration
intraventricular conduction block
intraventricular conduction defect
intraventricular conduction delay
intraventricular cryptococcal cyst
intraventricular hemorrhage (IVH)
intraventricular meningioma
intraventricular right ventricular obstruction
intraventricular systolic tension
intravesical obstruction
intravesical stone
intravesical ureter
Intrepid PTCA catheter
intrinsic deflection
intrinsic disease

intrinsic foot muscles
intrinsic lesion
intrinsic minus deformity (clawhand)
intrinsic minus hallux
intrinsic plus deformity
intrinsic pulmonary disease
intrinsic sick sinus syndrome
intrinsic stenotic lesions
intrinsic vein graft stenosis
introducer
   Becton-Dickinson
   Bentson
   Check-Flo
   Cook
   Desilets-Hoffman catheter
   Hemaquet catheter
   Hemaquet sheath
   Littleford-Spector
   LPS Peel-Away
   Pacesetter
   peel-away
   Schwartz
   Terumo sheath
   Tuohy-Borst
introducer sheath
introitus
Intropaque contrast medium
intubated small bowel series
intubation
   endotracheal
   esophagogastric (EG)
   nasal
   nasogastric (NG)
   nasotracheal
   oral
   orotracheal
intussusception
   appendiceal
   bowel
   intestinal
   retrograde
   vein
   venous

invagination
  basilar
  ligament into joint
  stomal
invasion
  arterial
  exogenous
  mediastinal
  neoplastic (of meninges)
  neoplastic (of roots)
  perineural
  tumoral
  vascular
invasive angiomatous interstitial infiltration
invasive malignant sheath tumor
invasive radiological vascular procedures
inverse radiotherapy technique
inversion-eversion
inversion injury of the ankle
inversion recovery (IR)
inversion recovery image
inversion recovery sequence
inversion recovery technique
inversion sprain
inversion time (TI)
inversus, situs
inverted Meckel diverticulum
inverted pelvis
inverted V sign
inverted Y block
inverted Y complex
inverted Y configuration
in vitro evaluation of coils
in vitro labeling
in vivo balloon pressure
in vivo correlation
in vivo disposition study
in vivo He-3 MR images
in vivo imaging
in vivo labeling

in vivo proton MR spectroscopy
involucrum
involuntary guarding
INVOS 2100 optical spectroscopy
Ioban prep
iobitridol imaging agent
iocetamic acid contrast medium
iodamine meglumine contrast medium
iodinated nanoparticles
iodine (I)
  $^{123}$I ABZM
  $^{125}$I brachytherapy
  $^{123}$I BMIPP SPECT
  $^{125}$I fibrinogen scan
  $^{123}$I heptadecanoic acid
  $^{131}$I Hippuran
  $^{123}$I IBZM
  $^{123}$I IBZP
  $^{192}$I high-dose-rate remote afterloader
  $^{123}$I IMP (iodomethyamphetamine)
  $^{125}$I interstitial radiation implant
  $^{131}$I iodocholesterol
  $^{123}$I IPPA (pentylpentadecanoic acid)
  $^{131}$I-labeled anti-CEA MoAb (CC49) and IFN-alpha
  $^{131}$I-labeled human MoAb
  $^{131}$I-labeled monoclonal Fab fragment directed against a tumor antigen
  $^{131}$I-MIBG
iodine-deficiency goiter
iodine dose
iodine radioactive source
iodipamide meglumine contrast medium
iodized oil imaging agent
iodoform gauze
Iodo-gen imaging agent

iodo-phenylated chelates
iodophenylpentadecanoic acid (I-123 IPPA) imaging agent
IOHDR (intraoperative high dose rate) brachytherapy
iohexol contrast medium
IOM (interosseous membrane)
ion exchange chromatography
ionic contrast medium
ionic paramagnetic contrast media
ionic potassium
ionic property
ionics, intrathecal
ionization chamber
ionizing radiation
iopamidol radiopaque medium
iopanoic acid contrast medium
iopentol nonionic contrast medium
iophendylate contrast medium
iopydone contrast medium
IORT (intraoperative radiation therapy) (or radiotherapy)
iothalamate contrast medium
ioversol contrast medium
ioxaglate meglumine contrast medium
ioxaglate sodium contrast medium
ioxilan with iohexol imaging agent
IP (interphalangeal) joint
IPA (idiopathic pulmonary arteriosclerosis)
IPCS (infrapatellar contracture syndrome)
IPG (impedance plethysmography)
IPH (idiopathic portal hypertension)
IPH (intraplaque hemorrhage)
IPHP (intraperitoneal hyperthermic perfusion)
ipodate calcium contrast medium
IPPA (iodine-123 phenylpentadecanoic acid)
IPPB (intermittent positive pressure breathing)

ipsilateral antegrade site
ipsilateral approach
ipsilateral basal ganglia
ipsilateral cerebellar signs
ipsilateral cortical diaschisis
ipsilateral corticospinal tract signs
ipsilateral downstream arteries
ipsilateral hemisphere activation
ipsilateral hemispheric carotid TIA (transient ischemic attack)
ipsilateral nonreversed greater saphenous vein bypass
ipsilateral pleural effusion
IPSP (intrapixel sequential processing) neuron evaluation method
iPTH (immunoreactive parathyroid hormone)
IR (inversion recovery), arrhythmia-insensitive flow-sensitive alternating
Ir (iridium)
IRA (ileorectal anastomosis)
IRBBB (incomplete right bundle branch block)
Irex Exemplar ultrasound
Iriditope (iridium-192, $^{192}$Ir) radioactive agent
iridium (Ir)
$^{192}$Ir endobronchial implant
$^{192}$Ir-loaded stent
$^{192}$Ir seed therapy
iridium radioactive source
iridium ribbon
iridium seed
iridium wire implant
IRIS (intensified radiographic imaging system)
iron overload artifact
iron overloading
iron storage disease
irradiated zinc

irradiation
  convergent beam
  curative
  external beam
  gamma
  heavy-particle
  interstitial template
  low-intensity laser (LILI)
  neutron
  palliative
  partial brain
  phosphorus-32 intracavitary
  proton
  stereotactic proton
  template
  total body
  whole brain
irradiation chamber
irradiation pneumonia
irreducible dislocation
irreducible dorsal dislocation of the metatarsophalanageal joint
irreducible fracture
irregular blocks
irregular bone
irregular gallbladder wall thickening
irregular hazy luminal contour
irregular mass, polypoid calcified
irregularity
  diffuse
  intimal
  luminal
irreversible airways obstruction
irreversible compression of MR image
irreversible ischemia
irreversible narrowing of bronchioles
irreversible organ failure
irrigation, saline
irritability
  atrial
  muscle
  myocardial

irritability *(cont.)*
  nerve root
  ventricular
irritable bowel syndrome (IBS)
irritable colon
ISAH stereotactic immobilization frame
ISAH stereotactic immobilizing mask
ischemia
  brachiocephalic
  brain
  brain stem
  cardiac
  carotid artery
  cerebral
  chronic cerebral
  coronary
  exercise-induced myocardial
  exercise-induced transient myocardial
  global myocardial
  hypoxia-
  irreversible
  limb-threatening
  mesenteric
  myocardial
  neonatal intracranial
  nonlocalized
  peri-infarction
  provocable
  regional myocardial
  regional transmural
  remote
  reversible
  segmental
  silent
  silent myocardial
  subendocardial
  transient cerebral
  transient myocardial
  vertebral-basilar
  vertebrobasilar
  zone of

ischemic area
ischemic brain damage
ischemic changes, persistence of
ischemic contracture
ischemic decompensation
ischemic disease
ischemic episode
ischemic event
ischemic heart disease (IHD)
ischemic hypoxia
ischemic infarction
ischemic injury
ischemic instability
ischemic necrosis
ischemic-reperfusion injury
ischemic segment (on echocardiogram)
ischemic time
ischemic ulcer, hypertensive
ischemic viable myocardium
ischemic zone
ischial bone
ischial spine
ischial tuberosity
ischioacetabular fracture
ischiogluteal bursa
ischiorectal abscess
ischiorectal fossa plane
ischium
 ascending ramus of
 ramus of
ISDN connection
ISG medical imaging workstation
ISIS spectroscopy
island
 bone
 bony
 mucosal
 tissue
 Reil
Isocam scintillation imaging system
Isocam SPECT imaging system

isocapnic hyperventilation-induced bronchoconstriction
isocenter placement error
isocenter shift method
isocenter, single
isoclosed curve
isodense appearance
isodense enhancement
isodense mass
isodensity
isodose contour
isodose plan
isodose width
isoechoic
isoeffective bronchial mucosa
isoelectric at J point
isoelectric line
isoelectric period
isointense soft tissue on MRI
isolated clustered calcifications of breast
isolated dislocation of semilunar bone
isolated heat perfusion of extremity
isolated ventricular inversion
isomerism, atrial
isometric exercise stress test
isometric heart contraction
Isopaque contrast medium
isoperistaltic ileal reservoir
isoproterenol infusion
isosulfan blue contrast medium
isotope
isotope bone scan
isotope cisternography
isotope injected intravenously as bolus
isotope meal
isotope scan (scanning)
isotope, stable
isotope venogram
isotopic bone scanning
isotopic cisternography
isotopic dilution

isotopic ratio
isotopic skeletal survey
isotropic 3D or volume study
isotropic imaging
isotropic lung scan
isotropic voxels
isovolumetric contraction
isovolumetric period
isovolumic contraction time
isovolumic period
isovolumic relaxation
Isovue (iopamidol, injectable) non-ionic contrast agent
Isovue contrast series (128, 200, 300, 370), parenteral injection
Isovue-M contrast series (200, 300), intrathecal injection
Israel camera
ISS (inferior sagittal sinus)
ISS (Injury Severity Score)
ISSI (interspinous segmental spinal instrumentation)
isthmic coarctation, congenital
isthmus
  aortic
  stenotic
  temporal
isthmus aneurysm
isthmus of aorta
isthmus of femur
isthmus of Vieussens
IT (iliotibial) band
ITA (internal thoracic artery) graft
ITC (Interventional Therapeutics Corporation)
  ITC balloon catheter
  ITC radiopaque balloon catheter

iterative algorithm
iterative gradient optimzation
iterative halftoning
IUdR (idoxuridine, iododeoxyuridine) halogenated thymidine analogue, a radiosensitizer
IUGR (intrauterine growth retardation)
IV (interventricular) septum
IV, I.V. (intravenous)
  IV bolus
Ivalon embolization
Ivalon particles
Ivalon sponge
IVB (intraventricular block)
IVC (inferior vena cava)
IVC (intravenous cholangiogram)
IVC filter, percutaneous
IVDSA (intravenous digital subtraction angiography)
Ivemark syndrome
IVFA (intravenous fluorescein angiography)
IVH (intraventricular hemorrhage)
IVP (intravenous pyelogram)
IVR (idioventricular rhythm)
IVS (interventricular septum)
IVSD (interventricular septal defect)
IVST (interventricular septal thickness)
IVU (intravenous urogram)
IVUS (intravascular ultrasound)

# J, j

J (joule)
jackknife position
Jackman orthogonal catheter
Jackson-Pratt catheter
Jaffe-Lichtenstein disease
jagged bone fragments
jagged osteophytes
Jahss classification of metatarso-
   phalangeal joint dislocation
Janeway lesion
Jansen disease
Janus syndrome
Jarcho-Levin syndrome
jaw bone
JB1 catheter
JB3 catheter
J-coupled spins
J-curve movable core guide wire
Jefferson burst fracture
Jefferson cervical fracture
Jefferson fracture of atlas
Jeffery classification of radial fracture
jejunal loop interposition of Henle
jejunal motility
jejunoileal bypass (JIB)
Jelco intravenous catheter
jeopardize

jet area (JA)
jet, high-velocity
jet length (JL)
jet lesion
jet nebulizer
Jeune-Tommasi syndrome
J guide wire
J-hook deformity of distal ureter
JIB (jejunoileal bypass)
JL (jet length)
JL4 (Judkins left 4) catheter
JL5 (Judkins left 5) catheter
J loop technique on catheterization
Jobert fossa
Jod-Basedow phenomenon
Johnson-Jahss classification of
   posterior tibial tendon tear
joint
   AC (acromioclavicular)
   atlantoaxial
   bail-lock knee
   ball-and-socket
   basal
   calcaneocuboid
   capitate hamate
   capitolunate
   carpometacarpal (CMC)

**joint**

joint *(cont.)*
 carpophalangeal
 Charcot
 Chopart
 chronic recurrent dislocation of
 condyloid
 costochondral
 costotransverse
 costovertebral
 cubonavicular
 cuneiform
 distal interphalangeal (DIP)
 distraction of
 ellipsoid
 facet
 flail
 free knee
 Gaffney
 Gillette
 glenohumeral
 gliding
 hallux interphalangeal (IP)
 hinge
 hip capsule
 hyperextensibility of
 immovable
 intercarpal
 interchondral
 intermetatarsal (IM)
 interphalangeal (IP)
 intervertebral
 lesser metatarsophalangeal
 Lisfranc
 lunotriquetral (LT)
 Luschka
 manubriosternal
 metacarpal-phalangeal (MCP, MP)
 metacarpophalangeal (MCP, MP)
 metatarsal-phalangeal (MTP)
 metatarsocuneiform (MC)
 metatarsophalangeal (MPJ, MTP)
 midcarpal

joint *(cont.)*
 midtarsal
 mortise
 naviculocuneiform
 neuropathic tarsal-metatarsal
 occipital-axis
 proximal interphalangeal (PIP)
 pisotriquetral
 pivot
 radiocapitellar
 radiocarpal
 radioscaphoid
 radioulnar
 Regnauld degeneration of MTP
 sacroiliac (SI)
 saddle
 scaphocapitate
 scapholunate
 scaphotrapezoid-trapezial (STT)
 secondary cartilaginous
 sesamoidometatarsal
 SI (sacroiliac)
 Silastic finger
 SL (scapholunate)
 sternal
 sternoclavicular
 sternocostal
 STT (scaphotrapezoid-trapezial)
 subtalar
 surgeon's tarsal joint
 Swanson finger
 synovial
 talocalcaneal
 talocrural
 talofibular
 talonavicular
 tarsal-metatarsal
 tarsometatarsal
 temporomandibular
 thoracic
 tibiofibular
 tibiotalar

joint *(cont.)*
  transverse tarsal
  trapeziometacarpal
  trapezioscaphoid
  trapeziotrapezoid
  triquetrohamate
  uncovertebral
  unstable
  weightbearing
  xiphisternal
joint arthrography
joint capsule
joint congruency
joint congruity
joint debris
joint depression fracture
joint dislocation
joint effusion
joint fracture
joint fulcrum
joint hyperextendability
joint incongruity
joint interface
joint kinematics
joint laxity
joint mice (or mouse)
joint morphology
joint photographic experts group (JPEG) algorithms
joint play, excessive
joint segment
joint space
  cartilage
  narrowed
  widened
joint survey
joint swelling
Joliot method for sorption studies
Jones classification of diaphyseal fractures
Jones fracture
joule (J)
joule radiation absorbed dose
joule shocks
JPEG (joint photographic experts group) algorithms
J pouch, two-loop ileal
J-shaped tube
J-shaped ureter
Jude pelvic x-ray
Judkins cardiac catheterization
Judkins coronary angiography
Judkins coronary arteriography
Judkins 4 diagnostic catheter
Judkins left 4 coronary catheter (JL4)
Judkins right 4 coronary catheter (JR4)
Judkins selective coronary arteriography
Judkins USCI catheter
jugular bulb, internal
jugular catheter
jugular foramen syndrome
jugular triangle, internal
jugular vein distention (JVD)
jugular veins filled from above
jugular veins filled from below
jugular venous distention (JVD)
jugular venous excursions
jugular venous impulse
jugular venous pressure (JVP)
jugular venous pressure collapse
jugular venous pulsation (pulse)
jugulodigastric chain
jugulodigastric node
jugulovenous distention (JVD)
jump vein graft
jumped facet
jumper's knee
junction
  anorectal
  aortic sinotubular
  atriocaval
  atrioventricular

junction *(cont.)*
  cardioesophageal (CE)
  cardiophrenic
  caval-atrial
  cervicomedullary
  cervicothoracic
  choledochopancreatic ductal
  chondrosternal
  corticomedullary
  costochondral
  craniocervical
  craniovertebral
  cystic-choledochal
  duodenojejunal
  esophagogastric (EG)
  fundic-antral
  gastrocnemius-soleus
  gastroesophageal (GE)
  gray-white matter
  ileocecal
  J
  meniscosynovial
  metaphyseal-diaphyseal
  mucocutaneous
  musculotendinous
  myoneural
  myotendinous
  neuromuscular
  occipitocervical
  pancreaticobiliary ductal
  pelviureteral
  phrenovertebral
  pontomedullary
  pontomesencephalic
  pyloroduodenal
  saphenofemoral
  sinotubular

junction *(cont.)*
  squamocolumnar
  sternoclavicular
  sylvian/rolandic
  temporal-occipital
  tracheoesophageal (TE)
  ureteropelvic
junctional defect
junctional focus (pl. foci)
junction separation, costochondral
juvenile ossifying fibroma
juvenile Paget disease
juvenile Tillaux fracture
juxta-anastomotic stenoses
juxta-arterial ventricular septal defect
juxta-articular osteoid osteoma
juxta-articulation
juxtacortical chondroma
juxtacortical sarcoma
juxtacrural
juxtaductal coarctation of aorta
juxtapapillary diverticulum
juxtaphrenic peak
juxtaposed leftward
juxtaposed rightward
juxtaposition
juxtapyloric ulcer
juxtarenal aortic aneurysm
juxtarenal aortic atherosclerosis
juxtarenal cava
juxtatricuspid ventricular septal defect
juxtavesical
JVD (jugulovenous or jugular venous distention)
JVP (jugular venous pressure)
J wire

*Karyorrhexis*

# K, k

Kager triangle
Kahler disease
Kalamchi-Dawe classification of congenital tibial deficiency
Kalman filter
Kaplan-Meier method
Kaposi sarcoma
   endobronchial
   epicardial
   intracolonic
   intrathoracic
   myocardial infiltration by
   pulmonary
Karplus sign of pleural effusion
Kartagener syndrome
Kartagener triad
Kasabach-Merritt phenomenon
Kashin-Bek disease
Kast syndrome
Katayama syndrome
Katzman infusion of radionuclide cisternography
Katz-Wachtel phenomenon
Kawai bioptome
Kawasaki disease
Kayexalate enema
k-capture

KCD (kinestatic charge detector)
KDA profile
Kearns-Sayre syndrome
keel of glenoid component
keel-like ridge
keeled chest
Keith bundle of fibers in heart
Keith-Flack sinoatrial node
Kellock sign of pleural effusion
Kellogg-Speed lumbar spinal fusion
Kelly-Goerss Compass stereotactic system
keloid scar
Kemp-Elliot-Gorlin syndrome
Kennedy area-length method
Kennedy ligament technique
Kennedy method for calculating ejection fraction
Kensey atherectomy catheter
Kent-His bundle
keratocyst
Kerckring fold
Kerckring nodule
Kerley A lines
Kerley B lines
Kerley C lines
kernel size

Kernig sign
Kernohan classification of astro-
 cytomas and glioblastomas
Kernohan notch phenomenon
Keshan disease
Kety equation
keV or kev (kiloelectron volt)
keV gamma ray
Key-Conwell classification of pelvic
 fracture
keyboard, Cherry
keyhole deformity
keystone of calcar arch
kg (kilogram)
kHz (kilohertz)
kick, atrial (AK)
kidney arteriovenous fistula
kidney
   abdominal
   arteriosclerotic
   atrophic
   cicatricial
   congenital absence of
   congested
   contracted
   contralateral
   cortical scarring of
   crush
   cyanotic
   cystic
   disk
   distended
   double
   doughnut
   duplication of left
   duplication of right
   dysfunctional
   ectopic
   edematous
   enlarged
   fatty
   fibrotic

kidney *(cont.)*
   floating
   Formad
   fused
   Goldblatt
   granular
   hilum of
   hilus of
   horseshoe
   hydronephrotic
   hypermobile
   infundibulum of
   irregular
   lobe of
   lobulated
   long axis of
   lumbar
   medullary sponge
   movable
   multicystic dysplastic
   mural
   myeloma
   nonfunctioning
   pelvis of
   polycystic
   porous
   ptotic
   Rose-Bradford
   sacciform
   scarred
   sclerotic
   shriveled
   sigmoid
   sponge
   supernumerary
   suspension of
   thoracic
   wandering
kidney function study
kidney-pancreas transplant
kidney rest
kidney scan

kidney shadow
kidney stone, passing of
kidney-to-background ratio
kidney tomography
kidney transplant
kidney transplantation
kidneys, ureters, and bladder (KUB)
Kienböck disease
Kienböck dislocation
Kiernan spaces in liver
Kikuchi-Fujimoto disease
Kilfoyle classification of condylar
    fracture
Kilian line
Kilian pelvis
Killip-Kimball classification of heart
    failure
kiloelectron volt (keV or kev)
kilohertz (kHz)
Kim-Ray Greenfield inferior vena
    caval filter
Kimura disease
kinematic MRI studies
kinestatic charge detector (KCD)
kinetic energy
kinetic parameter analysis
kinetic perfusion parameters
kinetics
    elimination
    sorption
    washout
kinetocardiogram
Kinevac contrast medium
King multipurpose coronary graft
    catheter
kink artifact
kinking
    arterial
    blood vessel
    bowel
    carotid artery
    catheter

kinking *(cont.)*
    colon
    graft
    innominate artery
    intestinal
    Lane
    patch
Kinnier-Wilson disease
Kinsbourne syndrome
Kinsey atherectomy catheter
Kirchner diverticulum
Kirk distal thigh amputation
kissing atherectomy technique
kissing balloon technique
kissing-type artifact
Kistler classification of subarachnoid
    hemorrhage
Klatskin tumor
Klauder syndrome
Klein-Waardenburg syndrome
Klippel-Feil sequence
Klippel-Trénaunay-Weber syndrome
K-L transform
K-means clustering algorithm
K-means clusters
knee
    anterior cruciate deficit of
    breaststroker's
    Brodie
    corner of
    dislocated
    floating
    housemaid's
    internal derangement of the (IDK)
    jumper's
    locked
    motorcyclist's
    runner's
    wrenched
kneecap
knee knob of Osgood-Schlatter disease
knee-like bend in a structure

knee view
knife, roentgen
knob, blurring of aortic
knobby process
knock-knee (genu valgum) deformity
knuckle bone
knuckle of colon
knuckle-shaped
knuckle sign
Knuttsen bending roentgenograms
Kocher anastomosis
Kocher fracture
Kocher lateral J approach
Kocher-Lorenz classification of capitellum fracture
Kocher maneuver
Koch sinoatrial node
Koch triangle, apex of
Kock pouch
Kodak software
Koerber-Salus-Elschnig syndrome
Köhler disease
Köhler-Pellegrini-Stieda disease
Kohlrausch fold
Kohn, pores of 3334
Komai stereotactic head frame
Kommerell diverticulum
Konica scanner
Konstram angle
Kontrast U radiopaque contrast medium
Kontron balloon catheter
Kopans needle
Korányi-Grocco sign
Korányi-Grocco triangle
Korotkoff method in Doppler cerebrovascular examination
Korsakoff syndrome

Korotkoff test for collateral circulation
Kouchoukos method
Kr-81m (krypton) imaging agent
Krabbe diffuse sclerosis
Krukenberg tumor
krypton ($^{81m}$Kr) imaging agent
k-space
k-space matrix
k-space velocity mapping
KUB (kidneys, ureters, and urinary bladder)
Kubelka-Munk theory
Kugel anastomosis
Kugel artery
Kugel collaterals
Kugelberg-Welander juvenile spinal muscle atrophy
Kumeral diverticulum
Kümmell disease
Kurtz-Sprague-White syndrome
Kussmaul-Maier disease
Kveim test
kVp (kilovolts peak) meter
Kyle fracture classification system
kyllosis (clubfoot)
kymography
kyphoscoliosis
kyphoscoliotic heart disease
kyphosis
    Cobb method of measuring
    loss of
    lumbar
    lumbosacral
    postlaminectomy
    Scheuermann juvenile
    thoracic
kyphotic angulation
kyphotic pelvis

# L, l

L (liter)
L (lumbar vertebra)
LA (left atrium)
LAA (left atrial appendage)
LAA (left auricular appendage)
LA/AR (left atrium/aortic root) ratio
LABA (laser-assisted balloon angioplasty)
Labbé triangle
Labbé, vein of
label
    double
    long wavelength photolabel
    radioactive
    radionuclide
    single
    triple
labeled antibodies
labeled fibrinogen
labeled positron
labeled RBCs
labeled red blood cell sequestration
labeling
    antibody
    $^{111}$In (indium-111) WBCs
    in vitro
    in vivo

labeling *(cont.)*
    in vivo/in vitro
    microglobulin
    radioactive
    radioisotope
    site-specific
    technetium Tc-human serum albumin
    Tc-tagged RBCs
    white blood cell
labile blood pressure
labral injury
labral variant
labrum
    acetabular
    articular
    glenoid
    glenoidal
labyrinth
    artery of
    bony
    cochlear
    ethmoidal
    Ludwig
    membranous
    osseous
    renal

labyrinth (*cont.*)
   Santorini
   vestibular
labyrinthine artery
labyrinthine hydrops
labyrinthine structures
LACD (left apexcardiogram,
   calibrated displacement)
laciniate ligament of ankle
lack of clear-cut cerebral dominance
lacrimal bone
lacrimal canaliculus obstruction
lactulose enema
lacuna (pl. lacunae)
   bone
   cartilage
   intervillous
   osseous
   penis
   resorption
lacunar abscess
lacunar infarct
lacunar ligament
lacunar stroke
LAD (left anterior descending)
   coronary artery
Ladder diagram
LAE (left atrial enlargement)
LAID (left anterior internal diameter)
LAIS excimer laser for coronary
   angioplasty
Laitinen CT guidance system
Laitinen stereotactic head frame
lake
   bile
   capillary
   mucous
   lipid
   venous
Laks method
lambdoid suture
Lambert projection

lamella (pl. lamellae)
   articular
   circumferential
   concentric
   enamel
lamellar body density (LBD) count
lamellated bone
lamina
   medullary
   osseous spiral
lamina propria
laminar flow
laminated calcification
laminated intraluminal thrombus
lamination of gyrus
laminography, cardiac
Lancisi muscle
landmark
   anatomic
   bony
   bony skull
landmark registration
Landolfi sign
Landsmeer ligament
Lane disease
Lane kink
Lanex medium screen
Langenbeck triangle
Langer line
Lanier clinical reporting system
lanthanide-induced shifts
Lanz point
LAO (left anterior oblique)
   LAO position
   LAO projection
   LAO view
LAP (left atrial pressure)
laparoscopic contact ultrasonography
   (LCU)
laparoscopic Doppler probe
laparoscopic intracorporeal ultrasound
   (LICU)

laparoscopic ultrasound (LUS)
L/A (liver/aorta) peak ratio
Laplace effect
Laplace law
Laplace mechanism
large-caliber coronary guiding catheter
large clothing artifact
large colloidal particles
large-field radiotherapy
large hinge angle electron fields
large obtuse marginal branch
large thymus shadow obscuring cardiac silhouette
large venous tributaries
large-vessel disease of diabetic foot
large-vessel thrombosis
Larmor equation
Larmor frequency
Larmor precession
Larsen-Johansson disease
laryngeal cartilage
laryngeal fracture
laryngeal keel
laryngeal nodule
laryngeal vestibule
laryngeal web
laryngogram
laryngography
    contrast
    double-contrast
larynx
    appendix of ventricle of
    glottic
    infraglottic
    laryngeal
    supraglottic
    ventricle of
    vestibule of
laser-assisted balloon angioplasty (LABA)
laser-assisted microvascular anastomosis (LAMA)

laser balloon angioplasty (LBA)
laser biomicroscopy
laser desiccation of thrombus
laser Doppler velocimetry
Laserflo Doppler probe
laser-induced thermotherapy (LITT)
laser-polarized helium MRI
laser printer, Ektascan
Laserprobe-PLR Plus
LASH (left anterior-superior hemiblock)
Lasix renography
Laslett-Short syndrome
last menstrual period (LMP)
Lastac System angioplasty laser
lata, fascia
Latarjet, nerve of
LATC (lateral talocalcaneal angle)
late effect analysis
late effects of normal tissues (LENT) scoring system
late effects toxicity scoring
late film
late graft occlusion
late normal tissue sequelae
late-phase termination
lateral aspect
lateral bending views of spine
lateral bronchi
lateral cervical spine film
lateral column calcaneal fracture
lateral condyle
lateral corticospinal tract
lateral costotransverse ligament
lateral decubitus position
lateral decubitus view
lateral entrapment
laterality
lateralization
lateralizing deficit
lateralizing finding
lateralizing sign

laterally displaced fracture
lateral opposed beam
lateral position
lateral projection
lateral spring ligament of foot
lateral sulcus
lateral tomography
lateral ventricle
lateral view
lateral web
lateral wedge fracture of vertebral
   body
lateroconal fascia
late systolic posterior displacement on
   echocardiogram
LaTeX device-independent
latissimus dorsi muscle
LATS (long-acting thyroid stimulator)
lattice, fibrovascular
lattice model
lattice relaxation time
lattice vibrations
latticework
Laubry-Pezzi syndrome
Laue pattern
Laue photographic technique
Lauge-Hansen classification of ankle
   fracture
Laurence-Moon-Biedl-Bardet
   syndrome
Laurin angle
Laurin x-ray view
Lausanne stereotactic robot
law
   Bragg
   Courvoisier
   Hilton
Law view
laxity
   joint
   ligament
   varus stress

layer
   bright
   circumferential echodense
   echodense
   echo-free
   hypoechoic
   inner bright
   sonolucent
layering calcification
layering effusion
layering of contrast material
layering of gallstones
lazaroid U74389G
LBA (laser balloon angioplasty)
L/B (lesion-to-brain) ratio
LBBB (left bundle branch block)
LBCD (left border of cardiac
   dullness)
LBP (low back pain)
LC-DCP (low-contact dynamic
   compression plate)
LCA (left coronary artery)
LCF or LCX (left circumflex)
   coronary artery
LCL (lateral collateral ligament)
LCP (Legg-Calvé-Perthes disease)
LCT (liquid crystal contact
   thermography)
LCU (laparoscopic contact ultrasonography)
LDF (laser-Doppler flowmetry) probe
lead apron
lead eye shield
lead-pipe colon
lead-pipe fracture
lead-pipe rigidity
lead pellet marker
lead points
leaflet
leaf of diaphragm
leak
   air
   aortic paravalvular

leak *(cont.)*
  baffle
  blood
  capillary
  cerebrospinal fluid (CSF)
  chyle
  contained (of aortic aneurysm)
  current
  generalized capillary
  interatrial baffle
  light
  mitral
  paraprosthetic
  paravalvar
  paravalvular
  periprosthetic
  perivalvular
leakage
  blood-tumor-barrier
  cerebrospinal fluid (CSF)
  contrast media
leaking abdominal aortic aneurysm
leaking vein
leaky valve
lean mass
least-squares (LS) algorithms
leather bottle stomach
leaves of diaphragm
leaves of mesentery
Le Fort (I, II, or III) fracture
left anterior descending (LAD) artery, superdominant
left anterior oblique (LAO) projection
left atrial active emptying fraction
left atrial end-diastolic pressure
left atrial enlargement
left atrial maximal volume
left atrial pressure (LAP)
left atrium, giant
left auricle
left auricular appendage (LAA)
left border of heart

left bundle branch block (LBBB)
left bundle branch hemiblock
left circumflex (LCX) coronary artery
left common femoral artery
left coronary artery arising from pulmonary artery
left coronary cusp
left coronary plexus (of heart)
left heart failure
left heart pressure
left iliac system
left internal mammary artery (LIMA)
left Judkins catheter
left main coronary artery (LMCA)
left main stem bronchus
left mid lung
left posterior oblique (LPO) position
left pulmonary artery
left pulmonary cusp
left respiratory nerve (phrenic)
left-right asymmetry
left-sided heart failure
left-side-down decubitus position
left sternal border
left-to-right shift
left-to-right ventricular shunt
left ventricle
  double-inlet
  hypoplastic
  morphologic
left ventricular afterload
left ventricular assist device (LVAD),
left ventricular chamber
left ventricular ejection fraction (LVEF)
left ventricular ejection fraction by acoustic quantification
left ventricular end-diastolic pressure (LVEDP)
left ventricular end-diastolic volume
left ventricular end-systolic volume
left ventricular hypertrophy (LVH)

left ventricular hypoplasia
left ventricular loading
left ventricular maximal volume
left ventricular outflow tract
left ventricular preload
left ventricular pressure
left ventricular regional wall motion abnormality
left ventricular segmental contraction
left ventricular stroke work (LVSW)
left ventricular stroke work index (LVSWI)
left ventricular systolic pump function
left ventricular systolic time interval ratio
left ventriculogram
left ventriculography
leg
  baker
  bayonet
  postphlebitic
Legg-Calvé-Perthes disease
Legg-Calvé-Waldenström disease
Lehman ventriculography catheter
Leiner disease
Leitner syndrome
Leksell D-shaped stereotactic frame
Leksell-Elekta stereotactic frame
Leksell stereotaxic device used with CT scanner
length
  crown-heel
  crown-rump
  echo-train
  limb
  track cone
LENI (lower extremity noninvasive)
LENT (late effects of normal tissues) scoring system
lenticular bone of hand
lenticular nucleus
lenticulostriate artery

lentiform nucleus
LEOPARD syndrome
leptomeningeal cyst
leptomeningeal disease
leptomeninges
Leriche syndrome
LEs (lower extremities)
LES (lower esophageal sphincter)
Lesgaft hernia
Lesgaft triangle
lesion
  acute cerebellar hemispheric
  adrenal
  afferent nerve
  angulated
  annular
  anterior parietal
  anterochiasmatic
  aortic arch
  apical
  apple core
  Armanni-Ebstein
  atheromatous
  atherosclerotic
  atrophic
  Baehr-Lohlein
  Bankart shoulder
  Bennett
  bifurcation
  bilateral
  biparietal
  bird's nest
  blastic
  bleeding
  Blumenthal
  Bracht-Wachter
  brain stem
  Brown-Séquard
  bull's-eye
  calcified
  callosal
  cardiac valvular

lesion (*cont.*)
  cartilaginous
  cavernous sinus
  caviar
  cavitary
  central
  cerebral
  cervical cord
  chiasmal
  chiasmatic
  circular
  circumscribed
  coin (of lungs)
  cold
  complete nerve
  complex
  concentric
  constricting esophageal
  constrictive
  conus medullaris
  coronary artery
  cortical
  corticospinal pathway
  critical
  culprit
  cyclops
  cystic
  deep
  de nov
  deep-seated
  dendritic
  desmoid
  destructive
  Dieulafoy
  diffuse
  discrete
  disk
  dominant hemisphere
  dorsal root entry zone
  doughnut
  DREZ (dorsal root entry zone)
  dumbbell

lesion (*cont.*)
  Duret
  Ebstein
  eccentric
  eccentric restenosis
  echogenic
  ellipsoid
  endobronchial
  enhancing
  epicortical
  epileptogenic
  esophageal
  excitatory
  expansile lytic
  extra-axial
  extrinsic
  fibro-osseous
  fibromuscular
  fingertip
  florid duct
  flow-compromising
  flow-limiting
  focal
  focal hemispheric
  focal ischemic
  frank
  frontal lobe
  geographic
  Ghon primary
  gross
  hamartomatous
  hemodynamically significant
  hemorrhagic
  high cervical spinal cord
  high-density
  high-grade obstructive
  high pontine
  high-signal
  Hill-Sachs shoulder
  homogeneous
  hot
  hourglass-shaped

**lesion**

lesion *(cont.)*
  hyperintense
  hypodense
  hypothalamic
  impaction
  indiscriminate
  infiltrating
  infranuclear
  intra-axial brain
  intracerebral
  intracranial vascular
  intramedullary spinal
  intrasellar
  intraspinal
  intrinsic stenotic
  invasive
  irregular-shaped
  irregularly shaped
  ischemic
  isointense
  Janeway
  jet
  Kidner
  lateral temporal epileptogenic
  left lower lobe (LLL)
  left upper lobe (LUL)
  lipomatous
  local
  localized
  Löhlein-Baehr
  low-density
  lower motor neuron
  lytic (osteolytic) bone
  malignant
  Mallory-Weiss
  mass
  medial longitudinal fasciculus
    (MLF)
  median nerve
  mesenteric vascular
  mesial temporal epileptogenic
  metabolic

lesion *(cont.)*
  metastatic bone
  midbrain
  midline
  mixed
  mongolian spot-like
  Monteggia
  multifocal
  multiple focal
  muscular
  nail bed
  napkin-ring annular
  necrotic
  neoplastic
  neurogenic
  neurologic bladder
  nidus of
  nodular
  nondominant hemisphere
  nonenhancing
  noninvasive
  nucleus basalis
  obstructive (of the CSF pathways)
  occipital
  occlusive
  occult
  onion scale
  onionskin
  organic
  osseous
  osteoblastic
  osteocartilaginous
  osteochondral (of the talus)
  ostial
  outcropping of
  papillary
  papular
  papulonecrotic
  parasagittal
  parasellar
  parietal cortex
  parietal lobe

lesion *(cont.)*
  parieto-occipital
  partial
  pedunculated
  periapical
  peripheral
  peripheral nerve
  periventricular
  permeative
  Perthes-Bankart
  photon-deficient
  plaquelike
  polyostotic bone
  polypoid
  pontine
  posterior column
  posterior compartment
  posterior fossa-foramen magnum
  posterior language area
  pretectal
  primary
  pulmonary
  purulent
  questionable
  radial sclerosing
  radiofrequency
  radiographic stability of
  radiopaque
  rectal
  rectosigmoid polypoid
  recurrent
  regurgitant
  renal mass
  resectable
  retrochiasmal
  retrochiasmatic
  rheumatic
  rib
  right lower lobe (RLL)
  right upper lobe (RUL)
  ring-enhancing (on CT)
  root

lesion *(cont.)*
  root entry-zone
  satellite
  secondary
  segmental
  serial
  sessile
  sharply demarcated circumferential
  signal characteristics of
  skip
  SLAP (superior labrum anterior posterior)
  slowly developing
  solitary
  sonolucent
  space-occupying
  spherical
  spinal cord
  spontaneous
  stacked ovoid
  Stener
  stenotic
  striatal
  structural
  subchondral
  subcortical intracranial
  submucosal
  subtentorial
  subtotal
  superficial
  supranuclear
  suprasellar
  supratentorial
  suspicious
  synchronous
  systemic
  tandem
  target
  tectal
  telangiectatic
  temporal
  temporal lobe

lesion *(cont.)*
   thalamic
   tight
   total
   transfer
   transverse cord
   trophic
   tuberculoid
   tuberculous
   tubular
   type A, B, or C
   ulcerated
   ulcerating
   ulcerative
   ulnar nerve
   uncommitted metaphyseal
   unilateral
   unresectable
   unstable
   upper motor neuron
   valvular regurgitant
   vascular
   vasculitic
   vegetative
   wedge-shaped
   well-defined
   white matter
   wide field
   wire-loop
   Wolin meniscoid
lesion in posterior fossa–foramen magnum
lesion in spinal cord
lesion localization
lesion-to-background ratio
lesion-to-cerebrospinal fluid noise
lesion-to-muscle ratio
lesion-to-nonlesion count ratio
lesion-to-white matter noise
lesion with increased blood pool
LESP (lower esophageal sphincter pressure)

lesser atrophy of disuse
lesser curvature of stomach
lesser metatarsophalangeal joint
lesser multangular (trapezoid) bone
lesser omentum
lesser saphenous vein
lesser sciatic notch
lesser trochanter
lethal consequences
lethal midline granuloma
lethal myocardial injury
Letterer-Siwe disease
lettering artifact
LeukaScan imaging agent
leukemia infiltrate
leukoencephalopathy, multifocal
leukomalacia, periventricular (PVL)
leukopenia, radiogenic
Leung thumb loss classification
Leur-par collimator
levator ani muscle
LeVeen catheter
LeVeen plaque-cracker
level
   air-fluid
   fluid
   fluid-fluid
   gas-fluid
   ring shadows with air-fluid
   window
levoposition
levorotatory
levoscoliosis
levotransposition (L-transposition)
levoversion
Levovist (SHU 508A) imaging agent
Lewis angle
L5-S1 vertebral interspace
LFV (large field of view)
LGA (low-grade astrocytoma)
LGV (lymphogranuloma venereum)
Lhermitte-Duclos disease

Lhermitte sign
LHV (left hepatic vein)
Lian-Siguier-Welti venous thrombosis syndrome
Libman-Sacks endocarditis disease
LICS (left intercostal space)
LICU (laparoscopic intracorporeal ultrasound)
Liddle syndrome
lidocaine
Lido-Pen Auto-Injector
lie
  horizontal
  longitudinal
  posterior
  transverse
Liebel-Flarsheim CT 9000 contrast delivery system
Lieberkühn crypt
lienography
LiF (lithium fluoride)
LiF thermoluminescence dosimeter
Life-Pack 5 cardiac monitor
ligament
  accessory
  acromioclavicular
  acromiocoracoid
  alar
  annular
  anococcygeal
  apical (of dens)
  Arantius
  arcuate
  arterial
  atlantal
  attenuated
  auricular
  avulsed
  axis
  Bardinet
  Barkow
  beak

ligament *(cont.)*
  Bellini
  Berry
  Bertin
  Bichat
  bifurcated
  Bigelow
  Botallo
  Bourgery
  broad (of uterus)
  Brodie
  Burns
  calcaneoclavicular
  calcaneocuboid
  calcaneofibular (CF)
  calcaneonavicular
  calcaneotibial
  Caldani
  Campbell
  Camper
  capsular
  Carcassonne
  cardinal
  caroticoclinoid
  carpometacarpal
  Casser
  casserian
  caudal
  ceratocricoid
  cervical
  check
  check rein
  cholecystoduodenal
  chondroxiphoid
  ciliary
  Civinini
  Clado
  Cleland
  Cloquet
  collateral
  Colles
  congenital laxity of

**ligament**

ligament *(cont.)*
  conjugate
  conoid
  conus
  coracoacromial
  coracoclavicular
  coracohumeral
  corniculopharyngeal
  coronary
  costoclavicular
  costocolic
  costotransverse
  costoxiphoid
  cotyloid
  Cowper
  cricopharyngeal
  cricosantorinian
  cricothyroid
  cricotracheal
  cross
  crucial
  cruciate
  cruciatum cruris
  cruciform
  Cruveilhier
  cuboideonavicular
  cuneocuboid
  cuneonavicular
  cystoduodenal
  deep collateral
  deltoid (of shoulder, of ankle)
  Denonvilliers
  dentate
  denticulate
  Denucé
  diaphragmatic
  Douglas
  duodenal
  duodenorenal
  epihyal
  extracapsular
  falciform

ligament *(cont.)*
  fallopian
  femoral
  Ferrein
  fibular collateral
  fibulotalar
  fibulotalocalcaneal
  flaval
  floating
  Flood
  fundiform
  gastrocolic
  gastrodiaphragmatic
  gastrohepatic
  gastrolienal
  gastropancreatic
  gastrophrenic
  gastrosplenic
  genital
  genitoinguinal
  Gerdy
  Gillette suspensory
  Gimbernat
  gingivodental
  glenohumeral
  glenoid
  glossoepiglottic
  Grayson
  Günz (Guenz)
  Günzberg (Guenzberg)
  Haines-McDougall medial
  hammock
  Helmholtz axis
  Henle
  Hensing
  hepatic
  hepatocolic
  hepatocystocolic
  hepatoduodenal
  hepatoesophageal
  hepatogastric
  hepatogastroduodenal

**ligament**

ligament *(cont.)*
 hepatophrenic
 hepatorenal
 hepatoumbilical
 Hesselbach
 Hey
 Holl
 Hueck
 Humphry
 Hunter
 Huschke
 hyalocapsular
 hyoepiglottic
 iliofemoral
 iliolumbar
 iliopectineal
 iliopubic
 iliotibial (of Maissiat)
 iliotrochanteric
 infrapatellar
 infundibulo-ovarian
 infundibulopelvic
 inguinal
 intercapital
 intercarpal
 interclavicular
 interclinoid
 intercornual
 intercostal
 intercuneiform
 interdigital
 interfoveolar
 intermetatarsal
 internal collateral
 interosseous
 intersesamoid
 interspinal
 interspinous
 intertransverse
 intervertebral
 intra-articular
 intrascapular

ligament *(cont.)*
 ischiocapsular
 ischiofemoral
 Jarjavay
 jugal
 Krause
 laciniate
 lacunar
 Landsmeer
 Lannelongue
 lateral arcuate
 lateral collateral (LCL)
 Lauth
 lienophrenic
 lienorenal
 limited proteoglycan matrix of
 Lisfranc
 Lockwood
 longitudinal
 LTC (lateral talocalcaneal)
 lumbocostal
 lunotriquetral
 Luschka
 Mackenrodt
 macroscopic hemorrhage
 Maissiat
 Mauchart
 Meckel
 medial collateral (MCL)
 median arcuate
 meniscofemoral
 meniscotibial
 metacarpoglenoidal
 metacarpophalangeal
 microscopic hemorrhage of
 mucosal suspensory
 natatory
 naviculocuneiform
 nuchal
 occipital-atlas-axis
 occipitoaxial
 odontoid

**ligament**

ligament *(cont.)*
  orbicular
  ovarian
  palmar
  pectinate
  pectineal
  peridental
  periodontal
  peritoneal
  Petit
  Pétrequin
  petroclinoid
  phalangeal glenoidal
  phrenicocolic
  phrenicoesophageal
  phrenicolienal
  phrenicosplenic
  phrenoesophageal
  phrenogastric
  phrenosplenic
  pisohamate
  pisometacarpal
  pisounciform
  pisouncinate
  plantar
  posterior cruciate (PCL)
  posterior longitudinal (PLL)
  posterior oblique (POL)
  Poupart
  pterygomandibular
  pterygospinal
  pterygospinous
  pubocapsular
  pubocervical
  pubofemoral
  puboprostatic
  pubovesical
  pulmonary
  quadrate
  radial collateral
  radial metacarpal
  radiate sternocostal

ligament *(cont.)*
  radiocarpal
  radiolunotriquetral
  radioscaphocapitate
  radioscaphoid
  radioscapholunate
  reflected inguinal
  reflecting edge of
  retinacular
  Retzius
  rhomboid
  right triangular
  ring
  Robert
  round
  Rouviere
  sacrodural
  sacrospinous
  sacrotuberous
  Santorini
  Sappey
  scapholunate
  Schlemm
  serous
  sesamoid
  sesamophalangeal
  sheath
  Simonart
  Soemmerring
  sphenomandibular
  spinoglenoid
  spiral
  splenocolic
  splenorenal
  spring
  Stanley cervical
  stellate
  sternoclavicular
  sternopericardial
  stretched out
  Struthers
  stylohyoid

**ligament** *(cont.)*
- stylomandibular
- stylomaxillary
- superficial dorsal sacrococcygeal
- superficial posterior sacrococcygeal
- superficial transverse metacarpal
- superficial transverse metatarsal
- superior costotransverse
- superior pubic
- superior transverse scapular
- suprascapular
- supraspinous
- suspensory
- sutural
- syndesmotic
- synovial
- talocalcaneal
- talofibular
- talonavicular
- tarsal
- tarsometatarsal
- tectoral
- temporomandibular
- Teutleben
- Thompson
- thyroepiglottic
- thyrohyoid
- tibial collateral
- tibial sesamoid
- tibiocalcaneal
- tibiofibular
- tibionavicular
- torn meniscotibial
- transverse atlantal
- transverse carpal
- transverse crural
- transverse genicular
- transverse humeral
- transverse intertarsal
- transverse metacarpal
- transverse metatarsal
- transverse perineal

**ligament** *(cont.)*
- transverse tibiofibular
- trapezoid
- Treitz
- triangular
- triquetrohamate
- Tuffier inferior
- ulnar collateral (UCL)
- ulnocarpal
- ulnolunate
- ulnotriquetral
- umbilical
- urachal
- uterine
- uterosacral
- uterovesical
- vaginal (of fingers and toes)
- venous
- ventral sacrococcygeal
- ventral sacroiliac
- ventricular
- vertebropelvic
- vesicoumbilical
- vesicouterine
- vestibular
- vocal
- volar
- volar carpal
- Walther oblique
- Weitbrecht
- Winslow
- Wrisberg
- xiphicostal
- xiphoid
- Y-shaped
- Zaglas
- Zinn

**ligament laxity**
**ligamentous bouncing**
**ligamentous box**
**ligamentous complex**
**ligamentous disruption**

ligamentous impingement
ligamentous insertion
ligamentous instability
ligamentous laxity
ligamentous luxation
ligamentous support
ligamentous thickening
ligand, neuroreceptor
light leak
light microscopy
light source, fiberoptic
lightbox, CCD
LILI (low-intensity laser irradiation)
Lilliequist membrane
LIMA (left internal mammary artery) graft
limb absence
limb asymmetry
limb bud
limb of bifurcation graft
limitation of joint motion
limitations, bandwidth
limited compression
limited films
limited view
limits, amplitude
line
  anorectal
  anterior humeral
  aortic
  axillary
  branching
  calcification
  central sacral (CSL)
  Correra
  costoclavicular
  costophrenic septal
  curvilinear subpleural
  CVP (central venous pressure)
  Ellis
  Ellis-Garland
  epiphyseal

line *(cont.)*
  fat
  Feiss
  fracture
  gas density
  gluteal
  growth arrest
  iliopectineal
  isodose
  isoelectric
  isopotential
  joint
  Kerley A
  Kerley B
  Kerley C
  Kilian
  Köhler
  lateral joint
  Linton
  Lorentzian
  lower lung
  low-intensity
  lucent
  medial joint
  median
  Meyer
  midaxillary
  midclavicular (MCL)
  midscapular
  midspinal
  midsternal
  Moyer
  Nélaton
  orthogonal tag
  parallel pitch
  pectinate
  photon therapy beam
  pleural
  popliteal
  posterior axillary
  pubococcygeal
  radiocapitellar

line *(cont.)*
   raster
   reference
   resonance
   Schoemaker
   semilunar
   Shenton
   soleal
   subcutaneous fat
   subpleural curvilinear
   Ullman
   vertebral body
   Wagner
   white (linea alba)
linea alba
linear absorption coefficient
linear accelerator isocenter motion
linear accelerator (LINAC, linac)
   radiosurgery
linear amplifier
linear and depressed skull fracture
linear array
   Acuson 5 MHz
   convex
   high-density
linear-array-hydrophone assembly
linear artifact
linear attenuation coefficient
linear band of maximal radiolucency
linear defect
linear density
linear fracture
linear infiltrate
linear interpolation
linearity
linearization, perceptual
linear lucency
linear markings
linear opacity
linear phased arrays
linear scanning
linear shadow

linear skull fracture
linear streaks en face
linear tomography
line imaging
line placement
line saturation
   gaussian
   Lorentzian
line scanning
line shadow
line-shape sensitivity
line width
lingual bone
lingual thyroid
linguine sign in breast
lingula pulmonis
lingular artery
lingular bronchus
lingular mandibular bony defects
   (LMBD)
lingular nodule
lingular orifice
link, musculotendinous-osseous
Linton shunt
Linx exchange guide wire
lipid-laden plaque
lipid-lowering therapy
lipid-rich material
lipid-sensitive MR
lipid signal
lipid zone
Lipiodol (iodized poppy seed oil)
   myelographic imaging agent
liplike projections of cartilage
lipofibroma
lipoid pneumonia
lipoma
   cardiac
   filar
   intratentorial
lipomatous hypertrophy of interatrial
   septum

liponecrosis
lipophilic contrast agents
lipophilic sequestration system
liposarcoma of heart
liposomes, antibody-conjugated
  paramagnetic (APCLs)
lipping, osteophytic
liquefactive emphysema
liquid crystal contact thermography
  (LCT)
liquid crystal thermogram
liquid pleural effusion
liquid scintillation analysis
liquid scintillation spectrometer
Liquipake contrast medium
Lisfranc dislocation
Lisfranc fracture
Lisfranc joint
Lissauer column
lissencephaly, cobblestone
list mode data collection
Lister tubercle
liters per minute per meter squared
  (L/min./m$^2$)
lithiasis, renal (also renolithiasis)
lithium
lithogenic bile
litholysis
Lithostar nonimmersion lithotriptor
lithotripsy
  laser
  ultrasonic
lithotriptor (also lithotripter)
lithotriptor with fluoroscopic and
  ultrasound localization
LITT (laser-induced thermotherapy)
Litten diaphragm phenomenon
Littre hernia
Litzmann obliquity
liver
  alcoholic fatty
  biliary cirrhotic

liver *(cont.)*
  capsule of
  caudate lobe of
  centrilobular region of
  cirrhosis of
  cirrhotic
  degenerative
  degraded
  diaphragmatic surface of
  dome of
  duodenal impression on
  echogenic
  enlarged
  fatty
  floating
  frosted
  hobnail
  infantile
  large-droplet fatty
  left lobe of
  metastasis to
  nodular
  noncirrhotic
  polycystic
  polylobar
  potato
  prominent
  pyogenic
  quadrate lobe of
  renal impression on
  right lobe of
  shrunken
  small-droplet fatty
  stasis (in cirrhosis)
  undersurface of
  visceral surface of
  wandering
  waxy
liver/aorta (L/A) peak ratio
liver bed
liver coil
liver edge

liver flap
liver function
liver hydatid disease
liver-jugular sign
liver, kidneys, and spleen (LKS)
liverlike lung
liver/liver peak (L/LP) ratio
liver parenchyma
liver scan, radionuclide
liver scintiphotograph
liver span
liver-spleen scan
Livingston triangle
LKS (liver, kidneys, and spleen)
LLD (leg length discrepancy)
LLD (limb length discrepancy)
LLE (left lower extremity)
LLQ (left lower quadrant)
L-loop heart
L-looping
L-loop ventricular situs
L/LP (liver/liver peak) ratio
L-malposition of aorta
LMCA (left main coronary artery)
L/min./m² (liters per minute per meter squared)
LMP (last menstrual period)
LMR (localized magnetic resonance)
LNV (last normal vertebra)
loading
    differential
    peripheral
    spike
    uniform
loading dose
lobar bronchus (pl. bronchi)
lobar cavitation
lobar consolidation
lobar emphysema
lobar lung atrophy
lobar pneumonia

lobe
    anterior tip of temporal
    azygos vein
    caudate (of liver)
    collapsed
    cuneiform
    falciform
    fetal
    flocculonodular (of cerebellum)
    frontal
    inferior
    insular
    left
    limbic
    lower
    medial temporal
    middle
    occipital
    orbital aspect of frontal
    parietal
    polyalveolar
    pulmonary
    pyramidal
    quadrate
    Riedel
    right
    sequestered (lung)
    superior
    temporal
    thyroid
    uncus of temporal
    upper
lobe of azygos vein
lobectomy
lobster-claw deformity
lobular architecture of liver
lobulated border
lobulated filling defect
lobulated saccular appearance
lobule
local compression fracture

localization
  autoradiographic
  CT-directed hook wire
  off-axis point
  wire
localization grid
localized H1 spectroscopy
localized magnetic resonance (LMR)
localized mass effect
localized obstructive emphysema
localizer, breast
localizing images
lock washer configuration
loco-regional hyperthermia
locomotor pattern
loculated effusion on chest x-ray
loculated fluid collection
loculated pleural effusion
locus, scanning
Loeffler (Löffler)
Loeffler endocarditis
Loehr-Kindberg syndrome
Löffler (Loeffler)
Löfgren syndrome
Lohlein diameter
LOM (low osmolar media)
L1-L5 (five lumbar vertebrae)
L1-APo cephalometric measurement
L1-L6 intervertebral disks
L1-NB cephalometric measurement
long ACE fixed-wire balloon catheter
long-acting thyroid stimulator (LATS)
long axial oblique view
long axis acquisition
long axis parasternal view
long axis slice
long axis view
Long Beach stereotactic robot
long bone
long bone fracture
long bore collimator
long fibers of the posterior talofibular ligament

long segment narrowing
Long Skinny over-the-wire balloon catheter
long taper/stiff shaft Glidewire (coronary artery imaging)
long TR, short TE
long TR/TE (T2 weighted image)
long tract signs
long wavelength photolabel
long-standing
Longdwel Teflon catheter
longitudinal arch of foot
longitudinal arteriography
longitudinal B-mode
longitudinal blood supply to ulnar nerve
longitudinal fasciculus, medial (MLF)
longitudinal fissure
longitudinal fracture
longitudinal lie
longitudinally
longitudinal magnetization
longitudinal muscles
longitudinal narrowing
longitudinal relaxation
longitudinal taenia musculature
longitudinal ultrasonic biometry
loop
  afferent
  air-filled
  alpha sigmoid
  bowel
  capillary
  cervical
  closed
  closed conducting
  colonic
  contiguous
  diathermic
  dilated bowel
  double reverse alpha sigmoid
  duodenal

loop *(cont.)*
  efferent
  flow-volume
  gamma transverse colon
  Gerdy interatrial
  Gerdy interauricular
  Henle
  intestinal
  J (on catheterization)
  jejunal
  lenticular
  Meyer
  Meyer-Archambault
  N-shaped sigmoid
  P (on vectorcardiography)
  peduncular
  pressure-volume
  puborectalis
  reentrant
  rubber vessel
  sentinel
  sigmoid
  small-bowel
  Stoerck
  subclavian
  T (on vectorcardiography)
  transverse colon
  vector
  ventricular
  vessel
  Vieussens
loop ostomy bridge
loopogram (ileostogram)
loose fracture
loose joint body
Looser-Milkman syndrome
Lo-Por tracheal tube
Lo-Profile and Lo-Profile II balloon
  catheter
Lorad M-II D mammographic system
Lorad StereoGuide stereotactic breast
  biopsy system

lordosis
  cervical
  lumbar
  reversal of
  thoracic
lordotic curve
lordotic position
lordotic view
Lorentzian line saturation
loss, electron equilibrium
loss of definition
loss of sigmoid curve
loss of thoracic kyphosis
lossy algorithm
Louis, sternal angle of
low angle scattering
low angle shot (flash) technique
low attenuation pulsation artifact
Low-Beers view
low cardiac output syndrome
low-contrast film
low-contrast structure
low-density lesion
low-density structure
low-dose film mammographic
  technique
low-dose folinic acid
low-dose screen-film technique
low-dose mammography
low-energy collimator
low-energy photon attenuation
  measurement
low-energy radiofrequency conduction
  hyperthermia treatment
lower esophageal sphincter (LES)
lower extremity noninvasive (LENI)
lower left sternal border
lower lobe lung mass
lower lung field
lower pole collecting system
lower pole of kidney
lower pole of patella

lower pole ureter
Lower (Richard Lower)
   Lower rings
   Lower tubercle
low-field MR angiography
low-field MR imaging
low-field-strength MR imaging
low-flow syndrome
low-intensity laser irradiation (LILI)
low-intensity pulsed ultrasound
low-level echo
low osmolality
low-osmolar contrast media
low-output heart failure
low-pressure cardiac tamponade
low signal intensity
low-speed rotational angioplasty
   catheter
low temperature diffraction
low urethral pressure (LUP)
low-velocity flow
Lown-Ganong-Levine syndrome
   (LGL)
LPA (left pulmonary artery)
LPO (left posterior oblique) position
LPS balloon catheter
LPS Peel-Away introducer
LPV (left pulmonary vein)
LRA (low right atrium)
LS (lumbosacral) spine
LSB (lower sternal border)
LSC background prediction
LSCVP (left subclavian central
   venous pressure)
LSD-image (line scan diffusion
   imaging)
L-transposition (levotransposition)
   of great arteries
L-tyrosine ($^{11}$C) imaging agent
lucency
   interspersed
   linear

lucent defect
Lucey-Driscoll syndrome
lucite beam spoiler
Ludovici angle
Ludwig angle
luetic aortitis
luetic arteritis
Lugol solution
Lukes-Collins classification of
   lymphoma
Lumaguide catheter
lumbar artery
lumbar pneumencephalography
lumbar scoliosis
lumbar spine view
lumbar transverse process
lumbar vertebra
lumbarization
lumbosacral kyphosis
lumbosacral series
lumbosacral spine
lumen (pl. lumens, lumina)
   aortic
   arterial
   attenuated
   bile duct
   bowel
   bronchial
   clot-filled
   cloverleaf-shaped
   crescentic
   cystic duct
   D-shaped vessel
   double-barrel
   duct
   duodenal
   eccentrically placed
   elliptical
   esophageal
   false
   gastroduodenal
   intestinal

lumen *(cont.)*
   occluded
   patent
   slitlike
   slit-shaped vessel
   star-shaped vessel
   true
   vascular
lumen-intimal interface
lumenogram
lumina (pl. of lumen)
luminal area
luminal caliber
luminal configuration, scalloped
luminal contour, irregular hazy
luminal cross-sectional area
luminal diameter
luminal dimension
luminal encroachment
luminal irregularity
luminal narrowing
luminal plaquing
luminal silhouette
luminal stenosis
luminal thrombosis
luminance
luminogram, air
luminol
Lumiscan scanner
lumpy appearance of lung
Lunar DPX densitometer
Lunar Expert densitometer
Lunar scanner
lunate bone
lunate dislocation
lunatomalacia
lung
   acquired unilateral hyperlucent
   air-conditioner
   airless
   arc welder's
   artificial
   atelectatic

lung *(cont.)*
   bauxite
   bird breeder's
   bird fancier's
   bird handler's
   black
   brown
   bubbly
   budgerigar-fancier's
   cardiac
   cheese handler's
   cheese washer's
   coal miner's
   coal worker's
   coffee worker's
   collapsed
   consolidated
   cork handler's
   cork worker's
   corundum smelter's
   dark and mottled
   drowned
   dynamic
   emphysematous
   empty collapsed
   eosinophilic
   expanded
   farmer's
   fibrinoid
   fibroid
   fibrosis of
   fish-meal worker's
   fissures of
   fresh
   furrier's
   gangrene of
   grain handler's
   hardened
   harvester's
   hemorrhagic consolidation of
   hen worker's
   hilum of
   honeycomb

**lung**

lung *(cont.)*
  humidifier
  hyperlucent
  hypogenetic
  hypoplastic
  light pink
  liverlike
  malt worker's
  maple bark-stripper's
  mason's
  meat wrapper's
  miller's
  mottled gray
  mushroom worker's
  pigeon-breeder's
  pigeon-fancier's
  premature infant's
  pump
  rheumatoid
  root of
  rudimentary
  septic
  shock
  shrunken
  silicotic
  silo-filler's
  silver finisher's
  silver polisher's
  smoker's
  static
  stiff noncompliant
  stretched
  subsegment of
  thatched roof worker's
  thresher's
  tropical eosinophilic
  underventilated
  unilateral hyperlucent
  vanishing
  welder's
  well-inflated
  wet
  white

lung abscess
lung agenesis
lung air spaces
lung apex (pl. apices)
lung architecture
lung base
lung calculus
lung carcinoma
lung cirrhosis
lung collapse
lung consolidation
lung count curve
lung disease, interstitial
lung expansion
lung field
lung fissure
lung/heart ratio of thallium 201 activity
lung hemangioma
lung hepatization
lung hypoplasia
lung infiltrate (infiltration)
lung inflammation
lung injury, penetrating
lung lobule
lung lymphoid hyperplasia
lung markings
lung mass with mediastinal invasion
lung necrosis
lung opacity
lung overexpansion
lung overinflation
lung parenchyma consolidation
lung periphery
lung reexpansion
lung scan, perfusion and ventilation
lung segment, infarcted
lung segmentation
lung stiffness
lung transplantation
lung underinflation
lung washout

lung zone
lunula (pl. lunulae)
LUP (low urethral pressure)
LUQ (left upper quadrant)
Luque rod used in spinal fusion for scoliosis
Luque sublaminar wire used in spinal fusion for scoliosis
LUS (laparoscopic ultrasound)
Luschka crypts of gallbladder mucosa
Luschka, joint of
Luschka muscle
Lutembacher complex
Lutembacher syndrome
luxated bone
luxation
Luxtec fiberoptic system for diagnostic and surgical visualization
luxury perfusion
LV (left ventricular) function pressure
LV (left ventricular) function wall motion
LVAD (left ventricular assist device), HeartMate
LVAS (left ventricular assist system), Novacor
LVdd (left ventricular diastolic dimension)
LVD (left ventricular dysfunction)
LVEDD (left ventricular end-diastolic dimension)
LVEDI (left ventricular end-diastolic volume index)
LVEDP (left ventricular end-diastolic pressure)
LVEF (left ventricular ejection fraction)
LVESD (left ventricular end-systolic dimension)
LVESVI (left ventricular end-systolic volume index)
LVET (left ventricular ejection time)
LVFS (left ventricular functional shortening)
LVFW (left ventricular free wall)
LVG (left ventriculogram)
LVH (left ventricular hypertrophy) with strain
LVID (left ventricular internal diameter) (or dimension)
LVIDd (left ventricular internal dimension at end-diastole)
LVIDD (left ventricular internal diastolic dimension)
LVIDs (left ventricular internal dimension at end-systole)
LVIV (left ventricular inflow volume)
LVM (left ventricular mass)
LVMI (left ventricular mass index)
LVOT (left ventricular outflow tract)
LVOTO (left ventricular outflow tract obstruction)
LVOV (left ventricular outflow volume)
LVP (left ventricular pressure)
LVP1 and LVP2 (left ventricular pressure on apex cardiogram)
LVPW (left ventricular posterior wall)
LVs (left ventricular systolic) dimension
LVS (left ventricular support) system
LVS (left ventricular systolic) pressure
LVSW (left ventricular stroke work)
LVSWI (left ventricular stroke work index)
LVW (left ventricular wall)
lym-1 monoclonal antibody labeled with iodine-131 ($^{131}$I)
Lyme carditis
Lyme disease
lymphangiographic contrast
lymphangiography
lymphangioma, cardiac

lymphangitic carcinomatosis
lymphangitic metastasis
lymphatic cachexia
lymphatic channels
lymphatic drainage
lymphatic duct
lymphatic malformation (LM)
lymphaticovenous malformation (LVM)
lymphatic system
lymphatic vessel
Lymphazurin (isosulfan blue) contrast medium
lymph capillaries
lymph gland
lymph node (see *node*)
lymph node enlargement
lymph node metastases
lymph node syndrome
lymphoblastoma
lymphocytic infiltrate
lymphocytic interstitial pneumonitis (LIP)
lymphocytic splenomegaly, postcardiotomy
lymphogenous dissemination
lymphogenous metastasis
lymphography, time-lapse quantitative computed tomography
lymphoid interstitial pneumonia
lymphoma
  adult T-cell
  African
  B-cell
  B-cell monocytoid
  Burkitt
  centrocytic
  cleaved cell
  diffuse
  diffuse large cell
  diffuse mixed small and large cell
  diffuse small cleaved cell

lymphoma *(cont.)*
  follicular center cell
  follicular mixed small cleaved
  follicular predominantly large cell
  follicular predominantly small cell
  giant follicle
  granulomatous
  histiocytic
  Hodgkin
  infiltrative
  intermediate lymphocytic
  large cell, immunoblastic
  large cleaved cell
  large noncleaved cell
  Lennert
  lymphoblastic
  lymphocytic plasmacytoid
  lymphocytic poorly differentiated
  lymphocytic well differentiated
  malignant
  mantle zone
  Mediterranean
  mixed lymphocytic-histiocytic
  multifocal
  nodular
  noncleaved cell
  non-Hodgkin
  pleomorphic
  polypoid
  primary of central nervous system
  small B-cell
  small cleaved cell
  small lymphocytic
  small noncleaved cell
  T-cell
    convoluted
    cutaneous
    small lymphocytic
  U-cell (undefined)
  ulcerative
  undefined
  undifferentiated

lymphonodular hyperplasia
lymphoproliferative disorder,
    intrathoracic
lymphosarcoma
LymphoScan nuclear imaging system
lymphoscintigraphy, radiocolloid
lymph vessels of thymus gland

Lynch and Crues Type 2 lesion on
    MRI scan
lyoluminescence
lytic (osteolytic) lesion
lytic area
lytic bone lesion
lytic change

# M, m

m (meta-stable) (in technetium $^{99m}$Tc)
m (meter)
m/sec (meters per second)
mA (milliampere)
mA/kV (milliamperes per kilovolt)
MAA ($^{99m}$Tc MAA) (macroaggregated albumin)
Mab-170 monoclonal antibody
MAC (mitral annular calcium)
Macalister muscle
machine, parallel virtual
Machlett collimator
Mackenzie point
MacLean-Maxwell disease
Macleod syndrome
macroadenoma, prolactin-secreting pituitary
macroaggregated albumin
macrocolon
macrofistulous AV (arteriovenous) communications
macromolecular contrast-enhanced MR imaging
macromolecular drugs
macronodular pattern
macroscopic magnetization vector
Macrotec imaging agent
MacSpect real-time NMR station
Maddahi method of calculating right ventricular ejection fraction
Madelung deformity
Maffucci syndrome
Magendie, foramen of
magic angle artifact
magic angle spinning NMR
Magna-SL scanner
Magnes biomagnetometer system
magnet
  doughnut
  GE Signa 1.5T
  Magnex
  non-enclosed
  open
  Oxford
  pancake MRI
  passively shimmed superconducting
  shim
  shimmed
  superconducting
  tubular
  2T large bore
magnet mode
magnet rate
magnet response

magnetic dipole
magnetic field gradients (MFG)
magnetic field, oscillating
magnetic moment
magnetic particulates
magnetic resonance (MR) (see also *magnetic resonance imaging*)
magnetic resonance angiography (MRA)
   echo planar
   gated inflow
   low-field
magnetic resonance angiography-directed bypass procedure
magnetic resonance arthrography
magnetic resonance catheter imaging and spectroscopy system
magnetic resonance cholangiography (MRC)
magnetic resonance cholangiography with HASTE
magnetic resonance cholangiopancreatography
magnetic resonance elastography (MRE)
magnetic resonance enhancement pattern
magnetic resonance epidurography
magnetic resonance H-1 stimulated-echo acquisition mode spectroscopy
magnetic resonance imaging (MRI) (see *imaging*)
   MRI-guided breast biopsy
   MRI-guided focused ultrasound transducer
   MRI-guided laser-induced interstitial
   MRI-guided thermotherapy
   MRI mapping
   MRI morphometry
   MRI prescan
   MRI probe head
   MRI segmentation
   MRI transducer

magnetic resonance mammography (MRM)
magnetic resonance myelography
magnetic resonance needle tracking
magnetic resonance neurography (MRN)
magnetic resonance phase velocity mapping
magnetic resonance phlebography
magnetic resonance receptor agents
magnetic resonance sialography
magnetic resonance signal
magnetic resonance simulator
magnetic resonance spectroscopy (MRS)
magnetic resonance spin incoherence
magnetic resonance system, open-configuration
magnetic resonance urography (MRU)
magnetic resonance velocity mapping
magnetic resonance venography
magnetic resonance volume estimation
magnetic source imaging (MSI)
magnetic susceptibility artifact (MRI)
magnetism
magnetite albumin contrast
magnetization
   longitudinal
   net tissue
   spatial modulation
magnetization and spin-lock transfer imaging
magnetization imaging
magnetization-prepared rapid gradient echo-water excitation (MRPRAGE-WE)
magnetization transfer (MT)
   high-power, thin-section quantitative
   quantitative
magnetization transfer contrast
magnetization transfer effect
magnetization transfer ratio (MTR)

magnetization-prepared 3D gradient-
    echo (MP-RAGE) sequences
magnetoacoustic MRI
magnetoencephalogram
magnetoencephalography (MEG)
magnetogyric ratio
Magnetom 1.5T scanner
Magnetom SP MRI imager
Magnetom SP63 scanner
Magnetom Vision MR system
magnetometer probe
magnetoresistive sensor circuit
Magnevist imaging agent
Magnex Alpha MR system
Magnex MR scanner
magnification
    high-resolution
    signal
magnification and spot compression
magnification error
magnification mammography
magnitude
Mahaim and James fibers
Mahaim bundles
Mahler sign
mahogany flush
main bronchus
main energy substrate
main fissure
main glow peak
main magnetic field inhomogeneity
    artifact
main portal vein peak velocities
    (MPPv)
main pulmonary artery
main sac
main stem bronchus
main stem carina
Maisonneuve fibular fracture
Majocchi disease
major fracture fragment
major histocompatability complex
    class II antigen (MHC-2)

Mal de Meleda syndrome
maladie de Roger (Roger disease)
malaligned atrioventricular septal
    defects
malalignment
malangulation
malar bone
Malcolm-Lynn C-RXF cervical
    retractor frame
maldevelopment
maldistribution of ventilation and
    perfusion
Malecot catheter
malformation
    adenomatoid
    anorectal
    Arnold-Chiari
    Arnold-Chiari (type II)
    arteriovenous (AVM)
    cavernous
    Chiari II
    congenital
    coronary artery
    cystic adenomatoid
    dancer foot
    Dandy-Walker
    Dieulafoy vascular
    Ebstein
    endocardial cushion
    familial cavernous
    fast-flow
    septal
    sink-trap
    slow-flow vascular
    valve
    vascular
malformed phlebectasia in the calf
Malgaigne fracture
malignancy
    aggressive
    borderline
    grading of

malignancy *(cont.)*
  high-grade
  low-grade
  metastatic
  primary
  secondary
  staging of
malignancy threshold
malignant acetabular osteolysis
malignant airway obstruction
malignant degeneration
malignant fibrous histiocytoma
malignant hemangioendothelioma
malignant lymphoma
malignant mesothelioma
malignant mixed tumor
malignant nephrosclerosis
malignant osteoid
malignant osteopetrosis
malignant pleomorphic adenoma
malignant pleural implants
malignant pleural mesothelioma
malignant teratoma
malleolar
malleolus (pl. malleoli)
  lateral
  medial
malleolus fibulae
malleolus tibiae
mallet finger
Mallinckrodt angiographic catheter
Mallinckrodt imaging agent
Mallinckrodt scanner
Mallory-Weiss mucosal tear
malperfused
malperfusion
malpighian vesicle
malposition of heart
malpositioned fetus
malrotation of intestine
malt worker's lung

malum coxae senile
malum perforans pedis
malunion of fracture fragments
malunited
Mamex DC mammography
mamillary body
mammalation
mammary-coronary artery bypass
mammary ductogram
mammary galactogram
mammary implant
Mammo QC
mammogram (see *mammography*)
mammographic features
mammographic-histopathologic
  correlation
mammographic measurement
mammographic parenchymal patterns,
  Wolfe
mammography
  baseline
  computed tomographic
  contoured tilting compression
  CT laser (CTLM)
  digital
  Egan
  high-resolution CT
  low-dose
  magnetic resonance (MRM)
  magnification
  Mamex DC
  Mammo QC
  Mammomat B
  microfocal spot
  radionuclide
  screen-film
  screening
  ultra-high magnification (UHMM)
  ultrasound augmented
  xero-
  x-ray (XMG)
Mammotest breast biopsy system

mandible
  alveolar border of
  angle of
mandibular canal
mandibular incisor angle, Frankfort
mandibular notch
mandibulofacial dysostosis
maneuver (pl. maneuvers)
  Adson
  costoclavicular
  flexion
  Heineke-Mikulicz
  hyperabduction
  Kocher
  Müller (Mueller)
  Osler
  Rivero-Carvallo
  scalene
  squatting
  transabdominal left lateral
    retroperitoneal
  Valsalva
mangafodipir trisodium imaging agent
manganese (Mn)
  Mn Cl (chloride) imaging agent
  Mn-DPDP (dipyridoxal diphos-
    phate) imaging agent
  Mn PcS4 imaging agent
  Mn-SOD
  Mn-TPPS
Mani catheter
manifest
manifestations, extrapulmonary
Mann-Bollman fistula
Mannkopf sign
Mann-Whitney test
manofluorography (MFG)
manometer-tipped cardiac catheter
manometric pattern
manometry
  anal
  aneroid

manometry *(cont.)*
  anorectal
  biliary
  ERCP
  esophageal
  rectosigmoid
  sphincter of Oddi
Mansfield Atri-Pace catheter
Mansfield orthogonal electrode
  catheter
Manson schistosomiasis-pulmonary
  artery obstruction syndrome
mantle
  anechoic
  hypoechoic
mantle block
mantle complex
mantle field
manual computed method
manual pressure over carotid sinus
manual subtraction films
manubriosternal joint
manubriosternal syndrome
manubrium
map
  acceleration
  bull's-eye
  bull's-eye polar
  color flow
  cylindrical
  cylindrical projection
  decimalized variance
  end-diastolic polar
  end-systolic polar
  sestamibi polar
  spherical
MAP (mean arterial pressure)
map-guided partial endocardial
  ventriculotomy
maple bark stripper's lung
maple bark worker's suberosis
maple syrup urine disease

mapper, brain
mapping
  activation-sequence
  body surface
  body surface potential
  brain
  catheter
  Doppler color flow
  electrophysiologic
  endocardial activation
  endocardial catheter
  epicardial
  FMRI
  homology
  ice
  intramural
  intraoperative electrocortical stimulation
  K-space velocity
  MR (magnetic resonance) velocity
  MRI (magnetic resonance imaging)
  pace
  parallel analog
  phase-shift velocity
  precordial
  retrograde atrial activation
  sinus rhythm
  spatial
  straight-line Hough transform (HT)
  2D pulsatility index
  2D resistance index mapping
mapping algorithms
mapping of cerebral sulci
mapping probe, hand-held
Marable syndrome
marantic clot
marantic thrombus
Marathon guiding catheter
march foot (fracture)
Marex MRI system
Marfan syndrome
marfanoid hypermobility syndrome

margin
  cardiac
  colon
  convex
  cortical
  costal
  disk
  obtuse
  scapular
  stomach
marginal artery of Drummond
marginal branch
marginal circumflex bypass
marginal osteophyte formation
marginal placenta
marginal serration
marginal spur
marginal ulcer
marginal vein
Marie-Bamberger disease
Marie-Tooth disease
Marie-Strümpell disease
Marine-Lenhart syndrome
markedly accentuated pulmonic component
marker
  implanted imaging opaque
  lead pellet
  nipple
  radioactive string
  radiopaque
marker-channel diagram
marker transit study
markings
  bronchovascular
  bronchovesicular
  coarse bronchovascular
  haustral
  increased pulmonary vascular
  linear
  peribronchial
  pulmonary vascular
  vascular

Markov chain Monte Carlo technique
Markov random field
Markov source model
Maroteaux-Lamy syndrome
marrow, bone
marrow edema pattern
Marshall, vein of
Martin disease
Martorell aortic arch syndrome
Martorell-Fabre syndrome
Martorell hypertensive ulcer
Mary Allen Engle ventricle
MAS (Morgagni-Adams-Stokes) syndrome
masculinizing tumor
mask (pl. masks)
  convolution
  ISAH stereotactic immobilizing
  Orfit
mask-based approach
masking
mask ventilation
mason's lung
masquerading effect
mass
  abdominal
  adnexal
  airless
  appendiceal
  apperceptive
  calcified
  cavitary
  conical
  cordlike
  cystic
  discrete
  doughy
  echogenic
  elongated
  encapsulated
  enhancing
  exophytic

mass *(cont.)*
  expansile
  extraovarian
  firm
  fixed
  fleecy
  fluctuant
  fluid
  fluid-filled
  focal
  high signal
  hilar
  hyperdense
  hyperintense
  hypodense
  ill-defined
  injection
  interbronchial
  intermediate signal
  intra-abdominal
  intracardiac
  intracavity
  intraluminal
  intraventricular
  irregular
  left ventricular (LVM)
  lobulated
  low attenuation
  low-density
  lower lobe lung
  low signal
  mediastinal
  mixed echogenic solid
  mixed signal
  molar
  nodular
  nonpulsatile abdominal
  paracardiac
  perirenal
  polypoid calcified irregular
  pulsatile
  relativistic

mass *(cont.)*
   right ventricular (RVM)
   saccular
   signal
   soft tissue
   solid
   solitary
   space-occupying
   spherical
   stony
   suspicious
   ventricular
mass attenuation coefficient
mass balance
mass effect
mass lesion
mass-like configuration
Massachusetts (General Hospital) Utility Multiprogramming System (MUMPS)
massage, carotid sinus
masseter muscle
massive ascites
massive edema
massive effusion
massive embolism (embolization)
Master syndrome
Master two-step exercise stress test
masticator muscle
masticator space
mastoid polytomography
mastoid sinus
match
   non-transmural
   transmural
   triple
match-line wedge
Match 35 PTA catheter
matched V/Q defect
matching
   atlas
   electron-photon field
   general pattern

mater (not *matter*)
   dura
   pia
material
   atheromatous
   contrast
   inspissated
matrix (pl. matrices)
   bone
   calcific
   cartilage
   chondroid
   germinal
   image
   solid
   transformation
Matrix LR3300 laser imaging
matter
   cortical gray
   cortical white
   gray
   white
maturation, disk
mature pseudocyst of pancreas
Maugeri syndrome
Max Plus MR scanner
maxillary sinus
maxillary spine
maximal volume (of left atrium)
maximal voluntary ventilation (MVV)
maximum amplitude constants
maximum diameter to minimum diameter ratio
maximum intensity pixel (MIP)
maximum intensity projection (MIP)
maximum intensity projection and source images
maximum likelihood algorithms
maximum predicted heart rate (MPHR)
maximum slew rate ramps
Maxwell 3D Field Simulator

Mayer view
Mazer stent
mazoplasia, cystic
MBF (myocardial blood flow)
MBIH catheter
MBq (megabecquerel)
McArdle syndrome
MCAT (myocardial contrast
   appearance time)
McBurney point
McCort sign
MCE (myocardial contrast
   echocardiography)
McGoon coronary perfusion catheter
mCi (millicurie)
McIntosh double-lumen catheter
MCL (midclavicular line)
MCLS (mucocutaneous lymph node
   syndrome)
MCP (metacarpophalangeal) joint
MCS (middle coronary sinus)
MCTC (metrizamide CT
   cisternogram)
MD-Gastroview contrast medium
MD-50 contrast medium
MD-60 contrast medium
MD-76 contrast medium
MEA syndromes IIa and IIb
Meadows syndrome
meal
   barium
   Boyden test
   double contrast barium
   Ewald test
   fatty
   isotope
   motor
   motor test
   opaque
   retention
   small bowel
   test

mean aortic pressure
mean arterial pressure (MAP)
mean atrial pressure
mean blood pressure
mean cardiac vector
mean circulatory filling pressure
mean circumferential fiber shortening
   rate (MCFSR)
mean free path
mean left atrial pressure
mean maximal expiratory flow
   (MMEF)
mean mitral valve gradient
mean pulmonary artery (MPA)
   pressure
mean pulmonary capillary pressure
   (MPCP)
mean pulmonary transit time
mean rate of circumferential
   shortening
mean right atrial pressure
mean-square error
mean time
mean vectors
mean venous pulsation
measurable endpoint
measure
   Hausdorff metric
   linear
   prophylactic
   root-mean-squared gradient
measurement
   attenuation (of photon)
   cardiac output
   cerebrospinal fluid flow
   Cerenkov
   diode
   excitation function
   4 T
   high-sensitivity
   intercomparison
   low-energy photon attenuation

measurement *(cont.)*
  mammographic
  morphometric
  nutation angle
  polarographic needle electrode
  rocking curve
  semiquantitative
  topographic
measurement and depiction in vivo
meatal segment
meat wrapper's lung
metacarpal-phalangeal (or metacarpo-phalangeal) (MCP) joint
mechanical augmentation
mechanical counterpulsation
mechanical dottering effect
mechanical insufflation
mechanical small bowel obstruction
mechanical thrombolysis
mechanical valve
mechanics, intramural
mechanism
  check-valve
  deglutition
  flap-valve
  Frank-Starling
  humeral
  internal retention
  pinchcock
  propulsive
  sphincteric
  swallowing
Meckel cave
Meckel diverticulitis
Meckel diverticulum
Meckel scan (scanning)
meconium plug
MEDDARS analysis system for cardiac catheterization
media (see *medium*)
media-adventitia interface
medial compartment
medially
medial rotation of viscera to right of midline
median arcuate ligament of diaphragm
median lethal dose
median level echos
median line
median sacral artery
mediastinal air
mediastinal border
mediastinal emphysema
mediastinal fat
mediastinal fibrosis
mediastinal fistula
mediastinal hernia
mediastinal invasion
mediastinal lung surface
mediastinal lymph node
mediastinal mass
mediastinal neoplasm
mediastinal node
mediastinal pleura
mediastinal prominence
mediastinal septum
mediastinal shift
mediastinal structures
mediastinal thickening
mediastinal tumor
mediastinal wedge
mediastinal widening
mediastinodiaphragmatic pleural reflection
mediastinum
  anterior
  deviated
  inferior
  middle
  posterior
  superior
  widened (or widening of)
mediastinum cerebelli
mediastinum cerebri

mediastinum displacement
medical cyclotron
medical linear accelerator
medication (see also *bowel prep*;
 *imaging agents*)
 ACE inhibitor
 AMI 227
 bromodeoxyuridine
 bromophenol blue
 Captopril
 Colonlite bowel prep
 CoLyte bowel prep
 dextrose 5% in water
 diazepam
 dihydroxyphenylalanine [DOPA]
 Dulcolax bowel prep
 EDTMP
 Emulsoil bowel prep
 enalaprilat ACE inhibitor
 etanidazole
 Ethiodol
 Evac-Q-Kit bowel prep
 Evac-Q-Kwik bowel prep
 ferric ammonium citrate-cellulose
  paste
 15-NH3
 5-chlorodeoxycytidine
 Fleet bowel prep
 furosemide
 glucagon
 GoLytely bowel prep
 indomethacin
 iophendylate
 isoflurane
 K4-81
 methyl methacrylate
 naloxone
 nicotinamide
 nimodipine
 nitrous oxide
 nonsteroidal antiphlogistics
 OCL bowel prep

medication *(cont.)*
 olsalazine
 P-32
 pentagastrin
 phenobarbital
 radiopharmaceutical
 Sincalide
 6FD
 somatostatin
 suppo-cire C
 tetramethylene
 Tridrate bowel prep
 U-235
 urokinase
 X-Prep bowel prep
 xylenol orange
medicine, photonic
Medigraphics analyzer
MedImage scanner
mediolateral oblique view
mediolateral stress
mediopatellar
MediPort implanted vascular access
 device
Medison scanner
Medi-Tech balloon catheter
medium (pl. media)
 contrast
 high osmolar (HOM)
 ionic contrast
 low osmolar (LOM)
 nonionic contrast media
 radiopaque
 tunica
Medrad contrast medium injector
Medrad Mrinnervu endorectal colon
 probe coil
medronate scan
Medspec MR imaging system
Medtronic balloon catheter
Medtronic Minix

Medtronic radiofrequency (RF)
  receiver
medulla (pl. medullas, medullae)
  adrenal
  lymphatic
  ovarian
  renal
  spinal
medulla oblongata
medullaris, conus
medullary canal
medullary nephrocalcinosis
medullary pyramids
medullary sponge kidney
medulloblastoma
Medweb clinical reporting system
MEDX gamma camera
Mees lines
MEG (magnetoencephalography)
megacolon
  acquired
  congenital
  idiopathic
  toxic
megacystis
megaduodenum
megaesophagus of achalasia
megahertz (MHz)
megalocystis
megaloureter
megarectum
megaureter
megavolt (MV)
megavoltage grid therapy
megavoltage radiation therapy
megavoltage treatment beams
meglumine diatrizoate imaging agent
meglumine imaging agent
meglumine iodipamide imaging agent
meglumine iothalamate imaging agent
meglumine iotroxate imaging agent
Meige lymphedema

Meigs capillaries
Meigs-Cass syndrome
Meigs disease
Meigs syndrome
Meissner plexus
melanin, leptomeningeal
melanoma, metastatic
melanosarcoma
melanosis, parenchymal neurocutaneous
melorheostosis of Leri
Melrose solution
Meltzer sign
membrane
  microporous
  mucous
  premature rupture of
  synovial
membranous septum
membranous subvalvular aortic
  stenosis
membranous urethra
membranous ventricular septal defect
memory-intensive algorithms
Memory-Vu angiographic catheter
MEN (multiple endocrine neoplasia)
Ménétrier disease
Mengert index in pelvimetry
meningeal hemorrhage
meningeal myelomatosis
meningioma
  cerebellopontine angle
  clival
  convexity
  cystic
  falcine
  falx
  fibroblastic
  fibrous
  malignant
  meningotheliomatous
  parasagittal

meningioma *(cont.)*
  posterior fossa
  suprasellar
  tentorial
  transitional
meniscal injury
meniscus
  articular
  diverging
meniscus (crescent) of contrast-saline mixture
meniscus articularis
meniscus lateralis
meniscus medialis
meniscus sign on upper GI study
meniscus (pl. menisci)
menses
menstrual age
menstrual date
mensuration algorithm
mental spine
mentoanterior
mentoposterior
mentum
Mercator projection
Mercedes Benz sign, reversed
mercury artifact
mercury-in-Silastic strain gauge
Meridian echocardiography
Merkell cell carcinoma cell lines
meroacrania
mesenchymoma
mesenteric angiography
mesenteric apoplexy
mesenteric arterial thrombosis
mesenteric artery occlusion
mesenteric infarction
mesenteric ischemia
mesenteric node
mesenteric rupture
mesenteric sclerosis

mesenteric tear
mesenteric venous thrombosis
mesenterium commune
mesentery
  fan-shaped
  fatty
  leaves of
  root of
  small intestine (SIM)
  ventral
mesial aspect
mesial hyperperfusion
mesial temporal sclerosis
meso-HMPAO
mesoappendix
mesoblastic nephroma
mesocardia
mesocaval anastomosis
mesocaval H-graft shunt
mesocolon
mesocolonic fat
mesocolonic vessels
mesocuneiform bone
mesoderm
  extraembryonic
  gastral
mesoderma
meson
mesorectum
mesosigmoid colon
mesosternum
mesothelial
mesothelioma
mesoversion of heart
Mester test for rheumatic disease
meta-analysis
metabolic 8-hydroxyquinolyl-glu-curonide
metabolic rate of oxygen
metabolic response
metabolic tracer uptake

metabolism
  cerebral
  fat
  fatty acid
  myocardial
metabolite
  $CMRO_2$ glucose
  phosphorus
metacarpal bone
metacarpophalangeal (or metacarpal-phalangeal) (MCP) joint
metaiodobenzylguanidine (MIBG) imaging agent
metal technetium target
metallic foreign body
metallic stent
metalloporphyrins
metaphyseal dysostosis
metaphyseal-epiphyseal angle
metaphyseal lucent bands
metaphysis (pl. metaphyses)
  agnogenic myeloid
  apocrine (of breast)
  autoparenchymatous
  celomic
  columnar
  fundic
  intestinal
  metaphyseal
  myeloid
  primary myeloid
  secondary myeloid
  squamous
metaplasia
  cartilaginous
  osteocartilaginous
metapneumonic empyema
metastasis (pl. metastases)
  air-space
  calcareous
  CX-1
  drop

metastasis *(cont.)*
  hematogenous
  local
  lymph node
  lymphangitic
  lymphatic
  micronodular
  neuroendocrine hepatic
  nodal
  osteoblastic
  osteolytic
  pulsating
  satellite
  white
  widespread
metastatic abscess
metastatic disease
metastatic tumor
metasynchronous tumor
metatarsal-phalangeal (or metatarso-phalangeal) (MTP) joint
metatarsal bone
metatarsal head
metatarsocuneiform joint
metatarsophalangeal (or metatarso-phalangeal) (MTP) joint
metatarsus adductocavus deformity
metatarsus adductus deformity
metatarsus atavicus deformity
metatarsus latus deformity
metatarsus primus varus deformity
metatarsus varus deformity
meter (m), rate
meter per second (m/sec; also mps) velocity
methionine
method (see also *technique*)
  Born
  calibration
  CHESS
  column extraction
  computer

method *(cont.)*
   DIET
   Dixon
   empirical
   Enhance deblurring
   error diffusion
   FBP (filtered back-projection)
   fixed grid stereologic
   fractal-based
   GLF lymphography
   in vivo
   IPSP neuron evaluation
   isocenter shift
   Joliot
   Kaplan-Meier
   manual computed
   multiple line scanning
   multiple sensitive point
   multisection
   NEUGAT (neutron/gamma transmission)
   neutron/gamma transmission (NEUGAT)
   PASTA
   Pfeiffer-Comberg
   phase-unwrapping
   radiotracer foil
   segmentation
   selective excitation
   selective saturation
   shock-monitoring
   spin-label
   stereologic
   sum-peak
   surface coil
   Syed-Neblett brachytherapy
   thresholding
   transvaginal US-guided drainage with trocar
   method/projection
      full-scan (FS)
      full-scan with interpolation (FI)

method/projection *(cont.)*
   half-scan (HS)
   half-scan with extrapolation (HE)
   half-scan with interpolation (HI)
   simulated annealing
   under-scan (US)
methoxy polyethylene glycol-L-lysine-DTPA imaging agent
methyl methacrylate
methyl protons
metrizamide cisternography
metrizamide computed tomographic cisternogram (MCTC)
metrizamide contrast material
metrizamide myelography
metrizoate acid contrast material
metrizoate sodium contrast medium
metrology
metroperitoneal fistula
"mets" (metabolic equivalents)
"mets" (slang for *metastases*)
MeV (megaelectron) dose
Mevatron 74 linear accelerator
MEVH (multiple exposure volumetric holography)
MFG (magnetic field gradients)
MFG (manofluorography)
mGy/MBq (milligray per megabecquerel)
MHC-2 (major histocompatibility complex class II antigen )
MHV (middle hepatic vein)
MHz (megahertz)
MI (mitral insufficiency)
MI (myocardial infarction)
MI adenosine thallium imaging
MIBG (metaiodobenzylguanidine) imaging agent
   MIBG scintigraphy
   MIBG SPECT scan
micelle
microabscess

microadenoma
microaneurysm
microbubble contrast imaging agent
microbubbles, Renografin-76
microcalcification, clustered
microcardia
Micro-CAST collimator
microcatheter (see also *catheter*)
   flow-directed
     UroLume flow-directed
     Wanderer
microcavitation
microcirculation, pulmonary
microculatory blood flow
microclusters, biodegradable magnetic
microcolon
microcurie
microcyst
microdactylia
microdistribution, heterogeneous
microdosimetry
microemboli
microencapsulated cisplatin
microerosion
microfiche
microfistulous AV (arteriovenous)
   shunt
microfluidization
microfocal spot mammogram
microfracture
microglobulin labeling
Micro-Guide catheter
microimaging
microinfarct
microlithiasis
micromanometer-tip catheter
micromelena
micronodular infiltrates
micronodular metastases
micronodular pattern
micronodule, centrilobular
microperforation

microporous membrane
microscope, scanning electron (SEM)
microscopic cortical dysplasia
microscopic imaging
microscopy
   differential interference contrast
     (DIC)
   electron
   in vivo
   light
   three-dimensional magnetic
     resonance (3D MR)
   ultrasound backscatter (UBM)
microsecond pulsed flashlamp pumped
   dye laser
Microsoft Access program
microsphere
   trisacryl gelatin
   ytterbium-90 ($^{90}$Yb)
microsphere perfusion scintigraphy
microtomography
Microtron, MM50 Racetrack
microvascular anastomosis
microvascular circulation
microvascular retrieval
microvasculature
Microvasive Rigiflex TTS balloon
   catheter
microvenoarteriolar fistula
microvesicular fat
microvillus (pl. microvilli)
microwave hyperthermia treatment
microwave imaging
microwave thermal balloon
   angioplasty
MID (multi-infarct dementia)
midabdominal wall
midaortic arch
midaortic syndrome
midaxillary line
midbody
MIDCAB (minimally invasive direct
   coronary artery bypass) procedure

midcircumflex
midclavicular line (MCL)
midcolon
mid-diastole
mid-distal
middle aortic syndrome
middle cardiac vein
middle lobe syndrome
middle third of the thoracic esophagus
middle-field-strength MR imaging
middorsal
midepigastrium
midesophageal diverticulum
midesophagus
midface, fetal
midface retrusion
midfemur
midfoot
midget MRI scanner
midgraft stenosis
mid-groove portion of lumina
midgut volvulus with malrotation
midlateral course
mid-left sternal border
midline, infracolic
midline mucosa-sparing blocks
midline shift
midline structures
midlung field
midlung zone
midmarginal branch of artery
midpelvis
midpole
midportion
midriff
midsagittal MR image
midscapular line
midshaft fracture
midshunt peak velocities (MSPv)
midsternum
midsystolic notching of velocity spectrum

mid-ventricular short-axis slice
midzone
migrational anomaly
migratory patchy infiltration
Mikro-tip micromanometer-tipped catheter
Mikulicz angle
Mikulicz syndrome
miliary lung disease
miliary pattern
miliary tuberculosis
milieu, therapeutic
milk leg syndrome
Milkman syndrome (also Looser-Milkman)
milky effusion
Millar catheter-tip transducer
Millar MPC-500 catheter
Miller-Abbott tube
Miller-Dieker syndrome
Miller disease
miller's lung
milliampere (mA)
millicurie (mCi)
millijoule (mJ)
Millikan-Siekert syndrome
millimeter (mm)
millimeters of mercury (mm Hg)
Millenia balloon catheter for percutaneous transluminal coronary angioplasty
milliroentgen
milliseconds (ms, msec)
millivolt (mV)
Milroy disease
Milton angioedema disease
mimic
mimicked
mimicking
mineral oil contrast
mineralization, bone
miner's lung

Ming classification of gastric
   carcinoma
Mini C-arm device
minimal luminal diameter (MLD)
minimally displaced fracture
minimal volume
minimum blood pressure
minimum intensity projection (MIP)
   image
mini-PACS
minipapillotome
Mini-Profile dilatation catheter, USCI
Minot–von Willebrand syndrome
minuscule
minute-sequence study
minute vessels
minute volume
MION (monocrystalline iron oxides)
   MION-gene complex
MIP (maximum intensity pixel)
MIP (maximum intensity projection)
   algorithms
MIPcor (coronal maximum-intensity
   projection)
Mirage over-the-wire balloon catheter
MIRI (myocardial infarction recovery
   index)
mirror image reversal
mirror, polygon
MIS (minimally invasive surgery)
misalign
misery perfusion
misleading images
mismatch
   perfusion-metabolism
   ventilation-perfusion (V/Q)
misonidazole (radiosensitizer)
missile wound
mitochondrial uncoupler CCCP
mitral annular calcification
mitral annulus
mitral apparatus

mitral arcade
mitral atresia
mitral configuration of cardiac shadow
mitral deceleration slope
mitral inflow velocities
mitral insufficiency
mitral leaflets
mitral leak
mitral orifice
mitral regurgitant signal area
mitral regurgitation
   congenital
   pansystolic
mitral regurgitation artifact
mitral regurgitation-chordal elongation
   syndrome
mitral ring calcification
mitral stenosis
   congenital
   relative
   true
mitral valve
   billowing
   cleft
   hammock
   parachute
   prosthetic
mitral valve atresia
mitral valve calcification
mitral valve commissures
mitral valve configuration, fishmouth
mitral valve echogram
mitral valve leaflet tip
mitral valve myxomatous degeneration
mitral valve prolapse, holosystolic
mitral valve regurgitation
mitral valve replacement
mitral valve septal separation
mitral valve stenosis (MVS)
Mitsubishi angioscopic catheter
mixed connective tissue disease
mixed echogenic solid mass

mixed lesion
mixed petal-fugal flow
mixed restrictive-obstructive lung
 disease
mixed signal mass
mixed tumor
mixed venous saturation
ml/min/100 g (milliliters per minute
 per 100 grams)
MLC (multileaf collimator)
MLD (minimal luminal diameter)
mm (millimeter)
mm Hg (millimeters of mercury)
MM50 Racetrack Microtron
MMCM (macromolecular contrast
 medium)
M-mode Doppler echocardiography
M-mode echocardiogram
M-mode echophonocardiography
M-mode transducer
M-mode ultrasound
mmol (millimoles)
mmol/kg (millimoles per kilogram)
mmol/L (millimoles per liter)
Mn (manganese)
MnCl2 (manganese chloride 2)
 imaging agent
MNP10 protocol
MO (mitral orifice)
MOAB, MoAb (monoclonal anti-
 body), radiolabeled
Mobetron electron beam system
mobile magnetic resonance (MR)
 imager
mobile thrombus
mobility
mode
  A-
  AAI (noncompetitive atrial
   demand)
  AAI rate-responsive
  active
  asynchronous transfer (ATM)

mode *(cont.)*
  atrial triggered and ventricular
   inhibited
  atrial-burst
  atrioventricular dual-demand
  B-
  bipolar pacing
  blink
  byte
  cine (high frame-rate)
  committed
  DDD pacing
  dual-demand pacing
  DVI (digital vascular imaging)
  fixed rate
  full-to-empty VAD
  inactive
  inhibited pacing
  M-mode
  multiplanar
  noncommitted
  pacing
  road-mapping
  semicommitted
  sequential
  64 x 64 byte
  stimulation
  triggered pacing
  underdrive
  unipolar pacing
  VAD (ventricular assist device)
  VVI (noncompetitive demand
   ventricular)
mode abandonment
model
  figure-of-eight
  lattice
  leading circle
  Markov source
  Renkin
  ring
  Shames
  xerography

modeler, solid
modeling
  Monte Carlo
  three-dimensional
moderately dilated ureter
Modic disk abnormality classification
modified birdcage coils
modified electron-beam CT scanner
modified vessel image processor (mVIP) software
modiolus
modulation
  off-center
  print reflectance
module, E-TOF detecting
Modulith SL 20
Moenckeberg ((Mönckeberg)
Mohr syndrome
moiré artifact
moiré fringes
molar pregnancy
mole, hydatidiform
molecular genetics
molecular recognition unit (MRU)
molecule
  ICAM-1
  intercellular adhesive (ICAM-1)
Molina needle-catheter
molybdenum cofactor deficiency
molybdenum-99 generator
moment, magnetic
Mönckeberg arteriosclerosis
Mönckeberg degeneration
Mönckeberg medial sclerosis
M1 (marginal branch #1)
monitor
  cardiac
  radiation
monitoring electrode
monitoring, ultrasound
monitoring wire
monoarticular

monochromatic radiation
monochromatic synchrotron radiation
monoclonal antibody (MoAb) imaging
monocrystalline iron oxide nanoparticles (MION)
monocular
monocusp valve
monodactylism
monodisk for septal defect closure
monoenergetic
monomalleolar ankle fracture
mononuclear infiltrate
monopolar RF electrocautery
Monorail balloon catheter
Monro bursa
Monro, foramen of
Monte Carlo calculation
Monte Carlo modeling
Monteggia fracture-dislocation
Montercaux fracture
Moore fracture
Morand spur
Morel syndrome
Morgagni
  appendix of
  column of
  crypt of
  foramen of
  hyperostosis of
Morgagni-Stewart-Morel syndrome
Morison pouch
morphine-augmented study
morphological and physiological image coregistration
morphological correlation
morphologic criteria
morphology
  enhancement
  morphologic
morphometric measurements
morphometry, magnetic resonance imaging

Morquio syndrome
Morris point
mortise, ankle
mortise joint
Morton neuroma
Morton toe
MOS capacitor
mosaic attenuation pattern
mosaic pattern of duodenal mucosa
Moschcowitz thrombotic thrombo-
  cytopenic purpura
MoSearch
moth-eaten appearance
moth-eaten pattern
motility
  colonic
  esophageal
  ileal
  jejunal
  small bowel
motility disorder
motility study
motion
  akinetic segmental wall
  anterior wall
  apical wall
  brisk wall
  catheter tip
  cusp
  discernible venous
  dyskinetic segmental wall
  forceful parasternal
  heaving precordial
  hyperkinetic segmental wall
  hypokinetic segmental wall
  inferior wall
  leaflet
  left ventricular regional wall
  linear accelerator isocenter
  paradoxical (of chest wall)
  paradoxical leaflet
  paradoxical septal

motion *(cont.)*
  photoreceptor
  posterior wall
  posterolateral wall
  regional hypokinetic wall
  regional wall
  rocking precordial
  segmental wall
  septal wall
  sustained anterior parasternal
  systolic anterior (SAM)
  trifid precordial motion
  ventricular wall
  visible anterior
  wall
motion artifact
motion-compensating format converter
motor cortex
motor meal barium GI series
motor task activation
mottled density
mottled echo texture
mottled gray lung
mottled pattern
mottled thickening
Mounier-Kuhn syndrome
movement
  basal
  bowel (BM)
  pendulum
  propulsive
  spontaneous fetal
movement artifact
movement pattern
moya moya ("puff of smoke") disease
Moynahan syndrome
MP-RAGE (magnetization prepared
  3D gradient-echo) sequences
MPA (main pulmonary artery)
MPAP (mean pulmonary artery
  pressure)
MPD (main pancreatic duct)

MPF catheter
MPGR (multiplanar gradient-recalled) echo
MPHR (maximum predicted heart rate)
MPPv flow
MPR (multiplanar reformation)
MPR (myocardial perfusion reserve)
mps (meters per second)
MR (magnetic resonance), 3D
MR (mitral regurgitation)
MRA (magnetic resonance angiography)
MRC (magnetic resonance cholangiography)
MRE (magnetic resonance elastography)
MRI (see *magnetic resonance imaging*; also *imaging*)
MRM (magnetic resonance mammography)
MRM (magnetic resonance myelogram)
MRN (magnetic resonance neurography)
MRS (magnetic resonance spectroscopy)
MRSA (pronounced "mer-suh") (methicillin-resistant MRU, magnetic resonance urography)
MRU (molecular recognition unit)
ms (milliseconds)
MS (mitral stenosis)
MS (morphine sulfate)
MS (multiple sclerosis) plaquing
MS Classique balloon dilatation catheter
MS-325 imaging agent
MSA (multiple system atrophy) syndrome
MSAD (multiple scan average dose)
MSAFP (maternal serum alpha fetoprotein)

msec (millisecond)
M-shaped pattern of mitral valve
MSI (magnetic source imaging), 3D
$MSO_4$ (morphine sulfate)
MT (magnetization transfer)
MTEs (main timing events)
MTP (metatarsophalangeal) joint
MTR (magnetization transfer ratio)
MTT (mean pulmonary transit time)
mu ($\mu$) rhythm ($\mu$, twelfth Greek letter)
mucinous tumor
mucocele
mucoid degeneration
mucoid impaction
mucoid plugging of airways
mucosa
  "burned out"
  cobblestone
  friable
  frothy
  isoeffective
  muscularis
mucosal abnormality
mucosal crinkling
mucosal folds
mucosal inflammation
mucosal island
mucosal pattern
mucosal relief
mucosa-sparing blocks
mucous fistula
mucous lake of stomach
mucous membrane
mucus hypersecretion
mucus plugging
Mueller (Müller) fibers
MUGA (multiple gated acquisition) blood pool radionuclide scan
mulberry gallstones
mulberry-type calcification
Müller (Mueller) fibers

Müller sign (aortic regurgitation)
multangular bone, accessory
multangular ridge fracture
multangulum
multiagent chemotherapy
multiangle, multislice acquisition
  magnetic resonance imaging
multibreath washout study
multicentric lytic lesions
multicentricity
multicolor flow cytometry
multicompartment clearance
multicoupled loop-gap resonator
multicrystal gamma camera
multicystic
multidetector system
multiecho axial
multiecho coronal image
multiecho image
multiecho sequence
multielemental neutron activation
  analysis
multiexponential relaxation
multifiber catheter
multifield beam
multifocal lesions
multifocal lymphoma
multifocal short stenosis
multiform ventricular complexes
multiforme, glioblastoma
multigated pulsed Doppler flow
  system
multigravida
multi-interval
multi-illuminant color correction
multi-infarct dementia (MID)
multilaminar bodies
multileaf collimator (MLC)
multilesion angioplasty
multilocular cyst
Multi-Med triple-lumen infusion
  catheter

multimodal image fusion technique
multimodality imaging
multinodular goiter
multinuclear magnetic resonance
  imaging
multiorgan imaging
multipara
multiparametric color composite
  display
multiparous
multiparticle cyclotron
multiphasic multislice magnetic
  resonance imaging technique
multiphasic renal computerized
  tomography (CT)
multiplanar gradient-recalled (MPGR)
  echo
multiplanar magnetic resonance
  imaging
multiplanar mode
multiplanar reformation (MRP) view
multiplanar reformatted radiographic
  and digitally reconstructed images
multiplanar transesophageal echocardiography
multiplane dosage calculations
multiple-beam interface spacing
multiple chord, center-line technique
  in echocardiogram
multiple endocrine neoplasia (MEN)
multiple exposure volumetric
  holography (MEVH)
multiple fractures
multiple gated acquisition (MUGA)
  blood pool radionuclide scan
multiple-gated acquisition (MUGA)
  scan
multiple jointed digitizer
multiple organ failure
multiple plane imaging
multiple scan average dose (MSAD)
multiple sclerosis plaquing

multiple slice acquisition
multiple trauma
multipulse nuclear magnetic resonance (NMR) imaging
multipurpose catheter
Multipurpose-SM catheter
multirod collimator
multisectional dose-volume histogram
multisection diffuse-weighted magnetic resonance imaging
multisection magnetic resonance imaging
multisection multirepetition acquisition
multisensor structured light range digitizer
multiseptate appearance
multishot echoplanar imaging
multislab magnetic resonance angiography
multislice first-pass myocardial perfusion imaging
multislice FLASH 2D
multislice mode
multislice multiphase spin-echo imaging technique
multislice spin echo sequence
multispin relaxation
multitracer study
multivessel angioplasty
MUMPS (Massachusetts [General Hospital] Utility Multiprogramming System)
Münchmeyer disease
mural aneurysm
mural architecture
mural clot
mural degeneration
mural dilatations
mural endomyocardial fibrosis
mural infiltration
mural leaflet of mitral valve
mural nodule

mural thrombosis
mural thrombus formation
muscle (pl. muscles)
  accessory
  adductor magnus
  Aeby
  Albinus
  anterior
  auricular
  axillary
  bipennate
  Bochdalek
  Bovero
  Bowman
  Braune
  Brücke
  bulbocavernosus
  canine
  cardiac
  Casser
  casserian
  cervical
  Chassaignac
  chin
  circular
  Coiter
  conal papillary
  Crampton
  deep
  detrusor
  digastric
  dorsal
  Dupré
  Duverney
  electrically conditioned and driven skeletal
  external
  fixation
  fixator
  Folius
  fused papillary
  Gantzer

**muscle**

muscle *(cont.)*
gastrocnemius
Gavard
greater
Guthrie
Hilton
Horner
Houston
iliococcygeal
iliocostal
inferior
intercostal
internal
interosseous
interspinal
intertransverse
intra-auricular
ischiocavernosus
Jung
Klein
Lancisi
lateral
latissimus dorsi
left ventricular
lesser
levator
longitudinal
Luschka
Macalister
major
Marcacci
masticator
medial
medial papillary
Merkel
middle
minor
Müller (Mueller)
multipennate
nonstriated
oblique
Ochsner

muscle *(cont.)*
Oddi
Oehl
omohyoid
opposing
organic
papillary
pectoralis major
pectoralis minor
peroneal
peroneus quartus
Phillips
plantaris
platysma
posterior
Pozzi
pubococcygeal
quadrate
Reisseisen
rhomboideus major
ribbon
rider
Riolan
Rouget
round
Ruysch
sacrospinalis
Santorini
sartorius
Sebileau
semimembranous
semispinal
semitendinous
serratus anterior
short
Sibson
skeletal
smaller
Soemmerring
soleus
somatic
sphenomandibularis

muscle *(cont.)*
   spindle-shaped
   sternocleidomastoid
   sternohyoid
   sternothyroid
   strap
   subaortic
   sucking (Bovero)
   superficial
   synergic
   tailor's
   Theile
   Tod
   Toynbee
   transverse
   trapezius
   Treitz
   triangular
   trigonal
   true back
   two-bellied
   unipennate
   Valsalva
   vastus medialis
   ventral
   vertical
   visceral
   vocal
   vocalis
   voluntary
   Wilson
   wrinkler
muscle artifact
muscle-fat boundary
muscle-fat interface
muscular atrioventricular septum
muscular branch
muscular bridging
muscular crus (of diaphragm)
muscular subaortic stenosis
muscular venous pump
muscularis mucosae
musculature
musculophrenic artery
musculophrenic branch
mushroom-shaped mass
mushroom picker's (or worker's) disease (or lung)
Musset sign (aortic aneurysm)
MUSTPAC (medical ultrasound 3D portable, with advanced communications) imaging
mutation, c-Ki-ras
MV (megavolt; not to be confused with mV, millivolt)
mV (millivolt)
MV (mitral valve)
MVA (mitral valve area)
MVD (mitral valve dysfunction)
MVO (maximum venous outflow)
MVO (mitral valve opening [or orifice])
$MVO_2$ (myocardial oxygen consumption)
MVP (mitral valve prolapse)
MVP over-the-wire balloon catheter
MVR (mitral valve replacement)
MVS (mitral valve stenosis)
myasthenia gravis
mycetoma
myelodysplasia
myelogram
myelography (with and without contrast)
   air
   cervical
   complete
   lumbar
   lumbosacral
   magnetic resonance (MRM)
   metrizamide
   positive contrast
   thoracic
myelographic contrast medium

myeloma
  indolent
  localized
  multiple
  sclerosing
  solitary
myenteric plexus of Auerbach
Myler catheter
mylohyoid ridge
myoblastoma, granular cell
myocardial blood flow (MBF)
myocardial blush
myocardial bridging
myocardial contractile dysfunction
myocardial contractility
myocardial contrast appearance time (MCAT)
myocardial contusion
myocardial degeneration
myocardial depression
myocardial dysfunction
myocardial fibers degeneration
myocardial fibrosis
myocardial granulomatous disease
myocardial hibernation
myocardial hypoperfusion, resting regional
myocardial incompetency
myocardial infarct imaging
myocardial infarction
myocardial infiltration by Kaposi sarcoma
myocardial injury
  lethal
  nonlethal
myocardial insufficiency, Sternberg
myocardial ischemia, exercise-induced transient
myocardial muscle
myocardial necrosis
myocardial oxygen consumption
myocardial oxygen demand
myocardial perfusion defect
myocardial perfusion scan
myocardial perfusion tomography
myocardial preservation
myocardial protection
myocardial recovery
myocardial reperfusion injury
myocardial revascularization
myocardial rupture
myocardial scan
myocardial shortening, fractional
myocardial-specific marker
myocardial stunning
myocardial tagging
myocardial thickening
myocardial tissue viability
myocardial tumor, metastatic
myocardial uptake of thallium
myocardial work
myocardium
  asynergic
  calcification of
  dilated
  hibernating
  hypertrophied
  ischemic reperfused
  ischemic viable
  jeopardized
  noninfarcted
  nonperfused
  perfused
  reperfused
  rupture of
  senile
  stunned
  ventricular
  viable
myofibril volume fraction
myofibroma
myoma
  pedunculated subserous
  submucous
  uterine

myometrium
Myoscint (monoclonal antibody Fab to myosin, labeled with indium-111)
myositis ossificans (MO)
myotendinous junction
Myoview imaging drug in scintigraphy
myxofibroma
myxoma
  atrial
  biatrial
  cardiac

myxoma *(cont.)*
  familial (of the heart)
  heart
  left atrial
  pedunculated
  vascular
  ventricular
myxomatous degeneration
myxomatous proliferation
myxomatous valve leaflet

# N, n

N (nitrogen)
NAA metabolite signal
Nagele obliquity
Nagele pelvis
naloxone
nanoparticles
nanoparticulate contrast agent
napkin-ring annular stenosis
napkin-ring annular tumor
Narco esophageal motility machine
naris (pl. nares)
narrow-band spectral-selective 90 RF
    pulse
narrow gating tolerance
narrowing
    arterial
    atherosclerotic
    diffuse
    disk space
    focal
    high-grade
    joint space
    large airway
    luminal
    neural foramen
    residual luminal
    subcritical
nasal sinus
nasal spine
nasion recession
nasobiliary drainage catheter
nasogastric (NG) tube
nasolabial cyst
nasopharyngeal atresia
nasopharyngeal carcinoma (NPC)
nasopharyngeal craniopharyngioma
nasotracheal tube
National Institutes of Health (NIH)
    catheter
native aortic valve, preservation of
native atherosclerosis
native coronary artery
native images
native kidney
native ventricle
native vessel
natural neon gas
Naughton-Balke treadmill protocol,
    modified
Navarre interventional radiology
    devices
navel string
navicular
    carpal
    tarsal

navicular view
naviculocapitate fracture
navigable echo signal
navigated spin-echo diffusion-weighted MR imaging
navigating heart structures
navigator echo-based real-time respiratory gating and triggering
navigator echo motion correction technique
navigator pulse
navigator shifts
NCC (normalized cross-section)
NCL-Arp monoclonal antibody imaging agent
NCL-ER-LHZ monoclonal antibody imaging agent
NCL-PGR monoclonal antibody imaging agent
NCPF (noncirrhotic portal fibrosis)
Nd:YAG (neodymium:yttrium-aluminum-garnet) laser
near anatomic position of joint
near field
near-infrared spectroscopy
near-resonance spin-lock contrast
nearest neighbor interpolation
neck
   aneurysmal
   bone
   dental
   femoral
   Madelung
   pancreatic
   surgical
   uterine
   wry
neck vessel engorgement
necroscopy, perinatal
necrosed tissue
necrosis
   acute sclerosing hyaline (ASHN)
   acute tubular

necrosis *(cont.)*
   alveolar septal
   aorta idiopathic
   arteriolar
   aseptic
   avascular
   bilateral cortical
   biliary piecemeal
   bloodless zone of
   bowel
   bridging
   caseous
   centrilobular
   coagulation
   colliquative
   colonic
   contraction band
   cystic medial
   diffuse
   embolic
   epiphyseal
   epiphyseal ischemic
   Erdheim cystic medial
   fat
   fatty
   fibrinoid
   fibrosing piecemeal
   focal
   focal hepatic
   frank
   heart muscle
   hemorrhagic
   hepatic
   hyaline
   indurative
   intestinal
   ischemic
   liquefaction
   localized
   lung
   massive
   massive hepatic

necrosis *(cont.)*
  medial cystic
  midzonal
  mucosal
  myocardial
  Paget quiet
  pancreatic
  papillary
  peripheral
  piecemeal
  postoperative
  postpartum pituitary
  pressure
  progressive emphysematous
  radiation
  renal cortical
  renal tubular
  septic
  strangulation
  stromal
  subacute hepatic
  subcutaneous fat
  subendocardial
  submassive
  submassive hepatic
  superficial
  total
  tracheobronchial mucosal
  ventricular muscle
  Zenker
necrotic myocardium
necrotizing emphysema
necrotizing pneumonia
necrotizing respiratory granulomatosis
necrotizing thrombosis
needle
  nonferromagnetic
  Quincke spinal
  stabilization
  Whitacre spinal
needle biopsy, CT-scan directed
needle hydrophone

needle tracking, real-time biplanar
Neer shoulder fractures (I, II, III classification)
NEFA (non-esterified fatty acid) scintigraphy
negative contrast agent
negative image
negative predictive value
negligible pressure gradient
Nélaton dislocation
Nélaton fold
NEMD (nonspecific esophageal motility disorder)
neoadjuvant chemotherapy
neoadjuvant hormonal therapy
neoaorta
neoaortic valve
neocerebellum
neocholangiole
neodymium:yttrium-aluminum-garnet (Nd:YAG) laser
neointimal hyperplasia
neointimal proliferation
neonatal adrenal ultrasound
neonatal cystic pulmonary emphysema
neonate
neon particle protocol
neopallium
neoplasia, multiple endocrine (MEN)
neoplasm
  benign
  encapsulated
  firm
  functioning
  gonadal
  lethal
  low-grade
  malignant
  ovarian
  primary
  spherical
  well-circumscribed

neoplastic fracture
neoplastic stenosis
Neoprobe radioactivity detector
neorectum
neovascularity
nephroblastoma
nephrogram
nephrographic phase (NP)
nephrolithiasis
nephroptosis
nephrosclerosis
   arterial
   senile
nephrosis
nephrotic
nephrostogram
nephrotic edema
nephrotomogram
nephrotomography
nephrotoxic contrast medium
nephrotoxicity
Neptune trident appearance
Nernst equation
nerve root compression
nerve root edema
nerve root sheath
nervous heart syndrome
net magnetization factor
net tissue magnetization
network
   articular
   lymphatic
   neural
   venous
network architecture
NEUGAT (neutron/gamma transmission) method
neural arch
neural crest origin
neural evaluation algorithm
neural foramen (pl. foramina)
neural network

neural tube defect
neurenteric cyst
neurinoma
neuritic plaque
neuritic plaquing
neuroangiography
neuroblastoma
neuroblockage
neurodiagnosis
NeuroEcho software
neuroendocrine carcinoma
neurofibrillary tangles
neurofibromatosis
neurogenic bladder
neurogenic dysfunction of the bladder
neurogenic fracture
neurogenic pulmonary edema
neurogenic sarcoma
neurogenic tumor
neurography, magnetic resonance (MRN)
neuroholography
neuroimaging
neurointerventional radiology
neuroleptic
Neurolite (technetium Tc 99m bicisate) imaging agent
Neuro Lobe software
neurologic signs, focal
neuroma
   Morton
   multicystic acoustic
neuromorphometry
neuromuscular blockade
Neuropac
neuropathic bladder
neuroradiologic examination
neuroradiology
   interventional
   pediatric
neuroreceptor ligand
NeuroScan 3D imager

NeuroSector ultrasound system
neurosonogram
neurosonology
Neuro SPGR software
neurosurgery, stereotactic
neurotoxic effect
neurotropic MR imaging contrast
   agents
neurovascular bundle
neurovascular compression
neutron activation analysis
neutron capture therapy
neutron/gamma transmission
   (NEUGAT) method
neutron
   slow
   thermal
neutron-deficient nuclei
neutron irradiation
neutron-rich biomedical tracer
neutron therapy
nevus (pl. nevi)
NEX (number of excitations) (on MRI
   scan)
NG (nasogastric) tube
NH region of AV (atrioventricular)
   node
Nicaladoni-Branham sign
niche
   Barclay
   Haudek
Nicolet NMR spectrometer
nicotinamide radiosensitizer
nidus demarcation
nidus, thrombus
Niemann-Pick disease
Niemeier gallbladder perforation
NIH (National Institutes of Health)
Nikolsky sign
nimodipine, intraarterial superselective
ninety-degree (or 90°) RF pulse (on
   MR spectroscopy)

91-41 MeV proton
Niopam contrast medium
nipple marker
NIPS (noninvasive programmed
   stimulation)
NIRS (near-infrared spectroscopy)
Nishimoto Sangyo scanner
Nissen antireflux operation
nitinol stent
nitrogen, body
nitrogen washout
nitrogen (N)
   $^{13}$N ammonia radioactive tracer
   $^{13}$N ammonia uptake on PET scan
nitrogen-nipple sign, aortic
nitrous oxide synthetase
NMIS (nuclear medicine information
   system)
NMR (nuclear magnetic resonance)
   imaging (see *imaging*)
no discernible findings
no therapy zone
NO (nitrous oxide)
no-carrier-added fluorine-18 imaging
   agent
no-gap technique
no-reflow phenomenon
nociceptive
nodal conduction
nodal contractions
nodal escape
nodal impulse
nodal metastases
nodal point
nodal premature contraction
nodal rupture
node
   abdominal lymph
   accessory lymph
   anorectal lymph
   aortic lymph
   aortic window

**node** *(cont.)*
  apical lymph
  appendicular lymph
  Aschoff
  Aschoff-Tawara
  atrioventricular (AV, AVN)
  auricular lymph
  AV (atrioventricular)
  axillary lymph
  bifurcation lymph
  Bouchard
  brachial lymph
  bronchopulmonary lymph
  buccal lymph
  buccinator lymph
  cardiac
  caval lymph
  celiac lymph
  central lymph
  cervical lymph
  cervical paratracheal lymph
  Cloquet inguinal lymph
  common iliac lymph
  companion lymph
  coronary
  cubital lymph
  cystic lymph
  Delphian lymph
  deltopectoral lymph
  diaphragmatic lymph
  Dürck
  epicolic lymph
  epigastric lymph
  epitrochlear lymph
  Ewald
  external iliac lymph
  facial lymph
  fibular lymph
  Flack
  Flack sinoatrial
  foraminal
  gastric lymph

**node** *(cont.)*
  gastroduodenal lymph
  gastroepiploic lymph
  gastro-omental lymph
  gluteal lymph
  gouty
  Haygarth
  Heberden
  hemal
  hemolymph
  Hensen
  hepatic lymph
  hilar lymph
  ileocolic lymph
  iliac circumflex lymph
  iliac lymph
  infraclavicular
  infrahyoid lymph
  inguinal lymph
  intercostal lymph
  interiliac lymph
  interpectoral lymph
  intramammary
  jugular lymph
  jugulodigastric lymph
  jugulo-omohyoid lymph
  juxtaintestinal
  Keith
  Keith-Flack sinoatrial
  Koch sinoatrial
  lacunar
  lumbar lymph
  lymph
  malar lymph
  mandibular lymph
  mastoid lymph
  medial supraclavicular
  mediastinal lymph
  mesenteric lymph
  Meynet
  nasolabial lymph
  NH region of AV (atrioventricular)

**node** *(cont.)*
  obturator lymph
  occipital lymph
  Osler
  pancreatic lymph
  pancreaticoduodenal lymph
  pancreaticolienal lymph
  pancreacticosplenic
  paracardial lymph
  paracolic lymph
  paramammary lymph
  pararectal lymph
  parasternal lymph
  paratracheal lymph
  parauterine lymph
  paravaginal lymph
  paravesicular lymph
  parietal lymph
  parotid lymph
  Parrot
  pectoral lymph
  pelvic lymph
  peribronchial
  pericardial lymph
  peroneal
  phrenic lymph
  popliteal lymph
  postaortic lymph
  postcaval lymph
  posterior mediastinal
  postvesicular lymph
  preaortic lymph
  precaval lymph
  prececal lymph
  prelaryngeal
  prepericardial lymph
  pretracheal lymph
  prevertebral lymph
  prevesicular lymph
  pulmonary juxtaesophageal lymph
  pulmonary lymph
  pyloric lymph

**node** *(cont.)*
  Ranvier
  rectal lymph
  regional lymph
  retroaortic lymph
  retroauricular lymph
  retrocecal lymph
  retropharyngeal lymph
  retropyloric
  retrorectal lymph node
  Rosenmüller
  Rotter
  SA (sinoatrial)
  sacral lymph
  satellite
  scalene
  Schmorl
  sentinel
  shotty lymph
  sick sinus
  sigmoid lymph
  signal
  singer
  sinoatrial (SAN)
  sinoauricular
  sinus
  Sister Mary Joseph
  solitary lymph
  splenic lymph
  subcarinal
  submandibular lymph
  submental lymph
  subpyloric
  subscapular lymph
  superficial inguinal lymph
  supraclavicular lymph
  suprapyloric
  supratrochlear lymph
  syphilitic
  Tawara
  teacher
  thyroid lymph

**node • nodule**

node *(cont.)*
   tibial
   tracheal lymph
   tracheobronchial lymph
   Troisier
   vesicular lymph
   vestigial left sinoatrial
   Virchow
   visceral lymph
nodo-Hisian (nodohisian) bypass tract
nodosum
   erythema
   polyarteritis (PAN)
nodoventricular bypass fiber
nodoventricular bypass tract
nodoventricular pathway
nodoventricular tachycardia
nodular aneurysm
nodular density
nodular enhancement
nodular fibrosis
nodular goiter
nodular-like
nodular lymphoid hyperplasia (NLH)
nodular mass
nodularity
   calcified
   coarse
   noncalcified
   surface
   vein
nodule (pl. nodules)
   air-space
   Albini
   aortic valve
   Arantius
   Aschoff
   autonomous
   Bianchi
   cold
   cortical
   Cruveilhier

nodule *(cont.)*
   cutaneous
   Dalen-Fuchs
   discordant
   enhancing
   fibrous
   Fraenkel typhus
   functioning
   Gamna
   Gamna-Gandy
   Gandy-Gamna
   Hoboken
   hot
   hypermetabolic
   Kerckring
   Koeppe
   Morgagni
   mural
   non-enhancing
   noncavitary
   nondelineated
   nonfunctioning thyroid
   ossific
   peripheral
   Picker
   regenerative
   rheumatic
   rheumatoid
   Schmorl
   semiautonomous
   siderotic
   silicotic
   singer's
   Sister Mary Joseph
   solitary
   surfer's
   teacher's
   tobacco
   toxic
   tuberculous
   typhoid
   typhus
   warm

nodulus Arantii (pl. noduli Arantii)
nodus arcus venae azygos
noise
    lesion-to-cerebrospinal fluid
    lesion-to-white matter
    pixel
    respiratory
    subtractive
    white
noise distribution, spectral
noise reduction intercom
NOMOS correction factor
nonablative heating
nonarticular radial head fracture
nonasbestos pneumoconiosis
noncalcified mitral leaflets
noncalcified nodule
noncardiac pulmonary edema
noncardiogenic pulmonary edema
noncaseating granuloma
noncaseating tubercles
noncavitary nodule
noncircularity degree
noncoaxial catheter tip position
noncollagenous pneumoconiosis
noncommunicating cyst
noncommunicating hydrocephalus
noncompensatory pause
noncompliant plaque
noncompressible appendix
noncontact imaging technology
noncontractile scar tissue
noncontrast phase (NCP)
non-coplanar arc technique
non-coplanar therapy beams
noncoronary cusp
noncoronary sinus
nondecremental
nondelineated nodule
nondependent lung
nondisplaced fracture
nondistensible balloon

nondominant vessel
nonenclosed magnet
nonenhanced CAT scan
nonenhancing nodule
nonenhancing lesion
nonferromagnetic needle
nonfilarial chylocele
nonfilling venous segment
nonforeshortened angiographic view
nonfunctioning thyroid nodule
non-Hodgkin lymphoma
nonhomogeneous consolidation
nonhyperfunctioning adrenal adenoma
nonimmunological fetal hydrops
noninducible tachycardia
noninfarcted segment
noninteger period
noninvasive diagnosis
noninvasive imaging study
nonionic contrast medium
nonionic paramagnetic contrast medium
nonisotropic gradient
nonlethal myocardial ischemic injury
nonlinear excitation profile
nonlingular branches of upper lobe
    bronchus
Nonne-Milroy lymphedema
non-nodular fibrosis
non-nodular silicosis
nonocclusive mesenteric arterial
    insufficiency
nonpeptide angiotensin II antagonist
nonpulsatile mass
nonradiopaque foreign body
nonresonance Raman spectroscopy
nonresponsive to TSH manipulation
nonrheumatic valvular aortic stenosis
nonsegmental areas of opacification
nonselective angiography
non-small cell lung cancer (NSCLC)
nonspecific bowel gas pattern
nonspecific changes

nonspecific esophageal motility
   disorder (NEMD)
nonspecific phenomenon
nonsteroidal antiphlogistics
nonstress test (NST)
nonsubtraction images
nonsyndromic bicoronal synostosis
nonsyndromic unicoronal synostosis
nontrabeculated atrium
nontransmural myocardial infarction
nontransmural match
nontraumatic dislocation
nontraumatic epidural hemorrhage
nontriggered phase-contrast MR
   angiography
nonuniform attenuation
nonuniform rotational defect (NURD)
nonunion of fracture fragments
nonunion, torsion wedge
nonvalved conduit
nonviable scar from myocardial
   infarction
nonvisualization of gallbladder
nonweightbearing view
Noonan syndrome
NoProfile balloon catheter
Norland bone densitometry
Norland pQCT XCT2000 scanner
Norland XR26 bone densitometer
normal
   borderline
   high
   low
normal anatomic variation
normalized average glandular dose
normalized cross-section (NCC)
normal-pressure hydrocephalus
normal-region pixel
normokalemic reperfusion
normotensive
normothermia
normovolemia
normovolemic
normoxia
NOS (not otherwise specified)
nose cone
nosocomial TB (tuberculosis)
   transmission
notch
   acetabular
   anacrotic
   angular
   antegonial
   aortic
   auricular
   cardiac
   cerebellar
   clavicular
   coracoid
   costal
   cotyloid
   craniofacial
   dicrotic
   digastric
   ethmoidal
   fibular
   frontal
   greater sciatic
   interclavicular
   intercondylar
   intercondyloid
   intervertebral
   Kernohan
   lesser sciatic
   radial sigmoid
   scapular
   sciatic
   sigmoid
   spinoglenoid
   sternal
   suprasternal
   trochlear
   ulnar
notched aortic knob

notching of pulmonic valve on echocardiogram
notching, rib
Nothnagel syndrome
Novopaque contrast medium
NOX (number of excitations) on MRI
NP (nephrographic phase)
$^{59}$NP (iodomethylnorcholesterol) scintigraphy
NPC (nasopharyngeal cancer)
NPC (nodal premature contraction)
NRH (nodular regenerative hyperplasia)
NSCLO (non-small cell lung cancer)
nubbin sign
Nuck
    canal of
    diverticulum of
nuclear bone imaging
nuclear electric quadripole relaxation
nuclear gated blood pool testing
nuclear hepatobiliary imaging
nuclear magnetic resonance (NMR)
    (see also *imaging*)
    NMR imaging
    NMR magnetometer probe
    NMR quadrature detection array
    NMR scan
    NMR spectography
    NMR spectrometer
    NMR spectroscopy
    NMR spectrum
    NMR station, MacSpect real-time
    NMR tomography of breast

nuclear medicine information system (NMIS)
nuclear parameters
nuclear perfusion imaging
nuclear relaxation
nuclear renal scintigraphy
nuclear signal
nuclear spin
nuclear spin quantum number
nuclear-tagged red blood cell bleeding study
nucleonics
nucletron applicator
nucleus (pl. nuclei)
    caudate
    dentate
    Kölliker
    lenticular
    lentiform
    neutron-deficient
    residual
nucleus globosus
nucleus pulposus
nuclide analysis
null point
number, clonogen
number of excitations (NEX) on MRI
NURD (nonuniform rotational defect)
nursemaid's elbow
nutation angle measurement
nutcracker esophagus
Nycomed contrast
Nycore angiography catheter

# O, o

O (oxygen) (see *imaging agent*)
OA (osteoarthritis)
OBD (organic brain disease)
oblique axial MR imaging
oblique diameter
oblique fracture
oblique radiograms
oblique vein
oblique view
obliquity
   Litzmann
   Nägele
   Roederer
   Solayrès
obliterans, atherosclerosis
obliteration
   costophrenic angle
   nidus
   psoas shadow
   surgical
obliterative arteriosclerosis
O'Brien classification of radial
   fracture
obscure
obscuration
obstetric ultrasound
obstipation

obstructing embolus
obstruction
   acute abdominal
   adynamic intestinal
   airway
   aortic arch
   aortic outflow
   aortoiliac
   arterial
   bilateral
   bile flow
   biliary
   bowel
   bronchial
   cardiac
   cerebrospinal fluid
   chronic airway
   closed-loop
   closed-loop intestinal
   colon
   colonic
   common bile duct
   common duct
   complete bowel
   congenital left-sided outflow
   congenital subpulmonic
   cowl-shaped

obstruction *(cont.)*
  duct
  endobronchial
  esophageal
  extrahepatic
  extrinsic malignant ureteral
  false colonic
  fecal
  fixed airway
  fixed coronary
  food bolus
  foreign body
  functional
  gastric
  gastric outlet
  hepatic
  hepatic venous outflow
  high-grade
  high small bowel
  hydrocephalic
  idiopathic
  infravesical
  interposed colon segment
  intestinal
  intrathoracic airway
  intraventricular right ventricular
  intravesical
  irreversible airway
  lacrimal canaliculus
  large bowel
  low small bowel
  lymphatic
  malignant airway
  mammary duct
  mechanical
  mechanical biliary
  mechanical duct
  mechanical extrahepatic
  mechanical intestinal
  mechanical small bowel
  neurogenic intestinal
  otic

obstruction *(cont.)*
  outflow
  outlet
  pancreatic duct
  paralytic colonic
  partial bowel
  preocclusive
  pulmonary artery
  pulmonary outflow
  pulmonary vascular
  pulmonary venous
  pyloric outlet
  pyloroduodenal
  rectal
  renal
  respiratory
  respiratory tract
  right ventricular outflow
  secondary
  simple mechanical
  small bowel (SBO)
  strangulated bowel
  strangulation
  subclavian artery
  subpulmonic
  subvalvular aortic
  subvalvular diffuse muscular
  superior vena caval
  supravesical
  upper airway
  ureteral
  ureteropelvic junction
  urethral
  urinary
  vascular
  venous
  vesical outlet
obstructive abnormality
obstructive airway disease
obstructive atelectasis
obstructive component
obstructive emphysema

obstructive hydrocephalus
obstructive hypopnea
obstructive jaundice
obstructive lesion
obstructive pneumonia
obstructive pulmonary disease (OPD)
obstructive pulmonary overinflation
obstructive renal dysplasia
obstructive thrombus
obstructive-type atelectasis
obstructive ventilatory defect
obturating embolus
obturator hernia
obturator internus muscle
obturator nodal chain
obturator node
obturator sign
obtuse marginal (OM) coronary artery
obtuse marginal branch (OMB)
occipital-atlas-axis ligaments
occipital-axis joint
occipital bone
occipital condyle
occipital fissure
occipital fracture
occipital gyrus
occipital lesion
occipital lobe
occipital pole
occipital-temporal sulcus
occipital tip
occipital vessels
occipital view of skull
occipitoanterior
occipitoatlantoaxial fusion
occipitocervical articulation
occipitofrontalis muscle
occipitoposterior
occipitotemporal gyrus
occipitotemporal sulcus
occipitotemporopontine tract

occiput
occlude
occluded graft
occluder
  ameroid
  radiolucent plastic
occluder delivered into left atrium
  under fluoroscopic control
occluding spring emboli
occluding thrombus
occlusal plane
occlusal segment
occlusion
  aqueductal
  arterial
  balloon
  basilar
  bilateral
  complete
  coronary
  deep venous
  ductus arteriosus
  embolic
  fallopian tube
  graft
  intermittent
  intracranial vascular
  late graft
  side branch
  snowplow
  subtotal
  tapering
  total
  traumatogenic
  unilateral
  ureteral
  vascular
  vein graft
  vertebrobasilar
  vessel
occlusion measurement
occlusive arterial thrombus

occlusive cerebrovascular insult
occlusive impedance phlebography
occlusive lesion
occult cerebral vascular malformation (OCVM)
occult fracture
occult lesion
occult, roentgenographically
occult subluxation
OCG (oral cholecystogram)
ochronosis
OCL bowel prep
O'Connor finger dexterity test
OCT (optical coherence tomography)
octagon board
octapolar catheter
OctreoScan radiologic imaging agent
Octreotide scintigraphy
ocular globe topography
ocular pneumoplethysmography (OPG)
oculoauriculovertebral (OAV)
oculomotor apparatus
oculomotor nerve (third cranial nerve)
oculomotor-trochlear nucleus
oculopharyngeal dystrophy
oculoplethysmography (OPG)
oculoplethysmography/carotid phonoangiography (OPG/CPA)
oculopneumoplethysmography
oculosubcutaneous syndrome of Yuge
Oddi, sphincter of
Oden classification of peroneal tendon subluxation
odontogenic fibromyxoma
odontoid bone
odontoid fracture
odontoid process
odontoid view
odontoma
ODQ (opponens digiti quinti) muscle
OEC Series 9600 cardiac system

off-axis dose inhomogeneity
off-axis factor
off-axis point localization
off-center cut
off-center modulation
off-resonance saturation pulse imaging
off-resonance spin-locking
offset, frequency
Ogden classification of epiphyseal fracture
Ogilvie syndrome (pseudo-obstruction of colon)
Ogston line
ohm (pl. ohms)
oil embolism
oil emulsions contrast
oil, peppermint (used with barium enema)
OKT3 monoclonal antibody
OKT4 monoclonal antibody imaging agent
OKT8 monoclonal antibody imaging agent
Okuda transhepatic obliteration of varices
olecranon
olecranon fossa
olecranon process
olecranon tip fracture
oleothorax
Olerud and Molander fracture classification
oligemic lobe
oligoclonal IgG bands in cerebrospinal fluid
oligodactylia
oligodendroglioma tumor
oligodendroma
oligohydramnios
olisthesis
olisthetic vertebra, wedging of
olive ring

Oliver-Cardarelli sign
olivopontocerebellar atrophy
olivopontocerebellar degeneration
Ollier disease
olsalazine
Olympus Gastrocamera GTF-A
Olympus GF-UM3 and CF-UM20 ultrasonic endoscope
Olympus UM-1W transendoscopic ultrasound probe
Olympus VU-M2 and XIF-UM3 echoendoscope
OM (obtuse marginal) coronary artery
OMB (obtuse marginal branch)
OMB1 (obtuse marginal branch #1)
omental cake
omentum
  colic
  gastric
  gastrocolic
  gastrohepatic
  gastrosplenic
  greater (omentum majus)
  incarcerated
  lesser (omentum minus)
  pancreaticosplenic
  splenogastric
omentum majus
omentum minus
Omniflex balloon catheter
Omnipaque (iohexol) nonionic imaging agent
Omnipaque contrast media
Omniscan (gadodiamide) nonionic contrast medium
omohyoid muscle
omphalic
omphalocele
omphaloma
on-column preparation
OncoScint breast imaging agent
OncoScint CR/OV (satumomab pendetide) contrast medium
OncoScint CR103 (colorectal) and OV103 (ovarian) (monoclonal antibody B72.3 labeled with indium-111)
OncoScint CR372 imaging agent
OncoScint-NSC (non-small cell) lung imaging agent
OncoScint PR356 imaging agent
OncoSpect imaging agent
OncoTrac imaging agent
one-part fracture
one-dimensional chemical shift imaging (1D-CSI)
one-shot echo planar imaging
onion bulb appearance of myelin sheaths
onion bulb changes on biopsy
onion-shaped dilatation of duodenum
onion peel appearance on x-ray
onionskin configuration of collagenous fibers
onlay graft
on-line anion exchange purification
on-line portal imaging
opacification
opacified
opacify
opacifying
opacity (pl. opacities)
  diffuse
  ground-glass
  linear
  patchy alveolar
  reticular
opaque media
opaque wire suture
OPD (obstructive pulmonary disease)
OPD4 monoclonal antibody imaging agent
open architecture system
open beam
open-break fracture

open-configuration magnetic
    resonance system
open dislocation
open fontanelle
open fracture
open magnet
open magnetic resonance imaging
open-mouth odontoid view
open neural tube defect
open pneumothorax
open systems interconnect (OSI)
open tuberculosis
opening, buttonhole
OpenPACS system
opera glass hand
operation, three-dimensional-connect
operative cholangiography
opercular
operculum, cerebral
OPG (ophthalmoplethysmography)
OPG/CPA (oculoplethysmography/
    carotid phonoangiography)
ophthalmic biometry by ultrasound
    echography
ophthalmoplethysmography (OPG)
opiate $\mu$ (mu) receptor
opiate receptor binding
opisthotonic position
Opitz thrombophlebitic splenomegaly
OPLL (opacification of posterior
    longitudinal ligament)
opposed GRE images
opposed loop-pair quadrature MR coil
opposed-phase GRE imaging
opposed-phase imaging
opposed-phase MRI
opposed-phase sequence
opposing pleural surfaces
optic chiasm
optic glioma
optic globe
optic nerve compression

optic pathway
optic recess
optic strut
optical coherence tomography (OCT)
optical imaging
optical isomer
optical localization fiber
optical surface imaging (OSI)
optimal imaging planes
optimally
optimization, interactive gradient
optimization parameters
Optiray (ioversol) nonionic contrast
    medium
Optiscope catheter
optokinetic nystagmus (OKN)
Orabilex contrast medium
Oracle Focus ultrasound imaging
    catheter
Oracle Megasonics high-pressure
    PTCA catheter
Oracle Micro Plus ultrasound imaging
    catheter
Oragrafin contrast medium
oral cholecystogram (OCG)
oral contrast agent
oral enhanced CT scan
oral magnetic particles
Oralex ultrasound imaging agent
orbit
    angular process of
    bony
orbit artifacts due to body contour
orbital apex
orbital bone
orbital mass compression
orbital pseudo-tumor
orbital rim stepoff
orbitofrontal region
orbitosphenoidal bone
Orca fluoroscopic C-arm

organ
  accessory
  annulospiral
  circumventricular
  Corti
  critical
  extraperitoneal
  floating
  poles of
  retroperitoneal
  Zuckerkandl
organic brain disease (OBD)
organic granulomatosis
organic liquid scintillator
organification defect
organoaxial
organomegaly
orientation
  coronal
  disk-to-magnetic field
  disturbed
  sagittal
  slice
  spatial
  temporal
  transverse
ORIF (open reduction and internal fixation)
orifice
  anal
  aortic
  atrioventricular
  cardiac
  coronary
  coronary sinus
  double coronary
  esophagogastric
  external urethral
  gastroduodenal
  golf-hole ureteral
  hypoplastic tricuspid
  ileocecal

orifice *(cont.)*
  inferior vena cava
  internal urethral
  lingular
  mitral
  narrowed
  pharyngeal
  pulmonary
  pyloric
  rectal
  regurgitant
  segmental
  slitlike
  tricuspid
  ureteral (or ureteric)
  urethral
  vaginal
  valve
orifice-to-annulus ratio
origin
  anomalous
  muscle
origin of artery
origin of vessel
Orion balloon catheter
oroendotracheal tube
orogastric tube
oropharyngeal airway
oropharynx
orotracheal intubation
Orthacor material
orthocephalic
Orthoclone
orthogonal angiographic projection
orthogonal RF coil
orthogonal tag lines
orthogonal view on angiography
orthonormal diameter
orthopantogram
orthoroentgenogram
orthotopic ureter
orthovoltage radiation therapy

Ortner syndrome
os (pl. ossa) (see also *bone*)
   cervical
   coronary sinus
   external cervical
   internal cervical
os acetabuli (acetabulum)
os calcis (calcaneus)
os coxae (hip bone; ilium, ischium, pubis)
os cuboides secondarium (cuboid bone)
os naviculare (navicular bone)
os pubis (pubic bone)
os trigonum (triangular bone of tarsus)
oscillating magnetic field
oscillography
oscilloscope tuning station
Osgood-Schlatter disease
OSI (open systems interconnect)
OSI (optical surface imaging)
Osler disease
Osler-Libman-Sacks syndrome
Osler nodes
Osler sign
Osler triad
Osler-Weber-Rendu telangiectasia
Osm (osmole)
osmotic blood-brain barrier disruption
osmotic demyelination syndrome
osmotic edema
osmotic effect
osseous bridge
osseous destructive process
osseous dysplasia
osseous graft
osseous metastases
osseous outgrowth
osseous remodeling
osseous spiral lamina
osseous structure

osseous survey
osseous union
ossicle, Riolan
ossiferous
ossific nodule
ossific nucleus of navicular
ossification
   abnormal
   enchondral
   endochondral
   heterotopic
   intracartilaginous
   intramembranous
   irregular enchondral
   muscle
   periarticular heterotopic (PHO)
   peripheral
   primary center of
   secondary center of
   soft tissue
ossification center
ossification variant
ossified body
ossifying fibroma of long bone
osteal stenoses
ostealgia
ostemia
ostempyesis
OsteoAnalyzer device
osteoaneurysm
osteoarthritic change
osteoarthritic spur
osteoarthritis (OA)
   degenerative
   erosive
   generalized
   post-traumatic
   traumatic
osteoarticular
osteoblastic bone regeneration
osteoblastic metastasis
osteoblastic tumor

osteocachexia
osteocalcin
osteocartilaginous lesion
osteochondral fracture
osteochondral lesion
osteochondritic loose body
osteochondritic separation of
 epiphyses
osteochondritis dissecans (OD)
osteochondrofibroma
osteochondrolysis
osteochondroma
 epiphyseal
 soft tissue
osteochondromatosis
 multiple
 synovial
osteochondromatous dysplasia,
 epiarticular
osteochondrophyte
osteochondrosarcoma
osteochondrosis deformans juvenilis
osteochondrosis dissecans
osteoclasis
osteoclastic
osteo condensans ilii
osteocystoma
osteocyte
osteodiastasis
osteodystrophy
osteoenchondroma
osteofibrochondrosarcoma
osteofibromatosis
osteogenesis, distraction
osteogenesis imperfecta
osteogenesis imperfecta tarda
osteogenic sarcoma
osteohalisteresis
osteoid osteoma
osteolipochondroma
osteolipoma
osteolysis, scalloping

osteolytic metastases
osteoma
 juxta-articular osteoid
 osteoid
 parosteal
 spongy
 ulcer
osteomalacia
 hematogeneous
 renal tubular
 senile
osteomatosis
osteomesopyknosis
osteomyelitic sinus
osteomyelitis
osteonal bone
osteonecrosis
 dysbaric
 Ficat classification of femoral head
osteopenia
osteopetrosis
osteophyte
 bony
 bridging
 cervical
 fringe of
 horseshoe
 jagged
 marginal
osteophyte formation
 beaklike
 hooklike
 marginal
 nipplelike
osteophytic bone lip
osteophytic lipping
osteophytic proliferation
osteophytosis
osteoporosis
 corticosteroid-induced
 disuse
 juvenile

osteoporosis *(cont.)*
   post-traumatic
   postmenopausal
   senile
osteoporotic bone
osteoradionecrosis
osteosarcoma
   cardiac
   classical
   extraosseous
   fibroblastic
   intracortical
   intraosseous
   juxtacortical
   osteoblastic
   parosteal
   periosteal
   telangiectatic
osteosclerosis
osteosis
osteospongioma
osteothrombosis
OsteoView desktop hand x-ray system
ostia (pl. of ostium)
ostial lesion
ostial stenosis
ostium (pl. ostia)
   aortic
   artery
   atrioventricular
   coronary
   coronary sinus
ostium abdominale tubae uterinae
   (abdominal orifice of uterine tube)
ostium primum defect
ostium secundum defect
Otto pelvis dislocation
out-of-phase GRE images
outcome, clinical
outcomes (radiology outcomes data)
outer table
Outerbridge ridge

Outerbridge scale (articular damage)
outflow
   hypoplastic subpulmonic
   maximum venous (MVO)
   subpulmonic
outflow anastomosis
outflow of ventricle
outflow tract
outgrowth, osseous patellar
outlet
   pelvic
   pyloric
   thoracic
   ventricular
   widened thoracic
outlet chamber, rudimentary
outlet view
outpocketings of mucosa
outpouching
output
   adequate cardiac
   augmented cardiac
   cardiac (CO)
   Dow method for cardiac
   Fick method for cardiac
   Gorlin method for cardiac
   Hetzel forward triangle method
      for cardiac
   inadequate cardiac
   low cardiac
   pulmonic
   reduced systemic cardiac
   stroke
   systemic
   thermodilution cardiac
   ventricular
output amplitude
output point
OV (ovarian)
Ovadia-Beals classification of tibial
   plafond fracture

ovale, foramen
ovalis
  annulus
  fossa
  limbus fossae
ovarian carcinoma
ovarian cyst
ovarian hernia
ovarian tumor
ovary (pl. ovaries)
  atrophied
  cystic
  embryonic
  ligament of
  mulberry
  polycystic
  suspensory ligament of
Ovation Falloposcopy System
overaeration
over couch view
overdistention
  alveolar
  pulmonary
overdrive suppression
overexpansion, pulmonary
overgrowth, bony
overhanging edges or margins
Overhauser effect
overhead film
overhead oblique view
overinflation
  pulmonary
  unilateral
overlapping images
overlie
overlying
overload (overloading)
  acute hemodynamic
  cardiac
  chronic hemodynamic

overload *(cont.)*
  diastolic
  fluid
  pressure
  right ventricular
  systolic ventricular
  volume
overlying attenuation artifact
over-read (noun)
overrelaxation factors
over-responsive programming
overriding of fracture fragments
overriding toes
oversampling (on MRI)
overstaged
over-the-wire balloon catheter
overuse injury
overuse syndrome
overventilation, alveolar
ovoid heart
ovoids, external beam with
ovoid-shaped
ovum (pl. ova)
Owen view
"ox heart" (cor bovinum)
oxalosis
Oxford magnet
oxidation, Baeyer-Villiger
oxidative metabolism
oxidized complex
Oxilan (ioxilan) imaging agent
oximetry, transcranial cerebral
oxycel
oxygen cisternography
oxygen extraction fraction (OEF)
oxygen, inhaled (MR contrast agent)
oxygen-15 labeled water ($^{15}$O-labeled water)
oxygen-17 NMR spectroscopy
oxygenation-sensitive functional MR

# P, p

P (posterior)
PA (posteroanterior or posterior-anterior)
PA and lateral films
PA and lateral views
PA (pulmonary artery)
Paas disease
PABP (pulmonary artery balloon pump)
pacchionian
pacemaker
pace mapping
Pace Plus System scanner
pack-a-day smoking history
packing
   cubic
   extraction, and calculation technique
   periodic
pack-year smoking history
pack-years of cigarette smoking
PACS (picture archive and communication system)
PACS, PBT Technologies
PACSRO (picture archiving and communications systems in radiation oncology)

pad
   abdominal
   antimesenteric fat
   fat
   fibrocartilaginous
   padding
   UltraEase ultrasound
PADP-PAWP (pulmonary artery diastolic and wedge pressure) gradient
pad sign of aortic insufficiency
PAEDP (pulmonary artery end-diastolic pressure)
Paget abscess
Paget-associated osteogenic sarcoma
Paget disease, "fluffy rarefaction" of pagetoid bone
Paget osteitis deformans
Paget-Schroetter venous thrombosis of axillary vein
Paget-von Schroetter syndrome
Pais fracture
PALA enhancement
palatal
palate
   bony
   Byzantine arch

palate (cont.)
   cleft
   hard
   high arched
   soft
palatine bone
palatopharyngeal fold
paleopathologic and radiologic study
palladium (Pd)
   $^{103}$Pd isotope used in brachytherapy
   $^{103}$Pd prostatic implant
   $^{103}$Pd radioactive material
palliation of pain
palliative irradiation
palliative radiation therapy
palmar metacarpal ligament
palmar plate
Palmaz balloon-expandable iliac stent
Palmaz-Schatz coronary stent
Palmaz vascular stent
palpability
palpation
palpatory
palpebral fissure
PAM (pulmonary artery mean) pressure
panacinar emphysema
panaortic
pancake MRI magnet
pancarpal destructive arthritis
panchamber enlargement
Pancoast syndrome
Pancoast tumor
pancreas
   aberrant
   accessory
   annular
   anterior surface of
   Aselli
   CT scan of
   degeneration of
   dorsal

pancreas (cont.)
   head of
   heterotopic
   interior surface of
   lesser
   neck of
   posterior surface of
   tail of
   uncinate process of
   ventral
   Willis
   Winslow
pancreatic angiography
pancreatic duct
   accessory
   disruption of
   duodenal end of dorsal
   duodenal end of main
   main
   obstruction of
   proximal part of dorsal
pancreatic duct cannulation, endoscopic retrograde
pancreatic-enteric continuity
pancreatic fistula
pancreaticobiliary common channel
pancreaticohepatic syndrome
pancreatic pseudocyst
pancreatic scan
pancreatitis
pancreatocholangiogram, retrograde
pancreatogram
pancreatography
   endoscopic retrograde
   intraoperative
   retrograde
pancreatolithiasis
panda sign
panfacial fracture
panlobular emphysema
pannus deformity of odontoid
pannus of synovium

panoramic CT scan
panoramic image
panoramic radiography
Panorex x-ray
pansystolic mitral regurgitation
pantalar fusion
pantaloon embolus
pantaloon hernia
Pantopaque contrast medium
Pantopaque myelography
PAP (pulmonary artery pressure)
papilla
    acoustic
    bile
    duodenal
    major duodenal
    minor duodenal
    renal
    Santorini
    urethral
    Vater
papillary epithelial neoplasm
papillary fibroelastoma
papilloma
    choroid plexus
    cockscomb
    Hopmann
    ventricular tumor
PAPVR (partial anomalous pulmonary venous return)
para-aortic region
para-articular bone remodeling
para-articular calcification
parabola, metatarsal
paracardiac mass
paracardiac-type total anomalous venous return
paracentral lobule
paracervical region
parachute deformity of mitral valve
paracicatricial emphysema
paracoccidioidomycosis
paracolic gutter
paracorporeal
paracostal
paradoxical embolus
paradoxical hyperconcentration of contrast medium
paradoxical motion
paradoxical suppression
paraesophageal hernia
paraesophagogastric devascularization
parafascicular nucleus
paraganglioma
paragangliomatosis
parahilar (also perihilar)
parallel analog mapping
parallel and spiral flow patterns
parallel hole image
parallel hole medium sensitivity collimator
parallel opposed ports
parallel opposed unmodified ports
parallel-tagged MR images and field-fitting analysis
parallel tag planes
Parallel virtual machine
paralysis of diaphragm
paralytic chest
paralytic ileus
paramagnetic artifact
paramagnetic contrast media
paramagnetic Cr-labeled red blood cells
paramagnetic relaxation
paramagnetic shift
paramagnetic substances
paramagnetism
paramalleolar arteries
paramedian position
paramedian sagittal plane
paramediastinal glands
parameningeal

parameter
   clinical
   hematologic
   kinetic perfusion
   nuclear
   optimization
   parameters
   physiologic
   scan
   sonographic
   thermal treatment
   ventricular function
paranasal sinus
paraneoplastic cerebellar degeneration
paraneoplastic hypercalcemia
paraneoplastic process
parapatellar plica
parapelvic (also peripelvic)
parapelvic gutter
parapharyngeal abscess
parapharyngeal space
paraprosthetic-enteric fistula
paraprosthetic leakage
pararenal abscess
pararenal aortic aneurysm
pararenal aortic atherosclerosis
parasagittal head region
parasagittal intracranial mass
parasagittal meningioma
parasagittal region
parasellar mass
paraseptal emphysema
paraseptal position
paraspinal abnormality
paraspinal muscles
paraspinal musculature
paraspinal pleural stripe
paraspinal soft tissue mass
paraspinal soft tissue shadowing
paraspinous musculature
parasternal bulge
parasternal long-axis view

parasternal lymph nodes
parasternal motion
parasternal short-axis view
parasternal view of heart
parasternal window
parasympathetic nervous system
paratracheal soft tissues
paratracheal stripe
paratrooper fracture
paravalvar leak
paravalvular
paravertebral gutter
paravertebral musculature
paravertebral nerve plexus
paravertebral region
paravertebral venous plexus
parchment heart syndrome
parchment right ventricle
parenchyma
   cerebral
   liver
   lung
   pulmonary
   spinal cord
parenchymal collaterals
parenchymal consolidation
parenchymal echogenicity
parenchymal fibrous band
parenchymal infarct
parenchymal infiltrates, pulmonary
parenchymal lung disease
parenchymal neurocutaneous
   melanosis
parenchymal tracer accumulation
parenchymal transit
parenchymatous atrophy
parenchymatous cerebellar
   degeneration
parenchymatous hemorrhage
parenchymatous neurosyphilis
parenchymatous phase
parent vein

paresis, hemilingual
parietal band
parietal bone
parietal branches
  paired
  unpaired
parietal cephalohematoma
parietal cortex lesion
parietal cortex, post-rolandic
parietal extension of infundibular
  septum
parietal gyrus
parietal layer
parietal lobe lesion
parietal lobe sign
parietal pericardial calcification
parietal pericardium
parietal pleura
parieto-occipital lesion
parieto-occipital sulcus
parietotemporal area
Paris system
Park Medical Systems scanner
Parks bidirectional Doppler flowmeter
Parks ileal reservoir
Parona space
parosteal chondrosarcoma
parosteal osteogenic sarcoma
parosteal osteosarcoma
parotid gland
parotid pleomorphic adenoma
paroxysmal crisis, hypertensive
parrot-beak meniscus tears
parry fracture
pars interarticularis
Parsons, third intercondylar
  tubercle of
partial anomalous pulmonary venous
  return (PAPVR)
partial-brain radiation therapy
partial collapse of lung
partial dislocation

partial dislodgement
partial K-space sampling
partial liquid ventilation with
  perflubron
partial obliteration of a lateral
  ventricle (on scan)
partial ossicular replacement
  prosthesis (PORP)
partial pericardial absence
partial saturation and spin-echo pulse
  sequence
partial saturation technique
partial-thickness tear
partial volume averaging
partial volume effect, artifact due to
particle (pl. particles)
  beta
  bone
  calcium/oxyanion-containing
  charged
  Ivalon
particle beam
particle debris
particle identification
particle masks
particle size determination
particulate debris
particulates, magnetic
partition
  atrial
  gastric
partition coefficient
parts, fetal small
PAS (pulmonary artery systolic)
  pressure
pascals of force (SI units)
passage of blind catheter
passages, narrowing of bronchiolar
passive clot
passive filling
passively congested lung tissue
passively shimmed superconducting
  magnet

passive pneumonia
passive track detector
passive vascular congestion
passive venous distention
PASTA (polarity-altered spectral-selective acquisition) imaging
patch crinkling
patch electrodes placed outside the pericardium
patch
  epidural blood
  kinking of
  pericardial
  periosteal
  Peyer
  transannular
  vein
patchy air-space consolidations
patchy alveolar opacities
patchy atelectasis
patchy atrophy of renal cortex
patchy consolidation
patchy distribution of the tracer
patchy infiltrate
patchy migratory infiltrates
patchy zones
patella
  apex of head of
  bipartite
  dislocated
  floating
  high-riding
  lower pole of
  skyline view of
  subluxing
  undersurface of
patella alta (high-riding)
patella baja
patellar button
patellar chondromalacia
patellar contour
patellar dislocation

patellar edge
patellar entrapment
patellar fat pad
patellar fossa
patellar groove
patellar subluxation
patellar tendinosis
patellofemoral articular cartilage
patellofemoral joint space
patellofemoral region
patency
  arterial
  coronary artery
  coronary bypass graft
  ductus arteriosus
  graft
  long-term
  short-term
  vein
patency and valvular reflux of deep veins
patency
patency of vein graft
patency of vessel
patency rate
patent bifurcation
patent ductus arteriosus (PDA)
patent foramen ovale
patent trifurcation
patent, widely
Paterson-Parker rules
Pathfinder catheter
pathognomonic sign
pathologic confirmation
pathologic correlation
pathologic diagnosis
pathologic dislocation
pathologic fracture
pathologic reflux
pathology, radiographic
pathophysiologic changes in airways obstruction

pathophysiology
pathway
  neural
  optic
  retrovestibular neural
patient motion artifact
pattern
  abdominal wall venous
  A fib (atrial fibrillation)
  air-space filling
  alveolar
  AM (associative memory)
  anhaustral colonic gas
  arterial deficiency
  bigeminal
  blood flow
  bowel
  bowel gas
  branching
  butterfly
  cobblestone
  cobweb
  contractile
  corduroy cloth (on myelogram)
  dP/dt upstroke
  ductal
  early repolarization
  echo
  electron and x-ray diffraction
  enhancement
  extended
  fibrotic cavitating
  filigree
  fine reticular
  fold
  gas
  gastric mucosal
  haustral
  helical
  hemodynamic
  heterogeneous perfusion
  hierarchical scanning

pattern *(cont.)*
  hole
  homogeneous
  honeycomb
  hourglass
  infiltration
  interstitial
  juvenile T wave
  Laue
  left ventricular contraction
  left ventricular strain
  lobular
  M (on right atrial waveform)
  miliary
  macronodular
  marrow edema
  micronodular
  mosaic
  mosaic attenuation
  mosaic duodenal mucosal
  moth-eaten
  movement
  MR enhancement
  M-shaped mitral valve
  mucosal
  nonspecific gas
  parallel
  pin
  P pulmonale
  pseudoinfarct
  pulmonary flow
  pulmonary vascular
  recurrence
  rheologic
  right ventricular strain
  rugal
  sigmoid hair (on spine)
  signet ring
  small bowel mucosal
  SMPTE test
  speckled
  spectral

pattern *(cont.)*
  spiral flow
  star
  stellate
  strain
  sulcal
  surface convexity
  task-rest
  temporal sawtooth
  thermal convection
  tree-in-bud (TIB)
  trigeminal
  ventricular contraction
  vesicular
patulous hiatus
pauciarticular
paucity of bowel gas
pause
  asystolic
  compensatory
  noncompensatory
  pauses
  postextrasystolic
  sinus
Pauwel angle of femoral neck fracture
Pauwel fracture classification
Pawlik trigone
PAWP (pulmonary artery wedge pressure)
Payr disease
Payr sign
Pb (lead)
Pb-212-labeled monoclonal antibody imaging agent
PBF (pulmonary blood flow)
PBPI (penile-brachial pressure index) to assess cardiac disease
PBT Technologies PACS
PBVI (pulmonary blood volume index)
PC (phase contrast) imaging
PC (posterior commissure)
PCA (posterior cerebral artery)
PCA (posterior communicating artery)
PCL (posterior cruciate ligament)
PCoA (posterior communicating artery)
PCP (pulmonary capillary pressure)
PCS (proximal coronary sinus)
PCVD (pulmonary collagen vascular disease)
PCWP (pulmonary capillary wedge pressure)
Pd (palladium)
PDA (patent ductus arteriosus)
PDA (posterior descending artery)
PDI (power Doppler imaging)
PDR (pulsed brachytherapy)
PE (pericardial effusion)
PE (pulmonary embolism)
peak
  airway pressure
  diffraction
  juxtaphrenic
  main glow
  pressure
  single
peak airway pressure
peak count density
peak dP/dt
peak early diastolic filling velocities
peak enhancement
peak expiratory flow (PEF)
peak expiratory flow rate (PEFR)
peak filling rate (PFR)
peak fitting
peak flow
peak flow variability
peak flow velocity
peak identification
peak-inflation pressures
peak late diastolic filling velocities
peak parenchymal activity

peak profile
peak regurgitant flow velocity
peak regurgitant wave pressure
peak systolic and diastolic ICA/CCA
　　ratios
peak systolic pressure
peak systolic velocity (cm/sec)
peak tidal expiratory flow
peak-to-peak pressure gradient
peak velocity of blood flow on
　　Doppler echocardiogram
pectoral
pectoralis major muscle
pectoralis major syndrome
pectoralis minor muscle
pectus carinatum
pectus excavatum deformity
pedal artery opacification
pediatric biplane TEE (transesophageal
　　echocardiography) probe
pediatric neuroradiology
pedicle
　　IMA (internal mammary artery)
　　musculofascial
　　phrenic
　　spinal
　　vascular
pedicle bone grafts
pedicle erosion
pedicle of vertebra
pedicle sclerosis
peduncle
　　cerebellar
　　cerebral
　　inferior cerebellar
peduncular segment of superior cere-
　　bellar artery
pedunculated myxoma
pedunculated polyp
pedunculated subserous myoma
pedunculated thrombus
pedunculated uterine myoma

pedunculated vesical tumor
pedunculation
PEG (pneumoencephalogram)
Pel-Ebstein disease
Pellegrini-Stieda disease
pellet
　　alanine-silicone
　　radiopaque
pellet artifact (shotgun pellets)
pellucidum
pelvic abscess
pelvicaliceal changes
pelvicaliceal distention
pelvic bone
pelvic brim
pelvic collateral vessel
pelvic diameter
pelvic floor
pelvic fracture frame
pelvic girdle
pelvic inlet
pelvic node
pelvic notching
pelvic obliquity
pelvic outlet
pelvic rim fracture
pelvic ring fracture
pelvic tilt, bent knee
pelvic traction
pelvic ultrasound
pelvic ultrasound CT scan
pelvic view
pelviectasis
pelvimetry, Mengert index in
pelvis
　　android
　　anthropoid
　　assimilation
　　beaked
　　bony
　　brachypellic
　　contracted

pelvis *(cont.)*
   cordate
   cordiform
   Deventer
   dolichopellic
   dwarf
   false
   female
   flat
   frozen
   funnel-shaped
   greater
   gynecoid
   hardened
   heart-shaped
   inverted
   juvenile
   Kilian
   kyphoscoliotic
   kyphotic
   lesser
   longitudinal oval
   lordotic
   male
   masculine
   mesatipellic
   Nägele
   osteomalacic
   Otto
   platypelloid
   portable film of
   Prague
   pseudo-osteomalacic
   rachitic
   reniform
   renal
   Rokitansky
   scoliotic
   small
   spider
   spondylolisthetic
   transverse oval

pelvis *(cont.)*
   true
   ureteral
   ureteric
pelviureteral junction
pelvocaliceal effacement
pencil beam approach
pencil-beam navigator echos
penciling of ribs
Pendred syndrome
pendulous urethra
pendulum movement
penetrating aortic ulceration
penetrating atherosclerotic ulceration
penetrating trauma
penetrating injury
penetrating ulceration
penile urethra
penis
   bulb of
   bulbospongiosus muscle of
   clubbed
   concealed
   corpora cavernosa
   corpus spongiosum
   crura of
   deep fascia of
   dorsal artery of
   dorsal nerve of
   dorsum of
   double
   glans
   ischiospongiosus muscle of
   root of
   suspensory ligament of
   webbed
penoscrotal
PenRad mammography clinical reporting system
Penrose drain
Pentagastrin
pentavalent DMSA

Pentax EUP-EC124 ultrasound gastroscope
Pentax-Hitachi FG32UA endosonographic system
pentetreotide indium-111 ($^{111}$In)
penumbra, dosimetric
penumbra zone
PEP (pre-ejection period)
PE Plus II balloon dilatation catheter
peppermint oil (used with barium enema)
peptic ulcer
    acute
    chronic
peptic ulcer disease (PUD)
peptide imaging agent
percentage signal intensity loss (PSIL)
Perception scanner
perceptual linearization
Perchloracap contrast medium
perchlorate washout test
Percor DL balloon catheter
Percor DL-II (dual-lumen) intra-aortic balloon catheter
Percor-Stat-DL catheter
percutaneous antegrade biliary drainage
percutaneous aortic balloon valvuloplasty
percutaneous automated diskectomy under fluoroscopy
percutaneous endoluminal placement of stent-graft
percutaneous fibrin glue
percutaneous gastrostomy, radiologic
percutaneous insertion via femoral vein
percutaneous interventional radiology
percutaneous intracoronary angioscopy
percutaneously cannulated
percutaneous pericardioscopy
percutaneous radiofrequency ablation
percutaneous retrograde transfemoral technique
percutaneous transcatheter ductal closure (PTDC)
percutaneous transhepatic biliary drainage with contrast monitoring
percutaneous transhepatic cholangiogram (PTHC)
percutaneous transhepatic liver biopsy
percutaneous transhepatic portography with hemodynamic evaluation
percutaneous transluminal angioplasty (PTA)
percutaneous transluminal coronary angioplasty (PTCA)
percutaneous transluminal renal angioplasty (PTRA)
percutaneous transperineal seed implantation
percutaneous transvenous embolization
perflubron contrast
perfluorocarbon F-19 ($^{19}$F) imaging agent
perfluoroctylbromide (PFOB) imaging agent
perfluoro-1H,-1H-neopentyl imaging agent
perforated diverticulum
perforating aneurysm
perforating arteries
perforating fracture
perforation
    bladder
    cardiac
    transseptal
    ulcer
perforator vessel
perfusate
perfuse
perfusion
    adequate coronary
    antegrade

perfusion *(cont.)*
  coronary
  diminished systemic
  homogeneous
  hypothermic
  intraperitoneal hyperthermic (IPHP)
  luxury
  misery
  mosaic
  myocardial
  peripheral
  poor
  pulsatile
  quantitative cardiac
  regional (by mixed venous blood)
  regional cerebral
  renal
  retrograde cardiac
  tissue
perfusion abnormality
perfusion agent
perfusion and ventilation lung scan
perfusion catheter
perfusion defect
perfusion deficit
perfusion gradient
perfusion lung scan
perfusion magnetic resonance imaging
perfusion-metabolism mismatch
perfusion pressure
perfusion scan
perfusion-weighted MRI
perialveolar fibrosis
periampullary diverticulum
periampullary duodenal tumor
periaortic area
periaortic fibrosis
periapical granuloma
periapical lesion
periappendiceal abscess
periaqueductal gray matter

periaqueductal region
periarticular calcification
periarticular fracture
periarticular heterotopic ossification (PHO)
peribronchial alveolar spaces
peribronchial connective tissue
peribronchial cuffing
peribronchial distribution
peribronchial fibrosis
peribronchial infiltrate
peribronchial lymph nodes
peribronchial markings
peribronchial thickening
peribronchiolar hemorrhage
pericallosal artery
pericardiacophrenic vein
pericardial absence
  congenital
  partial
pericardial cavity
pericardial constriction, occult
pericardial cyst
pericardial diaphragmatic adhesions
pericardial effusion
pericardial fat pad
pericardial fluid
pericardial fold
pericardial hematoma
pericardial infusion
pericardial reflection
pericardial sac
pericardial sinus
pericardial space
pericardiocentesis, ultrasonic guidance for
pericardium
  adherent
  autologous
  bread-and-butter
  calcified
  congenitally absent

pericardium *(cont.)*
   diaphragmatic
   fibrous
   parietal
   serous
   shaggy
   soldier's patches of
   veins of
   visceral
pericardium calcareous deposits
pericardium fibrosum
pericatheter thrombus (pl. thrombi)
pericecal abscess
pericholecystic edema
pericholecystic fluid
pericicatricial emphysema
pericolonic fat
pericystic edema
periductal calcification
periductal fibrosis
peridural fibrosis
perigastric deformity
perigraft hematoma
perihilar (also parahilar)
perihilar density
perihilar edema
perihilar fat
perihilar fibrosis
perihilar infiltrate
perihilar markings
perihilar region
peri-ileal
peri-infarction ischemia
peri-infarctional defect
perilesional bone
perilunate carpal dislocation
perilunate fracture dislocation (PLFD)
perimalleolar pain
perimedullary
perimembranous ventricular septal
   defect
perimuscular plexus

perimylolysis
perinatal respiratory distress syndrome
perineal descent
perineogram
perineoplastic edema
perinephric abscess
perinephric fat
perinephric space
perineural invasion
perineural tumor
perineural fibroblastoma tumor
period
   diastolic filling
   noninteger
   raster
   rapid filling (RFP)
   reduced ventricular filling
periodic packing
periodontal ligament
periorbital Doppler study
periosteal bone formation
periosteal creep
periosteal fibroma
periosteal new bone formation
periosteal osteosarcoma
periosteal reaction
periosteal sarcoma
peripancreatic arteries
peripancreatic fluid collection
peripelvic (also parapelvic)
peripelvic collateral vessel
peripheral air-space disease
peripheral arterial cannula
peripheral blood flow
peripheral circulatory vasoconstriction
peripheral consolidation
peripheral cutaneous vasoconstriction
peripheral embolus
peripheral fracture
peripheral gating technique
peripheral infiltrate

peripheral laser angioplasty (PLA)
peripheral lesion
peripheral loading
peripheral lung disease
peripherally inserted central catheter (PICC)
peripheral nerve
peripheral nodule
peripheral ossification
peripheral parenchymal atelectasis
peripheral pulmonary artery stenosis
peripheral pulmonic stenosis
peripheral quantitative computed tomography technology (pQCT)
peripheral resistance
peripheral small airways study
peripheral vascular disease, arteriosclerotic
peripheral vascular resistance, decreased
peripheral veins, absent
peripheral vessels
peripheral washout sign
periphery, echogenic
periportal area
periportal tracking of blood
periprosthetic bone resorption
periprosthetic leak (leakage)
periradicular nerve
periradicular sheath
perirectal abscess
perirenal fat
perirenal hematoma
perirenal hemorrhage
perirenal mass
perirenal septum
perirenal space
perirolandic cortex
perisigmoid colon
perisinusoidal space
peristalsing bowel
peristalsis
  absent
  accelerated
  decreased
  increased
  reversed
  visible
peristaltic contraction
peristaltic rush
peristaltic wave
peristriate cortex
peritoneal cavity
  greater sac of
  lesser sac of
peritoneal catheter
peritoneal enhancement
peritoneal effusion
peritoneal mouse
peritoneal-venous shunt patency test
peritoneogram
peritoneography, CT
peritoneovenous shunt (PVS)
peritoneum
  parietal
  pelvic
  visceral
periureteral fibrosis
perivalvular dehiscence
perivalvular disruption
perivalvular leak
perivascular canal
perivascular distribution
perivascular edema
perivascular fibrosis
perivascular plane
perivascular space of Virchow-Robin
periventricular density
periventricular gray (PVG) matter
periventricular halo
periventricular leukomalacia (PVL)
periventricular white matter
perivenular nodularity

perivesical
permanent brachytherapy
permeability
　capillary
　membrane
　tumor capillary
permeability-type pulmonary edema
permeative lesion
peroneal area
peroneal artery
peroneal muscles
peroneal obliterative thrombus
peroneal-tibial trunk
peroneal vein
peroneus tertius
Persantine thallium stress test
persistent common atrioventricular
　canal
persistent fetal circulation
persistent truncus arteriosus
perspective volume rendering (PVR)
Pertechnegas
pertechnetate sodium (technetium)
Perthes-Bankart lesion
Perthes disease
Perthes epiphysis
pertrochanteric fracture
pertubation, radiation dose
perusal
pervenous catheter
pes abductus
pes adductus
pes anserinus
pes arcuatus
pes calcaneocavus
pes calcaneovalgus
pes calcaneus
pes cavovalgus
pes cavovarus
pes cavus
pes contortus
pes equinovalgus

pes equinovarus
pes equinus
pes excavatus
pes malleus valgus
pes planovalgus
pes plantigrade planus
pes planus
pes pronation
pes pronatus
pes supinatus
pes valgus
pes varus
pessary
PET (positron emission tomography)
　PET balloon, USCI
　PET balloon with window and
　　extended collection chamber
　PET metabolic imaging
　PET myocardial fatty acid imaging
　PET perfusion imaging
　PET radioligands
　PET radiopharmaceuticals
　PET target material
petal-fugal flow on angiography
Petit disease
petroclinoid ligament
petroclival region
petromastoid
petro-occipital synchondrosis
petrosal bone
petrosal nerve
petrosal sinus
petrosphenoid
petrosquamosal
petrous bone
petrous carotid canal stenosis
petrous pyramid
petrous ridge
petrous segment of carotid artery
Peutz-Jeghers gastrointestinal
　polyposis
Peyer patch

Pezzer catheter
PF-PACS system
Pfeiffer-Comberg method
Pfeiffer syndrome
PFFD (proximal focal femoral deficiency)
PFOB imaging agent
P53-mediated radioresistance
PFR (peak filling rate)
PFWT (pain-free walking time) on treadmill
PGK (Panos G. Koutrouvelis, M.D.) stereotactic device
phagedenic ulcer
phagocytosis, MR imaging of
phakomatoses
phalangeal bones
phalangeal glenoidal ligament of hand
phalangeal herniation
phalanx (pl. phalanges)
   base of
   waist of
Phalen position
pharmacologic intervention
pharmacologic stress dual-isotope myocardial perfusion SPECT
pharmacologic stress echocardiography
pharmacoradiologic disimpaction of esophageal foreign body
pharyngeal area
pharyngoesophageal diverticulum
pharyngoesophageal function
pharynx
   laryngeal part of
   nasal part of
   oral part of
phase (see also *period*)
   corticomedullary (CP)
   delayed
   diastolic depolarization
   equilibrium
   expiratory

phase *(cont.)*
   hepatic arterial (HAP)
   inspiratory
   late
   NCP (noncontrast)
   NP (nephrographic)
   parenchymatous
   plateau (in cardiac action potentials)
   portal venous (PVP)
   prolonged expiratory
   prolonged inspiratory
   PVP (portal venous)
   rapid filling
   vascular
   ventilation
   wash-in
   washout
phase analysis
phase angle
phase cycling
phase-contrast angiography
phase-contrast imaging
phased-array surface coil
phased array, symmetrical
phase delay
phase difference
phase-encoded motion artifact
phase-encode pulse
phase encode time reduced acquisition sequence
phase identification
phase image (imaging)
phase relation
phase sensitive detector
phase shift
phase shifting interferometry
phase-shift velocity mapping
phase-unwrapping method
phase-velocity image
phasic contractions
phenomenological effective surface potential

phenomenon (pl. phenomena)
  A
  aliasing
  anniversary
  Aschner
  Ashman
  Austin Flint
  baked brain
  Bancaud
  Bell
  booster
  Bowditch staircase
  combined-flexion
  coronary steal
  crus
  Cushing
  dip
  dip and plateau
  Doppler
  embolic
  extinction
  flare
  flip-flop
  freezing
  Friedreich
  Gaertner (Gärtner)
  Gallavardin
  gap conduction
  Gibbs
  Goldblatt
  Gordon knee
  Gowers
  Hering
  Jod-Basedow
  Kasabach-Merritt
  Katz-Wachtle
  Kernohan notch
  kindling
  Litten diaphragm
  Marin-Amat
  no-reflow
  nonspecific

phenomenon *(cont.)*
  on-off
  Piltz-Westphal
  Robin Hood (steal syndrome)
  R-on-T
  Schellong-Strisower
  Schiff-Sherrington
  Schramm
  staircase
  steal
  steal syndrome
  stone heart
  treppe
  Uhthoff
  unilateral Raynaud
  V
  vacuum joint
  vertebral steal
  Wenckebach
  zone
phentetiothalein contrast medium
pheochromocytoma
Philips CT scanner
Philips DVI 1 system
Philips Gyroscan ACS scanner
Philips Gyroscan NT; NT5; NT15
  scanner
Philips Gyroscan S5 scanner
Philips Gyroscan T5 scanner
Philips linear accelerator (LINAC)
Philips 1.5T NT MR scanner
Philips scanner
Philips Tomoscan 350 CT scanner
Philips Tomoscan SR 6000 CT scanner
Philips ultrasound machine
phlebogram (phlebography), MR
  ascending
  ascending contrast
  direct puncture
  impedance
phlebolith

phleborheography (PRG)
phlebosclerosis
phlebostasis
phlebostenosis
phlebothrombosis
phlegmon
   Holz
   pancreatic
   periurethral
phlegmonous
phoenix abscess
phosphoric acid imaging agent
phosphorus metabolites
phosphorus nuclear magnetic resonance spectroscopy (P-MRS)
phosphorus-32 intracavitary irradiation
phosphorus-32 sodium phosphate
photo-plotter film
photoacoustic ultrasonography
photocell plethysmography
photodeficient region
photodetectors, CCD
photodiode
photodisruption
photoelasticity
photographic technique
   Debye-Scherrer
   Laue
photography, CT bone window
photolabel, long wavelength
photon attenuation measurement
photon deficiency
photon deficient lesion
photon densitometry
photon interaction depth
photon-neutron mixed-beam radiotherapy
photon, soft
photon therapy beam line
photonic medicine
photopeak
photopenia
photopenic area on film or scan
photopenic defect
photopenic region
photoplethysmographic digit
photoplethysmographic monitoring
photoplethysmography (PPG)
photoreceptor fractional velocity error
photoreceptor motion
photostimulable luminescence intensity
photostimulable phosphor dental radiography (PSP)
phrenic artery
phrenic pedicle
phrenoesophageal ligament
phrenogastric gastric
phrenovertebral junction
phrygian cap deformity
phthinoid chest
phthisis, aneurysmal
PHTN (pulmonary hypertension)
Phylax implantable cardioverter-defibrillator (Biotronik)
phyllodes tumor
physeal bar
physeal cartilage
physeal closure
physeal damage
physeal distraction
physeal fracture
physeal injury
physeal plate fracture
physicochemical speciation
physiologic flow
physiologic regurgitation
physiologic shunt flow
physis (pl. physes)
   distal tibial
   fibular
   fused
   medial
   unfused
phytobezoar

PI (pulmonic insufficiency)
pia arachnoid
pia mater
pial vessels
PIBC (percutaneous intra-aortic balloon counterpulsation)
pica artifact
PICA (posterior inferior communicating artery)
Pick body
Pick bundle
Pick disease
Picker camera
Picker CT scanner
Picker Magnascanner
Picker MR scanner
Picker PQ 5000 helical CT scanner
Picker PQ-2000 spiral CT scanner
Picker SPECT attenuation correction
Picket Fence fiducial localization stereotactic system
picture archive and communication system (PACs) for imaging
picture archiving and communications systems in radiation oncology (PACSRO)
picture element (pixel)
picture frame pattern of vertebral bodies
PIE (pulmonary interstitial emphysema)
piece, chin-occiput
Piedmont fracture
pigeon-breeder's lung
pigeon chest
pigeon-fancier's lung
Pigg-O-Stat x-ray chair for child
piggybacking
pigtail catheter
Pillar view
pillion fracture
pillow fracture

pilonidal cyst
pilonidal sinus
pin pattern
PIN (posterior interosseous nerve) entrapment
pinchcock mechanism at esophagogastric junction
pinched nerve
pincushion distortion, radiographic
pineal apoplexy
pineal body, calcified
pineal calcification displaced from midline
pineal gland, calcified
pineal gland tumor
pinealoma tumor
pineal region
pineoblastoma
pineocytoma
ping-pong fracture
pinhole, bone
pinhole collimator
pinhole image
Pinnacle 3 radiation therapy planning system
PION (posterior interosseous nerve)
PIP (proximal interphalangeal)
   PIP articulation
   PIP joint
pipestem arteries
pipe-stemming of ankle-brachial index
PIPIDA (P-isopropylacetanilide-iminodiacetic acid)
$^{99m}$TcPIPIDA hepatobiliary scan
PIPJ (proximal interphalangeal joint)
Pipkin classification of femoral fracture
Pirie bone
piriform muscle
pisiform bone of wrist
pisotriquetral joint
pistoning

piston sign
pit
　anal
　articular
　auditory
　central
　colonic
　costal
　cutaneous
　gastric
　postanal
pitch
　scan
　spiral CT
pitch ratio
pituitary fossa
pituitary gland
pituitary microadenoma
pituitary stalk distortion (PSD)
pituitary tumor
pivoting table
pixel (picture element)
　edge-region
　normal-region
pixel-block, 8 x 8
pixel noise
pixel-oriented algorithms
Pixsys FlashPoint camera
placement
　annular
　catheter
　intracoronary stent
　intrapericardial patch lead
　percutaneous endoluminal
　radiotherapy field
　shent
　shim
　subannular
　subject
placement of radiation therapy fields, ultrasonic guidance for

placenta
　abnormal adherence of
　accessory
　adherent
　annular
　battledore
　bilobate
　chorioallantoic
　chorioamniotic
　cirsoid
　deciduate
　Duncan
　fetal
　first-trimester
　fundal
　horseshoe
　incarcerated
　kidney-shaped
　marginal
　maternal
　nondeciduate
　panduriform
　retained
　Schultze
　second-trimester
　third-trimester
　velamentous
　villous
placenta previa
　central
　complete
　incomplete
　lateral
　marginal
　partial
　total
placental abruption (abruptio placentae)
placental localization
placental polyp
placental souffle
placentography

plafond fracture
plafond, tibial
plagiocephalic
plagiocephaly
plain film of abdomen
plain film radiography
plain tomogram
plain-paper image
planar (2D) imaging
planar exercise thallium-201
   scintigraphy
planar LAO image
planar spin imaging
planar thallium scan
planar thallium with quantitative
   analysis
planar view
Planck constant
plane (anatomical area)
   anatomic
   areolar
   auriculoinfraorbital
   axial
   axiolabiolingual
   axiomesiodistal
   bite
   buccolingual
   capsular
   circular
   coronal
   E
   eye-ear
   facial
   fat
   first parallel pelvic
   flexion-extension
   four-chamber
   fourth parallel pelvic
   Frankfort horizontal
   frontal
   gonion-gnathion
   Hensen
   Hodge

plane *(cont.)*
   horizontal
   imaging
   internervous
   interspinous
   intertubercular
   Ludwig
   median
   median sagittal
   mesiodistal
   midsagittal
   occlusal
   optimal imaging
   parallel tag
   paramedian sagittal
   pelvic
   perivascular
   sagittal
   sella-nasion
   semicoronal
   short-axis
   slicing
   spinous
   sternoxiphoid
   subadventitial
   subcostal (SCP)
   supracristal (SCP)
   subintimal cleavage
   suprasternal
   tag
   thoracic
   transaxial
   transmedial
   transpyloric
   transtrabecular (TTP)
   transumbilical (TUP)
   transverse
   tumor cleavage
   valve
   varus-valgus
   vertical
   XY
   ZY

plane of cleavage of tumor
planigram
planigraphy
planimeter
planimetry
planogram
planography
planovalgus foot deformity
plantar aponeurosis
plantar axial view
plantar calcaneal spur
plantar compartment
plantar flexion-inversion deformity
plantar hyperplasia
plantar spur
plantar vault
plantaris muscle
plantaris rupture
plantarward
plaque (also plaquing)
   arterial
   arteriosclerotic
   atheromatous
   atherosclerotic
   calcific
   calcified
   concentric atherosclerotic
   coral reef
   disrupted
   eccentric
   eccentric atherosclerotic
   echogenic
   echolucent
   endocardial
   fatty
   fibrofatty
   fibrotic
   fibrous
   fissured atheromatous
   gastrointestinal
   Hollenhorst

plaque *(cont.)*
   Hutchinson
   iliac
   infiltrating
   intraluminal
   Lichtheim
   lipid-laden
   luminal
   multiple sclerosis (MS)
   neuritic senile
   noncompliant
   obstructive
   pleural
   pulverized
   Randall
   residual
   sclerotic
   senile
   sessile
   stenotic
   talc
   ulcerated
   uncalcified
plaque cleaving
plaque compression
plaque-containing artery
plaque constituents
plaque erosion
plaque fracture (or fracturing)
plaquelike linear defect
plaque regression
plaque remodeling
plaque rupture
plaque splitting
plaque tearing
plaque vaporization
plaquing (see *plaque*)
plasma radioiron disappearance rate
plasma radioiron turnover rate
plasma volume
plastic clot

plate
- acetabular reconstruction
- alar
- anal
- auditory
- axial
- basal
- bone
- bone flap fixation
- bony
- budding
- cap-and-anchor
- cardiogenic
- cartilaginous growth
- chorionic
- clinoid
- cloacal
- cloverleaf
- coaptation
- compression
- condylar
- connecting
- cortical
- cranial bone fixation
- cribriform
- dorsal
- dual
- dynamic compression (DCP)
- end
- epiphyseal cartilage
- ethmovomerine
- femoral
- fibrocartilaginous
- flat
- flexor palmar
- foot
- frontal
- fusion
- growth
- hilar
- interfragmentary
- intertrochanteric

plate *(cont.)*
- localization-compression grid
- meningioma of cribriform
- microfixation
- nail
- neutralization
- occipitocervical
- orbital
- orthotic
- overlay
- palmar
- pedicle
- planar
- plantar
- pterygoid
- skull
- stabilization
- stainless steel
- stem base
- subchondral bone
- supracondylar
- tarsal
- tectal
- tendon
- 3-D or 3D (three-dimensional)
- titanium
- vertebral body
- volar

plate and screw system, MRI-compatible

plateau
- multiple sclerosis
- tibial

plateau fracture
platelet-activating factor inhibitor
platelet-rich thrombus
platelet survival study
platelike atelectasis
platform, Cemax PACS
platinum coil
platybasia
platycephaly

platypellic pelvis
platypelloid pelvis
platypodia
platyspondylosis
platyspondyly
PLC (posterolateral corner) of knee
pleating of ligamentum flavum
pleating of small bowel
pleomorphic xanthoastrocytoma
pleomorphism, nuclear
plesiography (brachytherapy)
plethora of findings
plethoric
plethysmogram
plethysmography
  air
  body box
  digital
  Doppler ultrasonic velocity
    detector segmental
  exercise strain gauge venous
  impedance (IPG)
  Medsonic
  photocell
  strain-gauge
  venous
pleura (pl. pleurae)
  cervical
  congested
  costal
  costodiaphragmatic recess of
  diaphragmatic
  edematous
  mediastinal
  parietal
  pericardiac
  pulmonary
  silicotic visceral
  visceral
  wrinkled
pleural adhesions, fibrous
pleural apical hematoma cap

pleural-based area of increased
  opacity
pleural cap
pleural cavity
pleural cupula (pl. cupulae)
pleural effusion
  ipsilateral
  liquid
  loculated
pleural empyema
pleural exudate
pleural fibrosis, asbestos-induced
pleural fistula
pleural flap
pleural fluid
pleural implants, malignant
pleural line
pleural margins
pleural plaque
pleural reflection
  costal
  mediastinodiaphragmatic
  sternal
  vertebral
pleural rind
pleural sac
pleural space
pleural thickening
pleurisy
  acute
  blocked
  chronic
  circumscribed
  costal
  diaphragmatic
  diffuse
  double
  dry
  encysted
  exudative
  fibrinous
  hemorrhagic

pleurisy *(cont.)*
   ichorous
   indurative
   interlobular
   latent
   mediastinal
   metapneumonic
   plastic
   primary
   proliferating
   pulmonary
   pulsating
   purulent
   sacculated
   secondary
   serofibrous
   serous
   single
   suppurative
   typhoid
   visceral
pleurocutaneous fistula
pleuroparenchymal plaque
pleuroperitoneal canal
pleuropulmonary adhesion
plexiform
plexus
   abdominal aortic
   anterior coronary
   anterior pulmonary
   aortic
   Auerbach mesenteric
   autonomic
   axillary
   basilar
   Batson
   biliary
   brachial
   calcification of choroid
   cardiac
   carotid
   cavernous

plexus *(cont.)*
   celiac
   cervical
   choroid
   ciliary ganglionic
   coccygeal
   colic
   colonic myenteric
   common carotid
   coronary
   cystic
   deep cardiac
   deferential
   enteric
   esophageal
   Exner
   extradural vertebral
   facial
   femoral
   gastric
   gastroesophageal variceal
   great cardiac
   hemorrhoidal
   hepatic nerve
   hypogastric
   ileocolic
   inferior mesenteric
   intermesenteric
   lumbar
   lumbosacral
   lymph
   Meissner
   myenteric
   nerve
   pampiniform
   paravertebral nerve
   paravertebral venous
   pelvic
   perimuscular
   pharyngeal
   presacral
   prostatic venous

plexus *(cont.)*
  pulmonary
  rectal
  right coronary
  sacral
  sciatic
  solar
  spinal nerve
  submucosal venous
  superficial
  superior hypogastric
  superior mesenteric
  uterovaginal
  vaginal
  vascular
  venous
  vertebral
  vertebral venous
  vesical
  vesical venous
plexus injury
plica (pl. plicae)
  medial
  parapatellar
  suprapatellar
  synovial
plication defect
P-LINK software
PLL (posterior longitudinal ligament)
ploidy, DNA
P loop (on vectorcardiography)
plots, cluster
PLSA (posterolateral spinal artery)
plug
  meconium
  mucus
Plummer disease
Plummer-Vinson syndrome
plump vessel
plurality of slices
plutonium, environmental
PM (posterior mitral)

PMD (papillary muscle dysfunction)
PML (posterior mitral leaflet)
pmol (picomole)
P-MRS (phosphorus magnetic resonance spectroscopy)
PMT (pyridoxyl-5-methyl tryptophan) imaging agent
PMT robotic fulcrumless tomographic system
PMV (percutaneous mitral balloon valvuloplasty)
PMV (prolapsed mitral valve)
PMVL (posterior mitral valve leaflet)
PNC (premature nodal contraction)
PNET (primitive neuroectodermal tumor)
pneumatic bone
pneumatization
pneumatocele
pneumencephalography, lumbar
pneumoarthrogram
pneumocele
pneumocephalus
pneumoconiosis
pneumoconstriction
pneumocystic infection
pneumocystis pneumonia (PCP)
pneumocystography
pneumocystotomography
pneumoencephalogram (PEG)
pneumoencephalographic pattern
pneumoencephalography
pneumoencephalomyelogram
pneumoencephalomyelography
pneumogastrography
pneumogram
pneumography
  cerebral
  retroperitoneal
pneumogynogram
pneumohemothorax
pneumointestinalis

pneumolith
pneumomediastinography
pneumomediastinum
  postoperative
  radiolucent
pneumomyelography
pneumonia (see also *pneumonitis*)
  acute
  alcoholic
  allergic
  amebic
  anthrax
  apex
  apical
  aspiration
  asthmatic
  atypical bronchial
  atypical interstitial
  bacterial
  bilious
  bronchial
  Buhl desquamative
  capillary
  caseous
  catarrhal
  central
  cerebral
  cheesy
  chelonian
  chemical
  chronic eosinophilic
  classic interstitial
  consolidative
  contusion
  Corrigan
  deglutition
  delayed resolution of
  desquamative interstitial (DIP)
  diffuse
  double
  Eaton agent
  embolic

pneumonia *(cont.)*
  exogenous lipoid
  eosinophilic
  ephemeral
  exogenous
  fibrinous
  fibrous
  Friedländer
  fungal
  gangrenous
  giant cell
  granulomatous
  gray hepatization stage of
  Hecht
  hypersensitivity
  hypostatic
  incomplete resolution of
  indurative
  infantile
  inhalation
  interstitial plasma cell
  irradiation
  lingular
  lipoid
  lobar
  lobular
  lymphoid interstitial
  massive
  metastatic
  migratory
  mycoplasmal
  necrotizing
  nonbacterial
  nosocomial
  obstructive
  oil-aspiration
  parenchymatous
  passive
  pertussoid eosinophilic
  Pittsburgh
  plague

pneumonia *(cont.)*
   plasma cell
   pleuritic
   pleurogenic
   pneumocystis
   postobstructive
   postoperative
   post-traumatic
   primary atypical
   protozoal
   purulent
   radiation
   red hepatization stage of
   resolving
   respiratory syncytial viral
   rheumatic
   rickettsial
   right-sided
   secondary
   segmental
   septic
   staphylococcal
   streptococcal
   subacute allergic
   superficial
   suppurative
   terminal
   toxic
   toxemic
   traumatic
   tuberculous
   tularemic
   typhoid
   unresolved
   varicella
   viral
   walking
   wandering
   white
   woolsorter's
pneumonic infiltrate
pneumonitis (see also *pneumonia*)
   acid aspiration
   acute interstitial
   aspiration
   bacterial
   chemical
   cholesterol
   chronic
   congenital rubella
   cytomegalovirus
   early
   granulomatous
   hypersensitivity
   interstitial
   lipoid
   lymphocytic interstitial
   malarial
   manganese
   *Mycoplasma* (mycoplasmal)
   pigeon breeder's
   plasma cell (PCP)
   radiation
   staphylococcal
   trimellitic anhydritic
   uremic
   ventilation
pneumonocirrhosis
pneumopericardium
pneumoperitoneum
pneumopreperitoneum
pneumopyelography
pneumoradiography
pneumoroentgenogram
pneumoscrotum
pneumothorax
   artificial
   basilar
   closed
   congenital
   diagnostic
   extrapleural
   induced

pneumothorax *(cont.)*
　life-threatening
　open
　positive-pressure
　pressure
　simultaneous bilateral spontaneous
　　(SBSP)
　spontaneous tension
　sucking
　tension
　therapeutic
　traumatic
　tuberculous
　uncomplicated
　valvular
pneumoventriculography
PO$_2$ imaging
pocket (see also *pouch*)
　air
　regurgitant
　Zahn
pocket Doppler
point (pl. points)
　Addison
　alveolar
　apophysary
　apophyseal
　auricular
　bleeding
　Cannon
　Cannon-Boehm
　cardinal
　Chauffard
　Clado
　congruent
　Cope
　coplanar contour
　craniometric
　dorsal
　end
　entry
　equilibrium

point *(cont.)*
　frontopolar
　glenoid
　Hartmann
　lead
　Mackenzie
　midinguinal
　nodal
　output
　Pauly
　preauricular
　random
　re-entry
　saddle
　sample
　seed
　Sudek
　target
　white
point imaging
point-in-space stereotactic biopsies
point localization
point scanning
point spread functions
point-to-point protocol (PPP)
Poisson-distributed activity
　concentrations
POL (posterior oblique ligament)
Poland classification of epiphyseal
　fracture
polar coordinate system
polarity-altered spectral-selective
　acquisition (PASTA) imaging
polarization, chemically induced
　dynamic nuclear
polarographic needle electrode
　measurement
pole
　abapical
　cephalic
　fetal
　frontal

pole *(cont.)*
   germinal
   inferior
   kidney
   lower
   middle
   patellar
   scaphoid
   superior
   temporal
   upper
pole figure texture analysis
Polhemus 3 digitizer
pollex pedis
polyarticular symmetric tophaceous
   joint inflammation
polyclonal IgG
polycystic kidney disease
polydactyly
polygelin colloid contrast medium
polygon mirror
polygyria
polyhydramnios
polymer
   friction-reducing
   PLA (polyactic acid)
polymer-coated drug-eluting stent
polymeric endoluminal paving stent
polynomial step-wise multiple-linear
   regression
polyostotic bone lesion
polyostotic fibrous dysplasia
polyp
   adenomatous
   benign
   bleeding
   broad-based
   bronchial
   cardiac
   cervical
   choanal
   colon

polyp *(cont.)*
   colonic
   colorectal
   cystic
   dental
   duodenal
   endometrial
   fibrinous
   fibroepithelial
   fibrovascular
   gastric
   hamartomatous gastric
   Hopmann
   hydatid
   hyperplastic gastric
   inflammatory fibroid
   juvenile
   laryngeal
   lipomatous
   lymphoid
   malignant
   metaplastic
   metastatic
   mucous
   multiple
   myomatous
   nasal
   neoplastic
   osseous
   pedunculated
   Peutz-Jeghers
   placental
   postinflammatory
   rectal
   regenerative
   retention
   sessile
   sigmoid
   single
   stalk of
   tubular
   tubulovillous

polyp *(cont.)*
   uterine
   vascular
   villous
polypoid calcified irregular mass
polypoid filling defect
polypoid lesion
polypoid lymphoid hyperplasia
polyposis
   adenomatous
   diffuse mucosal
   familial adenomatous (FAP)
   familial colorectal
   familial gastrointestinal
   familial intestinal
   FAP (familial adenomatous)
   filiform
   gastric
   hamartomatous
   intestinal
   juvenile
   multiple
   Peutz-Jeghers gastrointestinal
polyp stalk
polysplenia
Polystan venous return catheter
polystyrene, cross-linked
polytomographic radiology
polytomography
polytrauma
polyurethane foam embolus
polyurethane stent
polyvinyl alcohol particle size
Pompe disease
pond fracture
P1-P4 segments of posterior cerebral artery (PCA)
pons (pl. pontes)
   caudal
   infarction of
pons and midbrain, tegmentum of
pontine angle

pontine contusion
pontine glioma tumor
pontine hemorrhage
pontine infarction
pontine-medullary levels
pontocerebellar fibers
pontocerebellar glioma
pontomedullary junction
pontomesencephalic junction
pool
   blood
   focal
   vascular blood
pooling of blood in extremities
pooling, venous
poor shimming of MRI magnet
popcorn calcification
popliteal aneurysm
popliteal artery entrapment syndrome
popliteal artery occlusive disease
popliteal bypass
popliteal fossa
popliteal in situ bypass
popliteal recess
popliteal space
popliteal to distal in situ bypass
popliteal trifurcation
popliteal vein
porcelain gallbladder
porencephalic cyst
porencephalous
porencephaly
porosis, cerebral
porous ingrowth
porous metallic stent
port
   BardPort implantable
   parallel opposed unmodified
   single
   tangential
   treatment
portable C-arm image intensifier fluoroscopy

portable x-ray
portable film
Port-A-Cath
portacaval anastomosis, end-to-side
portacaval shunt
portal-systemic shunt (or portosystemic)
portal-to-portal bridging
portal triad
portal vein thrombosis
portal venography
portal venous phase (PVP)
PortalVision radiation oncology
 system
Portnoy ventricular catheter
porto-azygos collaterals
portogram
portography
 arterial
 CT arterial
 double-spiral CT arterial
 percutaneous transhepatic
 splenic
portopulmonary shunt
portosystemic (or portal-systemic)
Posicam HZ PET scanner
POSICAM PET (positron emission
 topography) system
position (see also *projection*; *view*)
 anatomic
 anterior oblique
 antero-oblique
 barber chair
 bayonet fracture
 beach chair
 Bertel
 catheter tip
 decubitus
 dorsal
 dorsosacral
 erect
 Fowler

position *(cont.)*
 frogleg
 full lateral
 horizontal
 infragenicular
 infrapulmonary
 LAO (left anterior oblique)
 lateral
 left anterior oblique (LAO)
 left-side-down decubitus
 lordotic
 lotus
 LPO (left posterior oblique)
 near anatomic
 neutral hip
 normal anatomic
 park bench
 Phalen
 prone
 pulmonary capillary wedge
 RAO (right anterior oblique)
 rectus
 recumbent
 reverse Trendelenburg
 right anterior oblique (RAO)
 right posterior oblique (RPO)
 right-side-down decubitus
 side-lying
 steep Trendelenburg
 supine
 swimmer's
 three-quarters prone
 Trendelenburg
 upright
position confirmed by fluoroscopy
 with aid of radiopaque marking
positioning error
position of joint, near anatomic
positive GI contrast agent
positive predictive value
positive-pressure pneumothorax
positive tilt test

Positrol II catheter
positron emission computed tomography (PET) scan
positron emitters
positron imaging
positron scanning (see PET scan)
postablation
postangioplasty aortogram
postangioplasty mural thrombosis
postangioplasty stenosis
post beat filtration
postcapillary venules
postcardiotomy lymphocytic splenomegaly
postcentral (sensory) gyrus
postcentral sulcus
postcontrast MR imaging
postcricoid area
postcubital
postdilatation arteriogram
postdrainage cystogram
postdrainage projection
postductal type of coarctation
posterior-anterior (PA)
posterior-aorta transposition of great arteries
posterior apical segment
posterior axillary line
posterior cervical triangle
posterior circulation
posterior colliculus
posterior column deficits (of spine)
posterior commissure
posterior communicating artery (PCA)
posterior compartment lesion
posterior coronary plexus (of heart)
posterior cusp
posterior descending artery (PDA)
posterior fossa
posterior fracture-dislocation
posterior free wall
posterior gray column of cord
posterior gray horns of the spinal canal
posterior inferior cerebellar artery (PICA)
posterior inferior communicating artery (PICA)
posterior intercostal artery
posterior interventricular groove
posterior interventricular vein
posterior joint syndrome
posterior-lateral (posterolateral)
posterior lip
posterior lumbar interbody fusion (PLIF)
posterior mediastinum
posterior neck surface coil
posterior olive in brain
posterior papillary muscle
posterior pulmonary plexus
posterior root entry zone (PREZ)
posterior root ganglia
posterior segment
posterior skull view
posterior spine fusion (PSF)
posterior spinocerebellar tract
posterior tibial artery
posterior tibiofibular ligament
posterior tibiotalar ligament
posterior wall myocardial infarction
posterior wall thickness
posteroanterior (PA)
posterobasal wall myocardial infarction
posterolateral aspect
posterolateral spinal artery (PLSA)
posterolateral wall myocardial infarction
posteromedial
postevacuation film
postganglionic gray fibers
postglomerular arteriolar constriction
post-glucose loading exam

postictal cerebral blood flow scan
postinfarction ventricular aneurysm
postinfarction ventriculoseptal defect
postinflammatory pulmonary fibrosis
post-injection image
postirradiation vascular insufficiency
postischemic recovery
postlymphangiography
postmastectomy lymphedema syndrome
postmetrizamide CT scan
postmyocardiotomy infarction
postobstructive pneumonia
postoperative bronchopneumonia
postoperative chylothorax
postorchiectomy para-aortic radiotherapy
postpartum pituitary apoplexy
postperfusion lung syndrome
postphlebitic incompetence
postprimary tuberculosis
postprocedure nephrostogram
post-PTCA residual stenosis
post-pyelonephritis cortical scarring
postradiation fibrosis
postreduction x-ray
postsphenoidal bone
poststenotic dilatation
poststress ankle/arm Doppler index
poststress images
postsurgical
post-thrombolytic coronary reocclusion
post-tourniquet occlusion angiography
post-transplant acute renal failure (ARF)
post-transplant coronary artery disease
post-traumatic or posttraumatic
post-traumatic angulation
post-traumatic cavus
post-traumatic fibrosis
post-traumatic neuroma
post-traumatic osteoporosis
post-ulnar bone
postvenography phlebitis
postvoid residual (PVR)
postvoid residual urine volume
postvoid(ing) film
potassium perchlorate contrast medium
potassium-43 imaging agent (myocardial perfusion imaging)
potassium-perchlorate
potential
   electrostatic
   phenomenological effective surface sorption
potentiometer
Pott fracture
Pott puffy tumor
potter's asthma
pouce flottant (floating thumb)
pouch
   antral
   apophyseal
   blind
   blind upper esophageal
   branchial
   Broca pudendal
   celomic
   deep perineal
   Douglas rectouterine
   dural root
   endodermal
   gastric
   Hartmann
   haustral
   Heidenhain
   hepatorenal
   hypophysial
   ileoanal
   ileocecal
   jejunal
   Kock
   Morison

pouch *(cont.)*
  paracystic
  pararectal
  paravesical
  pendulous
  pharyngeal
  Physick
  Prussak
  Rathke
  rectal
  rectouterine
  rectovaginal
  rectovaginouterine
  rectovesical
  renal
  Seessel
  superficial inguinal
  superficial perineal
  suprapatellar
  ultimobranchial
  uterovesical
  vesicouterine
  Zenker
pouchogram
pouchography, evacuation
Poupart inguinal ligament
power
  scanning
  stopping
power Doppler imaging (PDI)
power Doppler sonography
power injection
power injector
PowerVision Ultrasound System
PPAS (peripheral pulmonary artery stenosis)
PPH (primary pulmonary hypertension)
PPLO (pleuropneumonia-like organisms)
PPM (posterior papillary muscle)
PPP (point-to-point protocol)

pQCT (peripheral quantitative computed tomography)
pQCT micro-scanner
preablation
preacinar arterial wall thickness
preampullary portion of bile duct
preangioplasty stenosis
preaortic space, retropancreatic
preauricular point
precatheterization
precentral gyrus
precentral sulcus
precessing protons
precessional frequency
precharred fiber
precirrhosis
precision, test-retest
precluding catheter passage, tortuosity
preclusionary cue
precommunicating segment of anterior cerebral artery
precontrast scan
precordium
  active
  anterior
  bulging
  lateral
precursor sign to rupture of aneurysm
predicted target heart rate
prediction, LSC background
predictive assay
predictive value
predictor
predominance
  anterior
  posterior
  predominant
  temporal
predominant flow loads
preductal coarctation of aorta
pre-ejection interval
pre-ejection period (PEP)

preferential shunting
preformed clot
preformed guide wire
prefrontal bone of von Bardeleben
pregnancy
  abdominal
  ampullar
  bigeminal
  broad ligament
  cervical
  combined
  compound
  cornual
  ectopic
  extrauterine
  fallopian
  false
  heterotopic
  hydatid
  gemellary
  heterotopic
  interstitial
  intraligamentary
  intraperitoneal
  intrauterine
  membranous
  mesenteric
  molar
  multiple
  mural
  ovarian
  ovarioabdominal
  oviductal
  parietal
  phantom
  plural
  post-term
  prolonged
  pseudointraligamentary
  sarcofetal
  sarcohysteric
  spurious

pregnancy *(cont.)*
  stump
  toxemia of
  tubal
  tuboabdominal
  tuboligamentary
  tubo-ovarian
  tubouterine
  twin
  uteroabdominal
  uterotubal
Preiser disease
preliminary film
premature atherosclerosis
premature closure of ductus arteriosus
premature mid-diastolic closure of mitral valve
premature rupture of membranes
premature valve closure
premedullary arteriovenous fistula
preoperative renal angiography
preoperative resting MUGA scan
prep (preparation)
  bowel
  kit
  on-column
  touch
prepared and draped (prepped and draped)
prepatellar bursa
prepectorally
preponderance
preponderant
prepontine cistern
prepped and draped
prepulse, spin-lock
prepyloric antrum
prepyloric atresia
prepyloric fold
prereduction x-ray
prerenal
presacral mass

presaturation
  fat-selective
  projection
  spatial
presbyesophagus
presbyophrenia
prescan, MRI
prescapula
presentation of fetus
  breech
  brow
  cephalic
  compound
  face
  footling
  frank breech
  parietal
  shoulder
  transverse
  vertex
presenting part
pre-slip changes on x-ray
presphenoidal bone
PRESS sequence
PRESS spectroscopy
pressure
  A wave (left or right atrial
    catheterization)
  alveolar
  ankle-arm
  ankle systolic
  AO or Ao (aorta)
  aortic
  aortic root
  arterial (ART or Art.)
  arterial peak systolic
  atmospheres of
  bile duct
  blood (BP)
  brachial artery
  brachial artery cuff
  brachial artery end-diastolic

pressure *(cont.)*
  brachial artery peak systolic
  C wave (right atrial catheterization)
  capillary
  capillary wedge
  cardiac filling
  central aortic
  central venous (CVP)
  coronary artery perfusion (CPP)
  coronary wedge
  cuff blood
  diastolic blood (DBP)
  diastolic filling (DFP)
  diastolic perfusion
  diastolic pulmonary artery
  distal coronary perfusion
  Doppler ankle systolic
  Doppler blood
  Doppler calf systolic
  Doppler thigh systolic
  elevated
  end-diastolic
  end-systolic (ESP)
  endocardial
  equalized diastolic
  esophageal peristaltic
  extravascular
  femoral artery (FAP)
  filling
  hepatic wedge
  high filling
  high interstitial
  high wedge
  in vivo balloon
  interstitial fluid hydrostatic
  intraluminal esophageal
  jugular venous
  LA (left atrium)
  left atrial (LAP)
  left atrial end-diastolic
  left subclavian central venous
    (LSCVP)

pressure *(cont.)*
 left ventricular (LV)
 left ventricular cavity
 left ventricular end-diastolic
  (LVEDP)
 left ventricular filling
 left ventricular peak systolic
 left ventricular systolic (LVS)
 left-sided heart
 LES (lower esophageal sphincter)
 maximum inflation
 mean
 mean aortic
 mean arterial (MAP)
 mean atrial
 mean blood
 mean brachial artery
 mean circulatory filling
 mean left atrial
 mean pulmonary artery (MPAP)
 mean pulmonary artery wedge
 mean right atrial
 minimum blood
 PA (pulmonary artery) systolic
 PAD (pulmonary artery diastolic)
 PAS (pulmonary artery systolic)
 passage
 peak
 peak regurgitant wave
 peak systolic
 peak systolic aortic (PSAP)
 peak-inflation
 perfusion
 phasic
 portal venous (PVP)
 pulmonary arterial wedge (PAWP)
 pulmonary artery (PAP)
 pulmonary artery diastolic (PAD)
 pulmonary artery end-diastolic
  (PAEDP)
 pulmonary artery mean (PAM)
 pulmonary artery peak systolic

pressure *(cont.)*
 pulmonary artery/pulmonary
  capillary wedge
 pulmonary artery systolic (PAS)
 pulmonary artery wedge (PAWP)
 pulmonary capillary (PCP)
 pulmonary capillary wedge
  (PCWP)
 pulmonary venous capillary (PVC)
 pulmonary venous wedge
 pulmonary wedge
 pulse
 PV (pulmonary vein)
 PVC (pulmonary venous capillary)
 RA (right atrial)
 recoil
 regional cerebral perfusion (rCPP)
 right atrial (RAP)
 right-sided heart
 right subclavian central venous
  (RSCVP)
 right ventricular (RVP)
 right ventricular diastolic (RVD)
 right ventricular end-diastolic
 right ventricular peak systolic
 right ventricular systolic (RVS)
 right ventricular volume
 RV (right ventricular)
 RVD (right ventricular diastolic)
 RVS (right ventricular systolic)
 segmental lower extremity Doppler
 stump
 subatmospheric
 supersystemic pulmonary artery
 SVC (superior vena cava)
 systemic
 systolic
 systolic blood (SBP)
 toe systolic
 transmyocardial perfusion
 transpulmonary (PTP)

pressure *(cont.)*
   V wave (left or right atrial catheterization)
   venous
   ventricular
   wedge
   wedged hepatic venous (WHVP)
   withdrawal
   X' (prime) wave (right atrial catheterization)
   Y wave
   Z point
pressure catheter
pressure cuff
pressure difference, aortic-left
pressure equalization
pressure flow gradient
pressure fracture
pressure gradient on pullback
pressure injector
pressure measurement
pressure overload
pressure perfusion study
pressure pneumothorax
pressure pullback
pressure readings
pressure study
pressure waveform
Pressurometer
pretectal lesion
pretectal nucleus (region of midbrain)
pretectal region
pretendinous bands (of hand)
pretendinous cord
pretherapy imaging
pretibial region
prevertebral fascia
prevertebral soft tissue
PREZ (posterior root entry zone)
PRG (phleborheography)
primarily pulmonary hypertension (PPH)

primary bronchi, right and left
primary, cancer of unknown (CUP)
primary complex
primary megaloureter
primary motor strip
primary neoplasm
primary pulmonary hypertension
primary pulmonary plasmacytoma
primary rhabdomyosarcoma
primary sarcoma
primary thrombus
primary tuberculosis
primary vesical calculus (pl. calculi)
primary visual cortex
primitive dislocation
primitive neuroectodermal tumor (PNET)
principal bronchus
principal eigenvector
principle, uncertainty
print reflectance modulation
printer
   Codonics color
   raster scanning
   Winprint laser
Priodax contrast medium
prism interpolation
prism method for ventricular volume
Pro-Flo XT catheter
probability
   absolute emission
   emission
probe
   AngeLase combined mapping-laser
   Chandler V-pacing
   Doppler flow
   echocardiographic
   electromagnetic flow
   gamma
   hand-held
   hand-held exploring electrode
   hand-held mapping

probe *(cont.)*
   high-frequency miniature
   laparoscopic Doppler
   magnetometer
   Medrad Mrinnervu endorectal
     colon
   NRM magnetometer
   nuclear
   oligonucleotide
   pediatric biplane TEE
   sapphire contact
   side-hole cannulated
   Siemens-Elema AB pulse transducer system, USCI
   Teflon
   truncated NMR
   ultrasound
Probe balloon-on-a-wire dilatation
probehead, MRI
PROBE-SV spectrometer
probing catheter, USCI
procedure (see *imaging*)
process (pl. processes)
   accessory
   acromial
   alar
   alveolar consolidative
   apical
   articular
   ascending
   auditory
   basilar
   bony
   calcaneal
   caudate
   clinoid
   cochleariform
   condyloid
   conoid
   consolidative
   coracoid
   coronoid

process *(cont.)*
   costal
   energy transfer
   ensiform
   ethmoidal
   falciform
   fibroplastic
   frontal
   frontonasal
   frontosphenoidal
   glenoid
   inflammatory
   jugular
   knobby
   left ventricular posterior superior
   lumbar transverse
   neoplastic
   odontoid
   olecranon
   osseous destructive
   pterygoid
   sacral
   spinous
   styloid
   transverse
   trochlear
   uncinate
   vermiform
   vertebrospinous (or vertebral spinous)
   vertebral
   xiphoid
   zygomatic
processor, sequence
proctogram
   balloon
   video
proctographic features
proctosigmoidoscopy
procurvature deformity
product cipher
product, daughter

production
    fast routine
    one-step
    remote controlled
    secondary electron
profile
    asymmetric metabolic
    excitation
    nonlinear excitation
    peak
    rectangular section
    section-sensitivity
    slice
    slice sensitivity
    three-dimensional dose
Profile Mammography System
Profile Plus dilatation catheter, USCI
Proflex 5 dilatation catheter
profunda femoris artery
progeny
prognathic dilatation
program
    Analyze software
    daemon
    ESOLAN
    Microsoft Access
    surveillance
progressive diaphyseal dysplasia
progressive hydrocephalus
progressive interstitial pulmonary
    fibrosis
progressive nodular pulmonary fibrosis
ProHance (gadoteridol) nonionic
    gadolinium contrast agent (MRI)
project
projection (see also *position*; *view*)
    anterior
    cartographic
    caudad
    caudal
    caudal-cranial angulation
    craniocaudad
    cylindrical map

projection *(cont.)*
    fan-beam
    filtered-back
    fingerlike
    Lambert
    LAO (left anterior oblique)
    lateral
    left lateral
    left posterior oblique
    Low-Beers
    maximum intensity (MIP)
    minimum intensity
    oblique
    posterior
    presaturation
    RAO (right anterior oblique)
    ray-sum
    right posterior oblique
    rotating tomographic
    saturation inversion (SIP)
    sliding thin-slab, minimum intensity
    sliding-thin-slab, maximum intensity
    steep left anterior oblique
    stereographic
    stereotaxic surface (SSP)
    three-dimensional stereotaxic
        surface
    Towne
projection binning
projector, white light pattern
prolactinoma
prolapse
    anterior leaflet
    holosystolic mitral valve
    intestinal
    intracranial fat
    mitral valve (MVP)
    mitral valve leaflet systolic
    posterior leaflet
    systolic
    tricuspid valve
    valve

prolapsed tumor through mitral valve
    orifice
prolapsing scallop
proliferation
    angiofibroblastic
    bile duct
    bony
    fibroplastic
    glandular
    myointimal
    nodular
    osteophytic
    papillary
    synovial
    villous
prolonged interval
prolonged left ventricular impulse
prominence
    aortic
    bony (spur)
    hilar
    mediastinal
    tibial tubercle
prominent rim of radiolucency
    surrounding ulcer
prominent septal lymphatics
prominent xiphoid process
promontory, sacral
prompt-gamma neutron activation
pronation
pronator quadratus
prone lateral view
prone position
prone view
properitoneal flank stripe
property (pl. properties)
    CTA dosimetric
    ferromagnetic
    ionic
proportional counter
propria
    lamina

propria (cont.)
    substania
    tunica
propulsive mechanism
propyliodone contrast medium
prospective analysis
ProSpeed CT scanner
ProstaScint diagnostic imaging agent
ProstaScint monoclonal antibody
    imaging agent
prostate
    apex of
    carcinoma of
    inferolateral surfaces of
    lateral lobe of
    lymph vessels of
    median lobe of
    posterior surface of
prostate implant
prostate seeding
prostatic urethra
prosthesis (pl. prostheses)
    acetabular
    aortic valve
    aortofemoral
    ball-and-cage valve
    ball-cage
    ball valve
    bifurcated aortofemoral
    bileaflet valve
    bilioduodenal
    closure
    collar
    convexo-concave valve
    disk valve
    esophageal
    femoral
    femorofemoral crossover
    intraluminal sutureless
    intravascular
    iridium
    monostrut cardiac valve

prosthesis *(cont.)*
  outflow tract
  tilting-disk aortic valve
  total hip replacement
  total knee replacement
prosthesis cup
prosthesis dehiscence
prosthetic femorodistal graft
prosthetic heart valve
protection
  myocardial
  radiation
protein kinase C localization (brain)
protein synthesis rate
protocol
  MNP10
  MPRAGE
  neon particle
  RTOG
  2D GRE dynamic
  UCLA imaging
  urokinase
protodensity MRI image
protodiastolic reversal of blood flow
proton density
proton density images (MRI)
proton density-weighted images
proton irradiation
proton magnetic resonance spectroscopy
proton MR spectroscopy
protons
  methyl
  91-41 MeV
  precessing
protrude
protruding atheroma
protrusion
  disk
  spicular
  spoonlike (of leaflets)
  vascular

protrusion of navicular
protuberance, occipital
proximal anastomosis
proximal and distal portion of vessel
proximal anterior tibial artery
proximal articular set angle (PASA)
proximal carpal row
proximal circumflex artery
proximal coil
proximal focal femoral deficiency (PFFD)
proximal interphalangeal (PIP) joint
proximal popliteal artery
proximal segment
proximally
Pruitt-Inahara balloon-tipped perfusion catheter
pruned appearance of pulmonary vasculature
PS (pulmonary sequestration)
PS (pulmonic stenosis)
PSA (power spectral analysis)
psammoma body
psammoma, Virchow
psammomatous meningiomas
pseudarthrosis
pseudoaneurysm
pseudoangiomatous stromal hyperplasia
pseudocapsule
pseudocirrhosis, cholangiodysplastic
pseudocoarctation of aorta
pseudocolor B-mode display
pseudocyst
  adrenal
  mature pancreatic
  pancreatic
  pulmonary
pseudodextrocardia
pseudodislocation
pseudodiverticulum

pseudodynamic MR imaging of the
    temporomandibular joints
pseudoepiphysis
pseudoextrophy
pseudofracture artifact
pseudogestational sac
pseudohaustration
pseudojoints
pseudoluxation
pseudolymphoma, gastric
pseudomembrane
pseudomeningocele
pseudomitral leaflet
pseudoneuroma
pseudo-obstruction
    bowel
    chronic idiopathic intestinal (CIIP)
    colonic
    familial intestinal
    idiopathic intestinal
    nonfamilial intestinal
pseudo-orbital tumor
pseudopolyp
pseudopolyposis
pseudopregnancy
pseudosac
pseudosacculation
pseudosclerosis, spastic
pseudosheath
pseudostone
pseudothrombosis
pseudotumor
    fibrosing inflammatory
    orbital
pseudotumor cerebri (PTC)
PSF (posterior spine fusion)
PSG (peak systolic gradient)
PSIL (percentage signal intensity loss)
P623-Gd imaging agent
psoas abscess
psoas muscle shadow, obliteration of
PSP (photostimulable phosphor dental
    radiography)

P, substance
pSV-b-Gal plasmid imaging agent
pT3 tumor
pT4 tumor
PTA (percutaneous transluminal
    angioplasty)
pTa-T2 tumor
PTBD (percutaneous transhepatic
    biliary drainage) catheter
PTBD (percutaneous transluminal
    balloon dilatation)
PTC (percutaneous transhepatic
    cholangiography)
PTC (pseudotumor cerebri)
PTCA (percutaneous transluminal
    coronary angioplasty)
PTCA catheterization
PTCA coronary angiogram
PTD (percutaneous transhepatic
    drainage)
PTDC (percutaneous transcatheter
    ductal closure)
pterion
pterygoid bone
pterygoid chest
pterygoideus hamulus
PTF (posterior talofibular) ligament
PTHC (percutaneous transhepatic
    cholangiogram)
P-31 MR spectroscopy
PTL (posterior tricuspid leaflet)
ptosis
ptotic
PTRA (percutaneous transluminal
    renal angioplasty)
PTT (pulmonary transit time)
PTV (posterior terminal vein)
pubic bone
pubic ramus (pl. rami)
    inferior
    superior
pubic symphysis

pubic tubercle
pubis
   mons
   pecten
   ramus of
   symphysis
pubococcygeal line
pubococcygeus muscle
puboischial area
puborectalis loop
PUD (peptic ulcer disease)
puddle sign
puddling of contrast
puddling on barium enema
pudendal blood supply
puff of smoke (moyamoya) on angiography
Pugh Child grading system for bleeding esophageal varices
Pugh classification of Child liver criteria
Pulec and Freedman classification of congenital aural atresia
pullback across aortic valve
pullback arterial markings
pullback from ventricle
pullback pressure recording
pullback study
pulmoaortic canal
pulmogram
pulmolith
pulmolithiasis
pulmonale, cor (c. pulmonale)
pulmonary abscess
pulmonary agenesis
pulmonary alveolar microlithiasis
pulmonary alveolus (pl. alveoli)
pulmonary angiogram (angiography)
   balloon occlusion
   digital subtraction
pulmonary arterial circulation
pulmonary arterial input impedance
pulmonary arterial markings
pulmonary arterial occlusion
pulmonary arterial pressure, increased
pulmonary arterial vent
pulmonary arterial wedge pressure
pulmonary arteriolar vasoconstriction
pulmonary arteriosclerosis
pulmonary arteriovenous aneurysm
pulmonary arteriovenous fistula
pulmonary artery
   aberrant left
   anomalous
   dilated
pulmonary artery agenesis
pulmonary artery apoplexy
pulmonary artery catheter, balloon-tipped flow-directed
pulmonary artery compression ascending aorta aneurysm
pulmonary artery end-diastolic pressure (PAEDP)
pulmonary artery pressure (PAP)
pulmonary artery stenosis, peripheral
pulmonary artery wedge pressure (PAWP)
pulmonary atresia
pulmonary AV $O_2$ difference
pulmonary barotrauma
pulmonary bed
pulmonary blood flow redistribution
pulmonary capillary endothelium
pulmonary capillary hemangiomatosis
pulmonary capillary permeability using Tc-DTPA
pulmonary capillary pressure (PCP)
pulmonary capillary venous wedge pressure
pulmonary capillary wedge position
pulmonary capillary wedge pressure (PCWP)
pulmonary capillary wedge tracing
pulmonary cartilage

**pulmonary** 446

pulmonary cavitation
pulmonary cavity
pulmonary circulation
pulmonary cirrhosis
pulmonary compliance, reduced
pulmonary compression by pleural fluid or gas
pulmonary confluence
pulmonary congestion
pulmonary consolidation
pulmonary contusion
pulmonary cyanosis
pulmonary cystic lymphangiectasis
pulmonary edema
  acute
  cardiogenic
  frank
  fulminant
  high-altitude
  interstitial
  negative image
  neurogenic
  noncardiac
  noncardiogenic
  permeability-type
  postoperative
  reexpansion
pulmonary embolism (embolus, pl. emboli) (PE)
pulmonary emphysema
pulmonary eosinophilic infiltrates
pulmonary failure
pulmonary fibrosis (see *fibrosis*)
pulmonary fistula, congenital
pulmonary flotation catheter
pulmonary gangrene
pulmonary gas exchange
pulmonary hemorrhage
pulmonary hilus
pulmonary histoplasmosis
pulmonary incompetence
pulmonary infarction

pulmonary infiltrate
pulmonary insufficiency
pulmonary interstitial emphysema (PIE)
pulmonary interstitial idiopathic fibrosis
pulmonary interstitium
pulmonary ligament
pulmonary microcirculation
pulmonary microvasculature
pulmonary nodule enhancement
pulmonary orifice
pulmonary outflow tract
pulmonary overdistention
pulmonary parenchymal changes
pulmonary parenchymal infiltrates
pulmonary parenchymal window
pulmonary perfusion and ventilation
pulmonary perfusion imaging
pulmonary pleura
pulmonary plexus
pulmonary quantitative differential function study
pulmonary regurgitation
pulmonary sarcoidosis
pulmonary scars
pulmonary scintigraphy
pulmonary sequestration (PS)
pulmonary stenosis
pulmonary/systemic flow ratio
pulmonary TB (tuberculosis)
pulmonary thromboembolism (PTE)
pulmonary thrombosis
pulmonary time activity curve
pulmonary trunk idiopathic dilatation
pulmonary tuberculosis (TB)
pulmonary valve annulus
pulmonary valve atresia
pulmonary valve deformity
pulmonary valve insufficiency
pulmonary valve stenosis
pulmonary vascular bed impedance

pulmonary vascular congestion
pulmonary vascular markings
pulmonary vascular obstruction
pulmonary vascular pattern
pulmonary vascular redistribution
pulmonary vascular reserve
pulmonary vascular resistance (PVR)
pulmonary vascular resistance index (PVRI)
pulmonary vasculature
pulmonary vasoconstriction, hypoxic
pulmonary vein apoplexy
pulmonary vein atresia
pulmonary vein, congenital stenosis of
pulmonary vein fibrosis
pulmonary vein stenosis
pulmonary vein wedge angiography
pulmonary veno-occlusive disease
pulmonary venous anomalous drainage
pulmonary venous anomalous drainage to right atrium
pulmonary venous congestion
pulmonary venous drainage
pulmonary venous hypertension
pulmonary venous obstruction
pulmonary venous system
pulmonary venous-systemic air emboli
pulmonary venous wedge pressure
pulmonary ventilation imaging
pulmonary vesicles
pulmonary vessels
pulmonary wedge angiography
pulmonary wedge pressure (PWP)
pulmonic atresia with intact ventricular septum
pulmonic infiltrate
pulmonic regurgitation
pulmonic stenosis-ventricular septal defect
pulmonic valve stenosis

pulposus, nucleus
pulsate
pulsatile flow, dampened
pulsatile perfusion
pulsatile tinnitus
pulsatility index (PI)
pulsation balloon
pulse (pl. pulses)
   adiabatic slice-selective rf (RF) (radiofrequency)
   DANTE-selective
   fat suppression
   narrow-band spectral-selective
   90 RF
   navigator
   phase-encode
   radiofrequency (rf or RF)
   section-select
   spatially selective inversion
   2D spatially selective RF
pulsed brachytherapy (PDR)
pulsed Doppler transesophageal echocardiography
pulsed Doppler ultrasound
pulse deficit
pulsed electron paramagnetic NMR
pulsed gradient
pulsed infrared laser
pulsed L-band ESR spectrometer
pulse Doppler interrogation
pulsed magnetization transfer contrast MRI
pulsed ultrasound
pulse duration
pulsed-wave Doppler echocardiography
pulse height spectral analysis
pulse indicator, xylol
pulse length
pulse reappearance time
pulse sequence, single-shot adiabatic localization

pulse sequencing
PulseSpray injector
PulseSpray pulsed infusion system
pulse voltage
pulse volume recording (PVR)
pulse volume waveforms
pulse wave
pulse width
pulsion
pulverized plaque particulate matter
pulvinar region
pump
  angle port
  balloon
  cardiac balloon
  intra-aortic balloon (IABP)
  ion
  pulmonary artery balloon (PABP)
punctate area
puncture
  fine-needle
  stereotactic
  venous
puncture fracture
puncture wound (types I-IV)
purification, one-line anion exchange
purified water contrast
purity, radionuclide
putamen
putaminal hemorrhage, nondominant
PV (pulmonic valve)
PVD (peripheral vascular disease)
PVG (periventricular gray) matter
PVL (periventricular leukomalacia)
PVP (portal venous pressure)
PVR (peripheral vascular resistance)
PVR (perspective volume rendering)
PVR (postvoiding residual)
PVR (pulmonary vascular resistance)
PVR (pulse volume recorder)
PVR fly-through viewing

PVRI (pulmonary vascular resistance index)
PW (posterior wall)
PW (pulse width)
PWT (posterior wall thickness)
pyelectasia
pyelectasis
pyelocaliceal
pyelocaliectasis
pyelocaliceal
pyelofluoroscopy
pyelogram
  antegrade
  excretory intravenous
  intravenous (IVP)
  retrograde
pyelographic appearance time
pyelography
pyelostogram
pyelotubular backflow
pyemia
  cryptogenic
  portal
pyknomorphous
pyloric channel
pyloric hypertrophy
pyloric insufficiency
pyloric outlet obstruction
pyloric ring
pyloric stenosis
pyloric string sign
pyloric ulcer
pyloric valve
pyloroduodenal junction
pylorospasm, persistent
pylorus, hypertrophic
pyocephalus
pyogenic granuloma
pyonephrosis
pyopneumothorax
pyothorax

pyoventricle
PYP (pyrophosphate) technetium myocardial scan
pyramid, petrous
pyramidal bone
pyramidal fracture (of maxilla)
pyramidal hemorrhagic zone
pyramidal layer of cerebral cortex
pyramidal lobe
pyramidal neurons
pyramidal tract
pyribenzamine
pyriform (piriform) sinus
pyriform cortex
pyriform sinus
pyrophosphate (PYP) myocardial scan
pyrophosphate crystals
pyruvate dehydrogenase complex deficiency

# Q, q

Q (cardiac output)
Q (quotient, as in V/Q, ventilation perfusion scan)
QCA (quantitative coronary arteriography)
Q-cath catheterization recording system
Q space
QCT (quantitative computed tomography) test for bone loss
QDR-1500 or QDR-2000 bone densitometer
QHS (quantitative hepatobiliary scintigraphy)
QM (quantization matrix)
$QO_2$ (oxygen consumption)
QPD (quadrature phase detector)
QR pattern
QRS interval
QRS loop, counterclockwise superiorly oriented frontal
QRS score
QRS synchronized shock
QRS vector
QRS vertical axis
QRS-T angle, wide
quad resonance NMR probe circuit
Quad-Lumen drain with radiopaque stripe
quadrangle cartilage
quadrangulation of Frouin
quadrant
  left lower (LLQ)
  left upper (LUQ)
  left upper outer
  right lower (RLQ)
  right upper (RUQ)
  right upper outer
quadrant of death (anterosuperior quadrant of hip)
quadrate lobe of liver
quadrature phase detector (QPD) artifact
quadrature RF receiver coil
quadrature setting
quadrature surface coil system
quadrature T/L surface coil
quadratus femoris muscle
quadratus, pronator
quadriceps muscle
quadrigeminal plate
quadrigeminy
quadrilateral brim
quadripolar catheter

451

Quain fatty degeneration of the heart
qualitative study
quality factor
quantification
   automated
   flow
quantify
quantitative analysis
quantitative cardiac perfusion
quantitative computed tomography (QCT)
quantitative coronary arteriography (QCA)
quantitative CT during expiration
quantitative Doppler assessment
quantitative electroencephalography (QEEG)
quantitative exercise thallium-201 variables
quantitative fluorescence imaging
quantitative gated SPECT (QGS)
quantitative hepatobiliary scintigraphy (QHS)
quantitative magnetization transfer
quantitative regional myocardial flow measurement
quantitative scan
quantitative spirometrically controlled CT
quantity, spectrophotometric
quantization
   sequent scalar (SSQ)
   wavelet scalar (WSQ)
quantization matrix (QM) scaling
quantizer-design algorithms
quantum number
quench
quenching
Quénu-Muret sign
Quervain fracture
quiescence
Quik-Prep, Quinton
Quincke angioedema disease
Quinton PermCath
Quinton Quik-Prep
Quinton vascular access port
quotient, Rayleigh
QW 3600 contrast agent

# R, r

R (roentgen)
RA (right atrial) pressure
RA (right atrium) oxygen saturation
RA (rheumatoid arthritis) factor
Raaf Cath (vascular catheter)
RAAPI (resting ankle-arm pressure index)
RAB (remote afterloading brachytherapy)
RACAT (rapid acquisition computed axial tomography)
rachioscoliosis
rachitic rosary sign
Racobalamin-57 radioactive agent
rad (radiation absorbed dose)
radiability
radial artery catheter
radial artery to cephalic vein fistula
radial bone
radial collateral ligament
radial deviation
radial drift
radial epiphyseal displacement
radial facing of metacarpal heads
radial forearm flap
radial fossa
radial head fracture
radial head subluxation (RHS)
radial ray defect
radial styloid process fracture
radial tuberosity
radial vascular thermal injury
radialized
radiate ligament
radiation (see also *radiation therapy*)
    adjuvant
    Cerenkov
    diagnostic
    external beam
    ionizing
    monochromatic
    synchrotron
    therapeutic
    ultraviolet
radiation-absorbed dose (rad)
radiation changes
radiation dosages
radiation dose pertubation
radiation dosimetry calculation
radiation fibrosis
radiation fistula
radiation-induced ulceration
radiation-induced up-regulation
radiation intensity

**radiation • radioactive**

radiation interrogation
radiation monitor
radiation necrosis
radiation osteonecrosis
radiation pericardial disease
radiation port
radiation protection
radiation scatter
radiation source
  intracavitary
  intrastitial
radiation therapy (also radiotherapy)
  accelerated hyperfractionated
  combined-modality
  concomitant boost
  conformal
  conformal neutron and photon
  conventionally fractionated stereotactic
  craniospinal axis
  dynamic
  external beam (EBRT)
  eye-view 3D-CRT
  fractionated external beam
  fractionated stereotaxic
  hyperfractionated
  hypofractionated
  I-B1 radiolabeled antibody injection
  ICRU 50
  interstitial
  intracavitary
  intraoperative (IORT)
  large-field
  megavoltage
  neuroaxis
  orthovoltage
  palliative
  partial-brain
  photon-neutron mixed-beam
  postorchiectomy para-aortic
  rotational

radiation therapy *(cont.)*
  short-distance (brachytherapy)
  split-course accelerated
  split hyperfractionated accelerated
  stereotactic or stereotaxic
  three-dimensional conformal
  3D-CRT
  upper mantle
  whole-brain
radiation therapy planning (RTP) system
radiation toxicity syndrome
radical mastectomy
radicle, biliary
radicular arteries
radicular compression
radicular cyst
radicular vessels to spinal cord
radiculomedullary artery
radiculospinal artery
radioactive aerosol
radioactive bolus
radioactive cancer-specific targeting agent
radioactive cobalt
radioactive emissions from heart
radioactive fibrinogen scan
radioactive iodinated serum albumin (RISA) imaging agent
radioactive iodine uptake test (RAIU)
radioactive isotope (see *imaging agent*)
radioactive label (labeling)
radioactively tagged
radioactive marker
radioactive material
radioactive source
radioactive string markers
radioactive thallium
radioactive tracer
radioactive xenon clearance
radioactive xenon gas inhalation

radioaerosol clearance
radioaerosol imaging studies
radioallergosorbent test (RAST)
radioccipital
radiobiological
radiobiology
radiocalcium
radiocapitellar joint
radiocarcinogenesis
radiocardiogram
radiocardiography
radiocarpal angle
radiocarpal dislocation
radiocarpal joint
radiocarpal portal
radiochemical study
radiochemistry
radiochromic film
radiocurable
radiode
radiodiagnosis
radiodiagnostics
radiodigital
radioelement application
 interstitial
 intracavitary
 surface
radioelement solution
radiofluorinated
Radiofocus Glidewire for angiography
radiofrequency (RF)
 RF ablation (RFA) therapy
 RF catheter ablation (RFCA)
 RF coil
 RF energy
 RF field
 RF-generated thermal balloon
  catheter
 RF hypertheramia
 RF magnetic shield
 RF overflow artifact
 RF period

radiofrequency (cont.)
 RF pulse
 RF saturation bands
 RF screen
 RF modification transcatheter
 RF spatial distribution problem
 RF spatial distribution problem
  reconstruction artifact
 RF transmitter
radiogenic leukopenia
radiogold
radiogram (radiograph) (see *imaging*)
radiographic control
radiographic hallmark
radiographic imaging system,
 intensified (IRIS)
radiographically firm synostosis
radiography (see *imaging*)
radiohumeral articulation
radioimmunity
radioimmunoassay (RIA)
radioimmunoassay, scintillation
 proximity
radioimmunodetection (RAID)
radioimmunodiffusion
radioimmunoelectrophoresis
radioimmunoimaging
radioimmunoscintigraphy
radioimmunoscintimetry
radioimmunosorbent
radioimmunotherapy
radioiodinated serum albumin (RISA)
radioiodination
 direct
 electrophilic
radioiodine
radioiron oral absorption
radioiron red cell utilization
radioisotope (isotope) (see *imaging*
 *agent*)
radioisotope assay, thyroxine ($T_4$RIA)
radioisotope cisternography

radioisotope clearance assay
radioisotope-labeled antibody
radioisotope-labeled antigen
radioisotope labeling
radioisotope lung scan
radioisotope (static) scanning
radioisotope stent
radioisotope uptake
radioisotope voiding cystography
radiolabeled antifibrin antibody
radiolabeled compound
radiolabeled estrogen analog F-18 ($^{18}$F) estradiol (FES)
radiolabeled fibrinogen
radiolabeled MoAb
radiolabeled peptide alpha-M2 imaging agent
radiolabeled platelets
radiolabeled water study
radiolabeled WBCs
radiolesion
radioligand
radiologic-anatomic correlation
radiologic gastrostomy
radiologic guidance
radiologic-histopathologic study
radiologic-pathologic correlation
radiologic percutaneous gastrostomy
radiologic protection
radiologist
radiology
    computed (CR)
    diagnostic
    interventional
    neurointerventional
    percutaneous interventional
    polytomographic
    skeletal
    storage phosphor
    therapeutic
radiology outcomes data
radiolucency, soap-bubble

radiolucent area
radiolucent center
radiolucent cleft
radiolucent focus (pl. foci)
radiolucent pneumomediastinum
radiolucent spine frame
radiolucent stone
radiolunotriquetral ligament
radiolymphoscintigraphy, intraoperative
radiomuscular
radionecrosis, cerebral
Radionics CRW stereotactic head frame
radionitrogen
radionuclear venography
radionuclide (see *imaging agent*)
    absorption of
    concentration of
    inhalation of
    inhaled
    injection of
    uptake of
radionuclide angiocardiogram
radionuclide angiogram (RNA)
radionuclide blood flow (dynamic) studies
radionuclide carrier system
radionuclide cineangiography
radionuclide cisternography
radionuclide cystography
radionuclide flow scan
radionuclide gated blood pool scanning
radionuclide injection
radionuclide label (labeling)
radionuclide liver scan
radionuclide mammography
radionuclide milk scan
radionuclide purity
radionuclide scan (scanning)
radionuclide shuntogram

radionuclide signals
radionuclide study, blood pool
radionuclide testicular scintigraphy
radionuclide ventriculogram
radionuclide voiding study
radiopacity
radiopaque calculus
radiopaque contrast medium
radiopaque density
radiopaque distal tip for location on fluoroscopy
radiopaque fluid, extravasation of
radiopaque marker
radiopaque medium
radiopaque nanoparticulate
radiopaque pellet
radiopaque suture
radiopaque urine
radiopaque vesical calculi
radiopaque wire of counteroccluder buttonhole
radiopaque xenon gas
radiopathology
radiopharmaceutical (see *imaging agent*)
radiopharmaceutical ablation
radiopharmaceutical dacryocystography
radiopharmaceutical localization
radiopharmaceutical therapy
radiopharmaceutical voiding cystogram
radiopharmaceutical volume-dilution technique
radiophobia
radiophotography
radiophylaxis
radiopotassium
radiopulmonography
radioreaction
radioresistance
radioscaphocapitate ligament
radioscaphoid joint

radioscaphoid ligament
radioscapholunate ligament
radioscintigraphy
radioscopically tagged antihuman antibody
radiosensibility
radiosensitive
radiosensitivity, fibroblast
radiosensitizer
  carbogen
  halogenated thymidine analogue
  nicotinamide
radiostereoscopy
radiostyloid process
radiosulfur
radiosurgery
  Bragg-peak
  charged-particle
  dynamic stereotactic
  gamma knife
  heavy-charged particle Bragg peak
  image-guided
  interstitial
  LINAC or Linac (linear accelerator)
  multiarc LINAC
  stereotactic or stereotaxic
radiosurgically
radiotherapeutic agent
radiotherapist
radiotherapy (see *radiation therapy*)
radiotherapy with hyperthermia
radiotherapy without hyperthermia
radiotherapy field placement
radiotoxemia
radiotoxicity
radiotracer activity
radiotracer foil method
radiotracer foil method for sorption studies
radiotracer technique
radiotracer uptake
radiotransparency

radiotropic
radioulnar joint
radioulnar subluxation
radioulnar surface
radium radioactive source
radius
RadNet radiology information system
radon seeds radioactive source
RADstation radiology workstation
radwaste radioactivity detection
RAE (right atrial enlargement)
Raeder-Arbitz syndrome
Raeder paratrigeminal syndrome
ragpicker's disease
RAID (radioimmunodetection)
railroad track pattern on x-ray in Sturge-Weber syndrome
railroad track sign
Raimiste sign
Raimondi ventricular catheter
raised intracranial pressure
RAIU (radioactive iodine uptake test)
rake retractor
rake ulcer
Raman spectroscopy
Ramesh and Pramod algorithms
rami (see *ramus*)
ramp, folded step
Ramsay Hunt cerebellar myoclonic dyssynergia
ramus (pl. rami)
    dorsal
    dorsal primary
    inferior
    inferior pubic
    ischiopubic
    pubic
    superior
    ventral
    ventral primary
ramus intermedius artery branch
ramus medialis artery branch
R&F camera
Rand microballoon
random field, Gibbs
randomly distributed cortical perfusion defects
Ranfac LAP-013 cholangiographic catheter
Ranfac ORC-B cholangiographic catheter
Ranfac XL-11 cholangiographic catheter
range
    absorbed dose
    grayscale
    normal
    reference
    therapeutic
range-gated Doppler spectral flow analysis
Ranke angle
Ranke complex
Ranvier groove
Ranvier node
RAO (right anterior oblique)
    RAO position for cardiac catheterization
    RAO projection
    RAO view
RAP (right atrial pressure)
raphe
    abdominal
    amniotic
    anococcygeal
    anogenital
    longitudinal
    median
    palpebral
    penile
    pterygomandibular
    scrotal
    tendinous

rapid acquisition with relaxation
    enhancement (RARE)
rapid axial MRI
rapid deceleration injury
rapid dephasing
rapid early repolarization phase
rapid filling phase
rapid filling wave
rapid image transfer
rapid inspiratory flow rates
rapid oscillatory motion
rapid repolarization phase
rapid sequence intravenous pyelogram
    (IVP)
rapid sequential CT scan
rapid thoracic compression technique
rapid ventricular filling phase
rapid ventricular rate
rapid ventricular response
Rappaport classification of gastric
    lymphoma
Rappaport disability rating scale
raptus of attention
RARE (rapid acquisition with
    relaxation enhancement) MRI
RARE-derived pulse sequence
rarefaction of cortex
rarefied area
Rashkind double umbrella device
Rashkind septostomy balloon catheter
Rasmussen mycotic aneurysm
Rastelli atrioventricular canal defect
    (type A, B, or C)
raster frequency
raster lines
raster period
raster scanning printer
raster spacing error
rate
    complication
    deposition
    instantaneous enhancement

rate *(cont.)*
    patency
    protein synthesis
    shear
    slew
    transverse relaxation
    valley-to-peak
rate meter
Rathke pouch
Rathke duct
Rathke pouch (in the brain)
rating scale
ratio
    AH:HA
    ankle-brachial pressure
    AO:AC (aortic valve opening to
        aortic valve closing)
    aortic root
    artery/aortic velocity
    brain-to-background
    C/N (contrast to noise)
    cardiothoracic (CT, CTR)
    CBV/CBF
    cerebral blood volume/cerebral
        blood flow
    chemical-shift
    CK:AST
    compression
    conduction (number of P waves to
        number of QRS)
    contrast-to-noise (C/N)
    E:A (on echocardiography)
    escape-peak
    ESP-ESV
    ESWI-ESVI (end-systolic wall
        stress index to end-systolic
        volume)
    FL/AC (femur length to abdominal
        circumference)
    gray to white matter activity (also
        gray/white matter activity)
    gray to white matter utilization

ratio *(cont.)*
  gyromagnetic
  HC/AC (head circumference to abdominal circumference)
  heart-to-background
  heart-to-lung
  Holdaway
  inferior-anterior (I-A) count
  Insall (in patella alta)
  Insall-Salvati
  inverse inspiratory–expiratory time
  isotopic
  I-E (inspiration to expiration, or inspiratory to expiratory)
  kidney-to-background
  LA–AR (left atrium/aortic root)
  L/A (liver/aorta) peak
  L/B
  L/LP (liver/liver peak)
  left ventricular systolic time interval
  lesion-to-background
  lesion-to-muscle
  lesion to non-lesion count
  liver/aorta (L/A) peak
  liver/liver peak (L/LP)
  magnetogyric
  maximum diameter to minimum diameter
  metatarsal length
  nasal-to-plasma radioactivity
  orifice-to-annulus
  P:A (peroneal to anterior compartment)
  PASP–SASP (pulmonary to systemic arterial systolic pressure)
  patellar ligament-patellar
  peak systolic and diastolic
  pitch
  Poisson
  P:QRS

ratio *(cont.)*
  P–S flow (pulmonic–systemic)
  pulmonary–systemic blood flow
  pulmonary to systemic flow
  R/S amplitude
  R/S wave
  risk–benefit
  RVP–LVP (right ventricular to left ventricular systolic pressure)
  RV6:RV5 voltage
  scatter-to-primary
  septal to free wall
  serum glucose:CSF glucose
  SI joint to sacrum
  signal-to-clutter
  signal-to-noise (S/N)
  spleen-to-liver
  stroke volume
  target-to-background
  thallium-to-scalp
  TME (trapezium-metacarpal eburnation)
  tumor-to-normal brain
  T–D (thickness to diameter of ventricle)
  VLDL-TG to HDL-C
Ratliff classification of avascular necrosis
rat-tail appearance on pancreatogram
Rau, apophysis of
Rauchfuss triangle
rauwolfia derivative
RAW (airway resistance)
ray (pl. rays)
  central
  digital
  grenz
  hypermobile first
  keV gamma
  long axis
  pollicized
ray amputation

ray-casting method
Rayleigh quotient
Rayleigh scattering law
Raymond-Cestan syndrome
Raynaud phenomenon
ray-sum projection
ray-sum views
Ray-Tec x-ray detectable surgical sponge
Ray TFC (threaded fusion cage)
Ray ventricular cannula
Rb (rubidium)
$^{82}$Rb-based cardiac imaging
RBBB (right bundle branch block)
RBC (red blood cell)
  labeled
  technetium-99m-labeled
RBG (red, blue, green)
RCA (retained cortical activity)
RCA (right coronary artery)
RCA (rotational coronary atherectomy)
rCBF (regional cerebral blood flow) PET scan
rCBV (regional cerebral blood volume) PET scan
rCMRO$_2$ (regional cerebral metabolic rate for oxygen)
rCPP (regional cerebral perfusion pressure)
RCT (retinocortical time)
rd (rutherford) radioactive unit
RDG (retrograde duodenogastroscopy)
RDW (red cell diameter width)
RE (reflux esophagitis)
RE (rehabilitation engineering)
Re (rhenium)
reabsorption, bony
reaccumulation
reaction
  endoergic
  exoergic

reaction *(cont.)*
  hilar
  hypersensitivity
  lamellar
  periosteal
  pleural
  sarcoid-like
reactivation tuberculosis
reactive airways disease (RAD)
reactive airways dysfunction syndrome
reactive arterioles
reactive disease of smooth muscle
reactive hyperemia
reactivity, bronchial
Reader paratrigeminal syndrome
reading
  batch-
  wet x-ray
readout wavelength
reagent, Wittig
real-time assessment
real-time biplanar needle tracking
real-time chirp Z transformer
real-time color flow Doppler imaging of blood flow
real-time CT fluoroscopy
real-time DAP (dose area product)
real-time equipment
real-time display
real-time edge enhancement
real-time format converter
real-time images
real-time MR imaging tracking
real-time respiratory feedback
real-time scan ultrasound
real-time sonogram (sonography)
real-time two-dimensional (2D) blood flow imaging
real-time ultrasound (ultrasonography)
real-time volume rendering
realign
realignment, patellofemoral

reapproximating
reapproximation
rebleeding of aneurysm
rebreathing ventilation scan
re-bypass
recalcitrant
recanalization technique
   angiographic
   argon laser
   laser
   percutaneous transluminal coronary
   peripheral laser (PLR)
recanalized artery
recanalized ductus
recanalizing
receiver coil
receiver operating characteristics (ROC)
receptor (pl. receptors)
   baro-
   benzodiazepine
   dopamine
   D2
   GABA
   serotonin
   S2
   transferrin
receptor antagonist
receptor binding
recess
   attic
   cecal
   cerebellopontine
   cochlear
   costodiaphragmatic
   costomediastinal
   duodenojejunal
   epitympanic
   hepatorenal
   ileocecal
   inferior duodenal
   infraglenoid

recess *(cont.)*
   intersigmoid
   optic
   popliteal
   paraduodenal
   peritoneal
   pleural
   prestyloid
   retrocecal
   retroduodenal
   sacciform
   splenorenal
   sublabral
   subphrenic
   subscapularis
   superior duodenal
recession, nasion
recheck
reciprocal changes
reciprocating conduction
recirculation peak
Recklinghausen disease of bone
recoarctation of aorta
recognition, high-order curve
recoil
   arterial
   catheter
recoil pressure
recombinant human granulocyte colony stimulating factor (r-metHuG-CSF)
recon pitch
reconstituted via collaterals
reconstitution of blood flow in artery
reconstitution via profunda artery
reconstitution via collaterals
reconstructed with a 1:1 pitch at 1 mm increments
reconstruction
   aortic
   Dor
   external gamma dose

reconstruction *(cont.)*
   fan-beam
   gated 3D
   image
   multiplanar
   patch graft
   renovascular
   respiration gated 3D
   three-dimensional
   transannular patch
   zygomaticomalar
reconstruction algorithms
reconstruction artifact
reconstruction of aorta
reconstruction study
recording
   color Doppler
   continuous-wave Doppler
   evoked-potential
   pullback pressure
   pulsed-wave Doppler
   simultaneous
recovery
   fluid-attenuated inversion
   saturation
   shape
   uneventful
recovery period of myocardium
recovery time, corrected sinus node
recrudescence
recruitment potential
rectal endoscopic ultrasonography (REU)
rectal fold
   inferior transverse
   superior transverse
rectal multiplane transducer
rectal polyp`
rectal shelf
rectal stump
rectal vault
rectangular section profile

rectilinear bone scan
rectilinear thyroid scan
rectosigmoid function
rectovaginal fistula
rectovaginal pouch
rectovaginal septum
rectovesical pouch
rectum
rectus abdominis muscle
rectus muscle flap
rectus position
rectus sheath
rectus sheath pocket
recumbency
recumbent position
recumbent view
recur
recurred
recurrence
   local
   pattern
   tumor
recurrent artery of Heubner
recurrent dislocation
recurrent laryngeal nerve
recurrent meningeal nerve
recurvatum deformity
recurvatum during gait
red, blue, green (RBG)
red cell diameter width (RDW)
Reddick cystic duct cholangiogram catheter
RediFurl TaperSeal IAB catheter
redirection of inferior vena cava
redistributed thallium scan
redistribution
   blood flow
   flow
   myocardial image
   pulmonary blood flow
   pulmonary vascular
redistribution image

redistribution study
Redi-Vu teleradiology system
red Robinson catheter
red rubber catheter
reduced cardiac output
reduced circulation
reduced compliance of chamber
reduced plasma volume
reduced prominence of pulmonary vessels
reduced pulmonary compliance
reduced signal intensity
reduced stroke volume
reducible hernia
reduction
  afterload
  anatomic
  blood viscosity
  closed
  concentric
  congruent
  electrolytic
  fracture
  manual
  manual fracture
  open
  stable
  surgical
  thoracic volume
  trial
redundancy of interposed colon segment
redundant aortic valve leaflets
redundant carotid artery
redundant mitral valve leaflets
redundant scallop of posterior annulus
reefing, capsular
reefing of medial retinaculum of knee
re-entry point
reexpansion of lung
reexpansion pulmonary edema
reexploration

reference coordinate system
reference line
reference site
reference standards, Wilmad
reference, sternospinal
referred pain
REFI (regional ejection fraction image)
refill, capillary
reflectant
reflected edge of Poupart ligament
reflection
  costopleural
  epicardial
  hepatoduodenal
  hepatoduodenoperitoneal
  mediastinal
  mediastinodiaphragmatic pleural
  pericardial
  peritoneal
  sternal pleural
  vertebral pleural
reflectivity, high
reflectometer tuning unit
reflex (pl. reflexes)
reflux
  abdominojugular
  acid
  bile
  duodenobiliary
  duodenogastric (DGR)
  duodenopancreatic
  free
  gastric
  gastroesophageal (GE, GER)
  hepatojugular (HJ)
  intra-renal
  nasopharyngeal
  nocturnal gastric
  vesicoureteral
reflux atrophy
reflux esophagitis

reflux gastritis
reflux grades I through V
refluxing spastic neurogenic bladder
reflux of activity
reflux regurgitation
reformation, multiplanar
reformatted planar "Christmas tree" MR appearance of endolymphatic sac
reformatting, multiplanar
refractoriness, ventricular
refractory congestive heart failure
refractory hypertension
refractory hypoxemia
refractory period of myocardium (see *period*)
refractory to treatment
refracture
region
   anesthesic
   Broca
   dark
   insular
   interseptal
   midfrontal
   periaqueductal
   photodeficient
   photopenic
   septal
   subfrontal
   task-activated brain
   temporal
   Wernicke
regional cerebral blood flow (rCBF) PET tomography
regional cerebral blood volume (rCBV) PET scan
regional cerebral metabolic rate for oxygen (rCMRO$_2$)
regional cerebral oxygen saturation
regional cerebral perfusion pressure (rCPP)
regional ejection fraction image (REFI)
regional left ventricular function
regional lymph nodes
regional myocardial uptake of thallium
regional oxygen extraction fraction (rOEF)
regional perfusion by mixed venous blood
regional pulmonary perfusion
regional tracer uptake
regional ventilation
regional ventricular function
regional wall motion abnormality, left ventricular
regional washout measurements
region of interest (ROI)
region-of-interest fluoroscopy
region-of-interest imaging technique
registration
   landmark
   robust
   spatial
   surface
   two-dimensional portal image
registration and alignment of 3D images
registry, STAR
Regnauld degeneration of MTP joint
regress
regression
   plaque
   polynomial step-wise multiple-linear
   spontaneous
   stepwise
regrowth delay
regular wedge
regulation, defective volume
regurgitant flow
regurgitant jet
regurgitant lesion

regurgitant pandiastolic flow
regurgitant pocket
regurgitant stream
regurgitant velocity
regurgitant volume
regurgitation
  aortic (AR)
  aortic valve
  congenital
  congenital aortic
  congenital mitral (CMR)
  Dexter-Grossman classification of mitral
  Grossman scale for
  ischemically mediated mitral
  massive aortic
  mitral
  mitral valve
  pansystolic mitral
  paravalvular
  physiologic
  pulmonary
  pulmonic (PR)
  pulmonic valve
  silent
  sour fluid
  transient tricuspid (of infancy)
  tricuspid (TR)
  tricuspid orifice
  tricuspid valve
  trivial mitral
  valvular (VR)
regurgitation index
rehabilitation (rehab), cardiac
rehydrated
Reichek method of calculating end-systolic wall stress
Reichert flexible sigmoidoscope
Reichert-Mundinger-Fischer stereotactic frame
Reid baseline
Reil, island of
reimplantation technique
reinfarction
reinjection thallium stress exam
reinnervation, motor
reinsertion
reintimalization
reintubation
re-irradiation
re-irrigation
Reiter disease
rejection
  accelerated acute
  acute
  acute renal
  allograft
  borderline severe
  chronic
  chronic humoral
  end-stage
  first-set
  focal moderate
  hyperacute
  low moderate
  resolved
  resolving
  second-set
  severe acute
  transplant
  vasculitic
rejection crisis
relapsing course
relation
  end-diastolic pressure-volume
  end-systolic pressure-volume
  force-frequency
  force-length
  force-velocity
  Frank-Starling (of heart)
relationship
  dentoskeletal
  dose-volume
  globe-orbit

relative hypoxia
relative refractory period (RRP)
relative shunt flow
relativistic mass
relaxation
  ferromagnetic
  longitudinal
  multispin
  nuclear
  nuclear electric quadrupole
  paramagnetic
  reciprocal agonist-antagonist
  spin-spin
  spin-lattice
  spin-spin
  T2 star
  tissue-based T2
  transverse
relaxation atelectasis
relaxation rate
relaxation techniques
relaxation time
  T1
  T2
relaxivity
relaxometer
  Bruker PC-10
  IBM Field-Cycling Research
Reliance urinary control stent
relief, mucosal
relief pattern
reloading, anode tube
remineralization
remitting course
remnant
  ductal
  heart
remodeling
  bone
  craniofacial
  para-articular bone
  regressive
  thrombus

remote afterloader
remote afterloading brachytherapy (RAB)
remote afterloading high intensity brachytherapy
remote control afterloading high-dose-rate intracavitary brachytherapy
remote control afterloading machines
remote-controlled implantation of radioactive source
remote-controlled production
remote diagnosis
remote history
remote lower motor neuron lesion
remyelination
renal agenesis
renal angiogram
renal angiography
renal angiomyolipoma
renal arteriography
renal artery aneurysm
renal artery occlusion
renal artery stenosis
renal atrophy
renal axis
renal calculus
renal capsule
  fatty
  fibrous
renal cocktail
renal cortex, patchy atrophy of
renal cortical isotope scanning agent
renal cortical necrosis
renal cross-fused ectopia
renal cyst study
renal duplex scan
renal dysplasia
renal failure
renal flow curve
renal function impairment
renal hemangiopericytoma
renal hypertension

renal impression on liver
renal injury
renal isthmus
renal lithiasis (renolithiasis)
renal mass lesion
renal osteodystrophy
renal parenchymal disease
renal pelvic urothelial carcinoma
renal pelvis
renal perfusion
renal pyramids
renal resistive index
renal scan, diuretic
renal scarring
renal sclerosis
renal shadow
renal shutdown
renal sinus echo
renal sinus fat
renal transplant
renal trauma
renal tubules
renal ultrasound
renal vascular damage
renal vascular hypertension (RVH)
renal vein
renal vein thrombosis
rendering
  perspective volume
  surface projection
  3D
  transparent
  volume
  voxel gradient
Rendu-Osler-Weber disease or syndrome (also Weber-Osler-Rendu)
reniform contour
renin-angiotensin dependent outer cortex
renin-angiotensin mechanism
renin-secreting tumor
Renkin model

Renografin contrast medium
Renografin 60
renogram curve
renography, DTPA
renolithiasis (renal lithiasis)
Reno-M contrast medium
Reno-M-Dip contrast medium
Reno-M-30 contrast medium
Reno-M-60 contrast medium
renovascular hypertension
renovascular reconstruction
renovascular stent
Renovist II contrast medium
Renovue-Dip contrast medium
Renshaw cell
rent (tear or rupture)
Rentrop infusion catheter
reocclusion, post-thrombolytic coronary
reoxygenation
repeatability
repeated FID (free induction decay)
repeated microtraumas
reperfuse
reperfusion
  acute myocardial infarction
  controlled aortic root
  coronary
  normokalemic
reperfusion injury of postischemic lungs
reperfusion therapy
repetition time (TR)
repetitive seizures
repetitive strain (or stress) injury (RSI)
rephasing gradient
replacement
  aortic root
  aortic valve (AVR)
  ascending aneurysm
  bone

replacement *(cont.)*
  fatty
  mitral valve (MVR)
  orthotopic total heart
replantation of amputated digit or extremity
repletion
reproducibility
reproducible baseline state
reproduction, colorimetric color
rerotation, varus
reroute, rerouted
rerupture of aneurysm
resampling, volumetric
rescue defibrillation
rescue shock
resected, surgically
resecting fracture
resection
reserve
  cardiac
  contractile
  coronary flow (CFR)
  diastolic
  left ventricular systolic functional
  myocardial perfusion (MPR)
  preload
  pulmonary vascular
  regional contractile
  stenotic flow (SFR)
  systolic
  vascular
  ventricular
reserve force
reserve mechanism, heart rate
reservoir (also pouch)
  Accu-Flo CSF
  Braden flushing
  continent ileal
  Cordis implantable drug
  CSF (cerebrospinal fluid)
  double bubble flushing

reservoir *(cont.)*
  double J-shaped
  double-barrel
  fecal
  flush
  flushing
  Foltz flushing
  ileal
  ileoanal
  intra-abdominal ileal
  J-shaped
  J-Vac suction
  Kock ileal
  lateral internal pelvic
  McKenzie
  Ommaya ventriculostomy
  Parks ileoanal
  peripheral venous
  Rickham intraventricular
  Salmon Rickham ventriculostomy
  Secor implantable drug
  S-shaped
  ventricular catheter
  W-stapled urinary
reservoir effect
residual
  fibrocalcific
  fibrocystic
  fibrotic
  gastric
  postvoid
  postvoiding (PVR)
residual cement
residual contrast material
residual deficit, significant
residual gradient
residual hemiparesis
residual interstitial changes
residual-limb shape change
residual plaque
residual pulmonary dysfunction
residual stress analysis

residual urine
residual urine accumulation
residual volume (RV)
residual volume/total lung capacity (RV/TLC)
residue, fecal
residuum morphology
resilient artery
resistance
  airway (RAW)
  arteriolar
  calculated
  coronary vascular
  decreased peripheral vascular
  decreased systemic
  expiratory
  fixed pulmonary valvular
  increased airways
  increased cerebral vascular
  increased outflow
  increased peripheral
  increased pulmonary vascular
  index of runoff
  nasal airway
  peripheral vascular (PVR)
  pulmonary arteriolar
  pulmonary vascular (PVR)
  systemic vascular (SVR)
  total peripheral (TPR)
  total pulmonary (TPR)
  vascular
  vascular systemic
  Wood units index of
resistance blood flow
resistive exercise table
resistive index (RI)
resistive magnet
resolution
  contrast
  high temporal
  interval
  spatial

resolution stage
resolved (or resolving) rejection
resolving time
resonance
  bandbox
  cough
  cracked-pot
  nuclear magnetic (NMR)
  skodaic
  tympanic
  vesicular
  vesiculotympanic
  vocal
  whispering
  wooden
resonance line
resonant frequency
resonant percussion note
resonator
  bridged loop-gap
  multicoupled loop-gap
resorbable pin
resorbable plate
resorbable rod
resorbable screw
resorption
  bone
  bony
  dependent edema fluid
  fluid
  osteoclastic
resorption phase of healing
respiration gated three-dimensional (3D) reconstruction
respiratory atrium
respiratory compensation
respiratory complications
respiratory compromise
respiratory decompensation
respiratory disturbance of acid base
respiratory embarrassment
respiratory excursions full and equal

respiratory frequency
respiratory gating technique
respiratory insufficiency
respiratory modulation of vascular
 impedance
respiratory motion artifacts
respiratory muscle weakness
respiratory ordered phase encoding
 (ROPE)
respiratory spasm
respiratory status, compromised
respiratory stridor
respiratory tract obstruction,
 mechanical
response
  abnormal ejection fraction
  cardioinhibitory
  controlled ventricular
  hemodynamic
  metabolic
  rapid ventricular
  regional cerebral blood flow
  slow ventricular
  therapeutic
  vagal
  vasoactive
  vasoconstrictor
  vasodepressor
  vasodilatory
  ventricular
responsive to TSH manipulation
responsiveness, airway
re-stenosis after angioplasty
restiform body
resting electrocardiogram
resting end-systolic wall stress
resting heart
resting imaging
resting MUGA scan, preoperative
resting perfusion
resting phase of cardiac action
  potentials
resting pulse
resting-redistribution thallium-201
  scintigraphy
resting regional myocardial blood
  flow
resting regional myocardial
  hypoperfusion
rest injection
rest LV (left ventricular) function
rest-redistribution exam
rest RV (right ventricular) function
rest thallium-201 myocardial imaging
restoration algorithm
restoration of sinus rhythm
restriction, unilateral flow
restrictive abnormality
restrictive bulbo-ventricular foramen
restrictive cardiac syndrome
restrictive defect
restrictive hemodynamic syndrome
restrictive lung disease
restrictive myocardial disease
restrictive-obstructive lung disease,
  mixed
restrictive pattern
restrictive ventilatory defect
result (pl. results)
  concordant
  false-positive
  false-negative
  suboptimal
resurrection bone
retained cortical activity (RCA)
retained foreign body
retained secretions
retained urine
retard premature rewarming
rete (pl. retia)
rete pegs
rete ridges
retention of barium
retention of stool

reticular activating formation (RAF)
reticular activating substance
reticular activating system (RAS)
reticular formation of brain stem
reticular infiltrate
reticular opacity
reticulation artifact
reticulocortical pathway
reticuloendothelial contrast agent
reticuloendothelial system
reticulogranular appearance
reticulogranular pattern
reticulonodular infiltrate
reticulospinal tract
reticulum
   hematopoietic (of marrow)
   arcoplasmic
reticulum cell sarcoma
retina, angiomatosis of
retinacular disruption
retinacular ligaments
retinaculum
   avulsed
   extensor
   flexor
   patellar
   superior peroneal (SPR)
retinal exudate
retinoblastoma
retraction (pl. retractions)
   chest-wall
   clot
   costal
   inspiratory
   intercostal
   late systolic
   leaflet
   midsystolic
   mild subcostal
   nipple
   postrheumatic cusp
   sternocleidomastoid

retraction (*cont.*)
   sternum
   substernal
   suprasternal
   systolic
re-treating
retrieval
   microvascular
   transvaginal oocyte
retroappendiceal fossa
retroareolar dysplasia
retrobulbar hemorrhage
retrocalcaneal bursa
retrocalcaneal exostosis
retrocalcaneal spur
retrocardiac density
retrocardiac infiltrate
retrocardiac space
retrocecal appendix
retroclavicular
retrocrural lymph nodes
retroesophageal subclavian artery
retroflexed scope
retroflexed view
retroflexion
retrograde aortogram
retrograde arterial catheterization
retrograde atherectomy
retrograde atrial activation mapping
retrograde blood flow across valve
retrograde blood velocity
retrograde conduction
retrograde coronary sinus infusion
retrograde duodenogastroscopy (RDG)
retrograde femoral arterial approach
retrograde flow on barium enema
retrograde imaging
retrograde injection
retrograde percutaneous femoral
   artery approach for cardiac
   catheterization
retrograde perfusion

retrograde peristalsis
retrograde pyelogram
retrograde pyelography
retrograde refractory period
retrograde transfemoral aortography
retrograde ureterogram
retrograde ureterography
retrograde ureteropyelogram
retrograde urethrogram
retrograde ventriculoatrial conduction
retrohepatic vena cava
retroileal appendix
retrolisthesis
retromammary space view in mammography
retromedullary arteriovenous malformation
retronuchal muscle
retroorbital space
retropancreatic preaortic space
retropancreatic tunnel
retropectoral mammary implant
retroperfusion
  coronary sinus
  synchronized
retroperitoneal actinomycosis
retroperitoneal approach
retroperitoneal area
retroperitoneal fibrosis
retroperitoneal hematoma
retroperitoneal region
retroperitoneal space
retroperitoneal tumor
retroperitoneal tunnel
retroperitoneally
retroperitoneum
retropharyngeal abscess
retropulsion of bone fragment into spinal canal
retrosellar region
retrosomatic cleft
retrosternal chest pain
retrosternal thyroid
retrotorsion, femoral
retroversion, femoral
retrovestibular neural pathway
retrusion, midface
return
  anomalous
  anomalous pulmonary venous
  central arterial
  infracardiac-type total anomalous venous
  paracardiac-type total anomalous venous
  pulmonary venous
  supracardiac-type total anomalous venous
  systemic venous
  total anomalous pulmonary venous
  total anomalous venous
  venous
return to baseline
Retzius
  ligament of
  line of
  space of
  system of
  vein of
REU (rectal endoscopic ultrasonography)
revascularization
  cerebral
  coronary
  coronary ostial
  endosteal
  foot
  graft
  heart
  infrainguinal
  myocardial
  percutaneous
  surgical
revascularized tissue

reverberation echos
reversal of blood flow
reversal of cervical lordosis
reversal, shunt
reversal sign
reverse Barton fracture
reverse Colles fracture
reverse distribution
reverse immunoassay
reverse redistribution
reverse transport
reversed coarctation
reversed differential cyanosis
reversed greater saphenous vein
reversed Mercedes-Benz sign
reversed peristalsis
reversed 3 sign
reversible (or resolving) ischemic neurologic deficit (RIND)
reversible airways disease (RAD)
reversible atrial pacing
reversible defect
reversible ischemia
reversible obstructive airway disease (ROAD)
reversible organic brain syndrome
reversible perfusion defects
revolving Ge-68 pins as transmission sources
Reye syndrome
Reynolds number
REZ (root exit zone)
RF (rapid filling)
RFA (radiofrequency ablation)
RFCA (radiofrequency catheter ablation)
RFP (rapid filling period)
RFW (rapid filling wave)
Rh (rhodium) isoimmunization
rhabdoid suture
rhabdoid tumor
rhabdomyolysis

rhabdomyoma of heart
rhabdomyosarcoma
  alveolar
  cardiac
  childhood
  primary
rhebosis
Rhees views of orbits
rhenium (Re)
  $^{186}$Re hydroxyethylidene diphosphate (HEDP)
  $^{188}$Re-labeled antibodies
rheologic pattern
rheumatic adherent pericardium
rheumatic aortic insufficiency
rheumatic aortic stenosis
rheumatic chorea
rheumatic fever (RF)
rheumatic heart disease (RHD)
rheumatic lesion
rheumatic mitral stenosis
rheumatic nodule
rheumatic pneumonia
rheumatic valvular disease
rheumatoid arthritis (RA) factor
rheumatoid arthritis-associated interstitial lung disease
rheumatoid nodule
rheumatoid spondylitis
rheumatologist
rhinocerebral mucormycosis
rhodium (Rh)
rhomboid fossa
rhomboid ligament
rhomboid major muscle
rhomboideus muscle
rhonchus (pl. rhonchi)
RHS (radial head subluxation)
RHV (right hepatic vein)
rhythmic segmentation
RI (resistive index) angiography
RIA (radioimmunoassay) test

rib (pl. ribs)
  angle of
  bed of
  bicipital
  bifid
  cervical
  facet for head of
  false
  first
  floating
  fused
  head of
  hypoplastic horizontal
  inferior margin of superior
  lumbar
  minced
  neck of
  notching of
  penciling of
  periosteum of
  retracted
  rudimentary
  shaft of
  slipping
  sternal
  Stiller
  superior
  superior margin of inferior
  true
  tubercle of
  vertebral
  vertebrocostal
  vertebrosternal
ribbon application
rib contusion
rib fracture from cough
rib guillotine
rib notching
rib recession
rib spaces, narrowed
rib view
Richet, tibio-astragalocalcaneal canal of

Richter hernia
Richter-Monroe line
rickets, familial hypophosphatemic
rickettsial pneumonia
Rickham reservoir
rider's bone
ridge
  alveolar
  alveodental
  apical ectodermal (AER)
  basal
  bicipital
  bisagittal
  broad maxillary
  buccocervical
  buccogingival
  bulbar
  cerebral
  cranial
  cutaneous
  dental
  dorsal
  epicondylar
  epidermal
  epipericardial
  fibrocartilaginous
  fibromuscular
  ganglion
  gastrocnemial
  genital
  gluteal
  greater multangular
  humeral
  interarticular
  interosseous
  intertrochanteric
  interureteric
  longitudinal
  marginal
  mesonephric
  mylohyoid
  oblique

ridge *(cont.)*
  Outerbridge
  palatine
  pectoral
  petrous
  radial
  ridging
  sagittal
  semicircular
  septal
  sphenoid
  supra-aortic
  supracondylar
  supracoronary
  supraorbital
  tentorial
  transverse
  triangular
  ulnar
  urethral
  vastus lateralis
  wolffian
riding embolus
Ridley sinus
Ridley syndrome
Riedel lobe
Riedel struma
Rieux hernia
RIF-1 tumor
right and left atrial phasic volumetric function
right and retrograde left heart catheterization
right-angle chest tube
right-angled telescopic lens
right anterior oblique (RAO) position
right aortic arch with mirror image branching
right atrial enlargement
right atrial extension of uterine leiomyosarcoma
right atrial patch positioned over the
right atrioventricular sulcus
right atrial pressure (RAP)
right atrium
right border of heart
right bundle branch block (RBBB)
right bundle branch block with left anterior (or posterior) hemiblock
right coronary artery, dominant
right heart catheter
right heart failure
right heart pressure
right inferior epigastric artery
right internal iliac artery
right internal jugular artery
right internal mammary anastomosis
right Judkins catheter
right lateral decubitus view
right-left disorientation
right lower lobe (RLL) of lung
right main stem bronchus
right middle lobe (RML) of lung
right middle lobe lingula
right posterior oblique (RPO) position
right side down decubitus position
right-sided empyema
right-sided heart failure
right-sided pneumonia
right subclavian artery, retro-esophageal
right-to-left shift
right-to-left shunt with pulmonic stenosis
right-to-left shunting
right to left shunt of blood
right upper lobe (RUL) consolidation
right upper quadrant (RUQ)
right ventricle
  augmented filling of
  double-outlet
  parchment
right ventricle adherent to posterior table of sternum

right ventricle outflow tract
right ventricle-pulmonary artery
 conduit
right ventricular assist device (RVAD)
right ventricular coil
right ventricular conduction defect
right ventricular ejection fraction
 (RVEF)
right ventricular end-diastolic volume
 (RVEDV)
right ventricular end-systolic volume
 (RVESV)
right ventricular failure
right ventricular hypertrophy (RVH)
right ventricular impulse,
 hyperdynamic
right ventricular obstruction,
 intraventricular
right ventricular outflow obstruction
right ventricular outflow tract
right ventricular overload
right ventricular pressure (RVP)
right ventricular stroke volume
right ventricular stroke work (RVSW)
right ventricular stroke work index
 (RVSWI)
right ventricular systolic time interval
rigid ureter
Rigiflex TTS balloon catheter
Rigler sign
RIGScan CR49
rim
 dark signal intensity
 glenoid
 high-density
 low-density
 sclerotic
 signal intensity
rimlike calcium distribution
rim sign
RIND (reversible or resolving
 ischemic neurologic deficit)

Rindfleisch, fold of
ring (pl. rings)
 abdominal
 Ace-Colles half
 amnion
 annular
 anorectal
 aortic subvalvular
 apex of external
 arc
 atrial
 atrioventricular
 Bickel
 Cannon
 Carpentier
 cartilaginous
 CBI stereotactic
 centering
 Charnley centering
 choroidal
 ciliary
 common tendinous
 congenital (of aortic arch)
 constriction
 Crawford suture
 crural
 distal esophageal
 double-flanged valve sewing
 doughnut
 drop-lock
 esophageal A
 esophageal B
 esophageal contractile
 esophageal mucosal
 esophageal muscular
 external
 external inguinal
 femoral
 fibrocartilaginous
 fibrous
 Fischer
 fracture

ring *(cont.)*
   fracture encircling foramen
      magnum
   half
   halo
   ilioinguinal
   iliopsoas
   Ilizarov
   inguinal
   internal abdominal
   internal inguinal
   intrahaustral contraction
   ischial weightbearing
   Kayser-Fleischer
   lymphoid
   mitral
   mitral valve
   Mose concentric
   Ochsner
   olive
   orthosis drop-lock
   pelvic
   perichondral
   periosteal bone
   pleural
   prosthetic valve sewing
   prosthetic valve suture
   proximal-to-distal
   pyloric
   retraction
   Schatzki
   sewing
   Silastic
   silicone elastomer
   sizing
   sodium iodide
   sphincter contraction
   stereotactic or stereotaxic
   superficial inguinal
   supra-annular suture
   supravalvar
   tricuspid valve

ring *(cont.)*
   tubal
   valve
   vascular
   vertebral
   Vieussens
   Waldeyer
   Zinn
ring apophysis
ring blush on cerebral arteriography
Ring catheter
ring enhancement
ring-enhancing lesion
ringlike configuration
ringlike contractions
Ring-McLean catheter
ring-type imaging system
ring shadows with air-fluid levels
Riolan, arch of
Riolan bone (ossicle)
Riordan finger pollicization
RISA (radioactive iodinated serum
   albumin)
Riseborough-Radin classification of
   intercondylar fracture
rise times
risk analysis
risk/benefit ratio
Ritchie index
Riva-Rocci manometer
Riviere sign
RLE (right lower extremity)
RLL (right lower lobe) of lung
RLQ (right lower quadrant)
R (roentgen) meter
r-metHuG-CSF (recombinant human
   granulocyte colony stimulating
   factor)
RML (right middle lobe) of lung
RNA (radionuclide angiogram), gated
RNS terminal
RNV (radionuclide ventriculogram)

R/O (rule out)
ROA (regurgitant orifice area)
ROAD (reversible obstructive airway disease)
road-mapping for interventional radiography
road-mapping mode
Robengatope radioactive agent
Robertson sign
Robicsek vascular probe (RVP)
Robin Hood phenomenon (steal syndrome)
Robinson catheter, red rubber
Robinson-Chung-Farahvar clavicular morcellation
robotics-controlled stereotactic frame
robust registration technique
ROC (receiver operating characteristics)
rocking curve measurement
rocking precordial motion
Rockwood classification of acromioclavicular injury
rod, TLD (thermoluminescent dosimeter)
RODEO (rotating delivery of excitation off-resonance), 3D
Rodriguez-Alvarez catheter
Roederer obliquity
rOEF (regional oxygen extraction fraction)
roentgen (R)
roentgen knife
roentgen stereophotogrammetric analysis (RSA)
roentgenkymography
roentgenogram
roentgenographic control
roentgenographic silhouette
roentgenography
roentgenologist
roentogenographically occult

Rogan teleradiology system
Roger syndrome
Roger ventricular septal defect
ROI (region of interest)
Rokitanski-Aschoff sinus
Rokitansky-Cushing ulcer
Rokitansky diverticulum
Rokitansky pelvis
Rolando angle
Rolando area
Rolando fissure
Rolando fracture
Rolando line
Rolando point
Rolando tubercle
roll, radiolucent
Rolleston rule for systolic blood pressure
Romano-Ward syndrome
Romberg-Wood syndrome
Romhilt-Estes score for left ventricular hypertrophy
ROMI (rule out myocardial infarction)
ROMIed
roof
  acetabular
  intercondylar
root
  anatomical
  cochlear
  coronary sinus
  cranial
  dental
  dilated aortic
  facial
  insula
  lingual
  lung
  motor
  nerve
  palatine

root *(cont.)*
   retained
   sensory
   spinal
   ventral
   ventricle
rootlets of nerve
root-mean-squared gradient measure
ROPE (respiratory ordered phase encoding)
rope-like cord (in thrombophlebitis)
ropy
Roques syndrome
Rosch catheter
rose bengal sodium $^{131}$I radioactive biliary agent
Rosenbach syndrome
Rosen-Castleman-Liebow syndrome
Rosenmüller, fossa of
Rosenthal, basal vein of (BVR)
rosette appearance of anus
rostral brain stem ischemia
rostral cervical nerve
rostral connection
rostral hypothalamus
rostral medulla
rostral pons
rostral spinal cord
rostral terminus
rostrally
rostrum of corpus callosum
rostrum sphenoidale
rotary instability
rotary scoliosis
rotary subluxation
rotary thoracolumbar scoliosis
rotatable pigtail catheter
rotating bur (or burr)
rotating delivery of excitation off-resonance), 3D (RODEO)
rotating frame imaging
rotating frame of reference
rotating gamma camera
rotating tomographic projection
rotating tourniquets for pulmonary edema
rotation
   360°
   tube position
rotation therapy
rotational alignment
rotational atherectomy system (RAS)
rotational coronary atherectory (RCA)
rotational flaps
rotational force
rotational radiotherapy
rotator cuff tear
rotatory loads on spine
Rotch sign in pericardial effusion
Roubin-Gianturco flexible coil stent
rough zone
roughened state of pericardium
roughened surface
rouleaux formation
round cell tumors
round pronator (pronator radii teres)
rounded border of lung
rounded convex borders
routine magnfication view
routine view
Rouviere, ligament of
Roux-en-Y anastomosis
Roux-en-Y limb
row, carpal
row mode sinogram images
Rowe calcaneal fracture classification
Rowe-Lowell fracture-dislocation classification system
Royal Flush angiographic flush catheter
Royer-Wilson syndrome
RPA (right pulmonary artery)
rpm (rotations per minute)
RPO (right posterior oblique) position

RPT (rapid pull-through) technique
RPV (right pulmonary vein)
RSA (roentgen stereophotogrammetric analysis)
Rsch-Uchida transjugular liver access needle-catheter
RSCVP (right subclavian central venous pressure)
RSI (repetitive stress injury)
RT (repetition time)
RT 3200 Advantage ultrasound scanner
RT 6800 ultrasound scanner
RTL cassette
RTOG protocol
RTP (radiation therapy planning) system
RTV cassette
rubidium (Rb)
   $^{82}$Rb-based cardiac imaging
Rubin test
Rubratope-57 radioactive agent
rubrospinal tract
rubrous
rudimentary bone
rudimentary ribs
rudimentary sinus
rudimentary ventricular chamber
RUE (right upper extremity)
Ruedi-Allgower tibial plafond fracture classification
ruga (pl. rugae)
rugal fold
rugal pattern
rugger jersey spine
RUL (right upper lobe) of lung
rule-based scheme
rule out (R/O)
rule out myocardial infarction (ROMI)
rules, Paterson-Parker
Rumel catheter

runoff
   absent
   aortic
   aortofemoral
   arterial
   digital
   distal
   inadequate
   peripheral
   single-vessel
   suboptimal
   three-vessel
   two-vessel
   vessel
runoff arteriogram
runoff resistance, index of
runoff vessel
runoff views, aortofemoral arteriography with
rupture
   abdominal aortic aneurysm
   aneurysma
   appendix
   Achilles tendon
   arch
   arterial
   buttonhole
   cardiac
   chordae tendineae
   chordal
   complete Achilles tendon
   contained aneurysmal
   forniceal
   interventricular septal
   myocardial
   nodal
   papillary muscle
   plantaris (tennis leg)
   plaque
   silicone implant
   ventricular free wall

rupture *(cont.)*
   ventricular septal
   vessel
rupture of membranes (ROM)
ruptured capillaries
ruptured chordae tendineae
ruptured disk
ruptured emphysematous bleb
ruptured intracranial aneurysm
ruptured thoracic duct
RUQ (right upper quadrant)
Russell-Rubinstein classification of cerebrovascular malformation
Russell-Silver syndrome
rutherford (rd) radioactive unit
Ruysch disease
RV (residual volume)
RV (right ventricle) pressure
RVA (right ventricular apical) electrogram
RVBF (reversed vertebral blood flow)
RVD (right ventricular diastolic) pressure
RVD (right ventricular dimension)
RVE (right ventricular enlargement)
RVFW (right ventricular free wall)
RVH (renal vasular hypertension)
RVH (right ventricular hypertrophy)
RVID (right ventricular internal diameter)
RVM (right ventricular mass)
RVOT (right ventricular outflow tract)
RVP (right ventricular pressure)
RVP–LVP (right ventricular to left ventricular systolic pressure) ratio
RVS (right ventricular systolic) pressure
RVSTI (right ventricular systolic time interval)
RVSW (right ventricular stroke work)
RVSWI (right ventricular stroke work index)
RV/TLC (residual volume/total lung capacity)

# S, s

SAA protein
SAB (sinoatrial block)
Sabathie sign
saber shin
sac
    abdominal
    abnormal gestational
    air
    alveolar
    amniotic
    aneurysmal
    aortic
    bursal
    chorionic
    common dural
    cystic
    decidual
    dental
    double decidual
    dural
    effacement of dural
    embryonic
    endolymphatic
    enterocele
    false
    fluid-filled
    gestational
sac *(cont.)*
    greater peritoneal
    heart
    hernia
    indirect hernia
    intrauterine
    lesser peritoneal
    narrowing of thecal
    pericardial
    peritoneal
    pleural
    spinal
    terminal air
    thecal
    tight dural
    wide-mouth
    wrapped aneurysmal
    yolk
sacciform recess
saccular aneurysm
saccular appearance, lobulated
saccular bronchiectasis
saccular collection
saccular mass
sacculated pleurisy
sacculation
saccule

sacculus ventricularis
Sack-Barabas syndrome
saclike spaces
sacral ala
sacral cyst
sacral dermatomes
sacral gutter
sacral insufficiency fracture (SIF)
sacralization of vertebrae
sacralized transverse process
sacral plexus
sacral promontory
sacroabdominoperineal pull-through
sacrococcygeal chordoma
sacrococcygeal joint
sacrococcygeal remnant tumor
sacrococcygeal teratoma
sacrococcyx
sacroiliac (SI)
sacroiliac articulation
sacroiliac disease
sacroiliac joint
sacroiliac sprain
sacroiliac subluxation
sacropubic diameter
sacrosciatic foramen
sacrosciatic notch
sacrospinalis muscle
sacrotuberous ligament
sacrouterine
sacrovertebral angle
sacrum (sacral spine)
   alae of
   assimilation
   cornua of
   promontory of
   scimitar
   tilted
SACT (sinoatrial conduction time)
saddle-area anesthesia
saddle coil
saddle embolism or embolus

saddle joint
saddle points
SADIA (small angle double incidence angiograms)
Sadowsky breast marking system
SaECG (signal-averaged electrocardiogram)
SAFHS (sonic-accelerated fracture-healing system)
Sage-Salvatore classification of acromioclavicular joint injury
sagittal gradient echo image
sagittal groove
sagittal image
sagittal oblique images
sagittal orientation
sagittal plane
sagittal plane faults
sagittal plane loop
sagittal roll spondylolisthesis
sagittal section
sagittal sinus
sagittal slice
sagittal suture
sagittal T-1 image
sagittal tomogram
sagittal transabdominal image
sagittal ultrasound
SAH (subarachnoid hemorrhage)
sail sign (of fat pad in elbow joint)
Sakellarides classification of calcaneal fracture
saline
   heparinized
   hypertonic
   sterile
saline-enhanced MR arthrography
saline-enhanced RF tissue ablation
saline loading
saline solution
saline torch
salivary gland function study

Salkowski test
salpingitis
  chronic interstitial
  follicular
  gonococcal
  hemorrhagic
  interstitial
  pseudofollicular
  purulent
  tuberculous
salpingogram
salpingography, selective osteal
salpinx (pl. salpinges)
Salpix contrast medium
salt and pepper duodenal erosion
salt wasting, cerebral
Salter-Harris classification of fracture (I through VI, or 1-6)
Salter-Harris-Rang classification of fracture
salvage, interventional limb
salvage of myocardium
salvage surgery
salvage therapy
salvo of echoes
salvo of premature ventricular complexes
SAM (scanning acoustic microscope)
SAM (systolic anterior motion) on 2-D echocardiogram
samarium (Sm)
  $^{153}$Sm ethylene diamine tetramethylene phosporic acid imaging agent
same-day microsurgical arthroscopic lateral-approach laser-assisted (SMALL) fluoroscopic diskectomy
sample points
sampling
  adrenal vein
  tissue
  zonal

SAN (sinoatrial node)
Sanchez-Perez automatic film changer
sandbag hazard
sandbagging fracture of long bones
Sandhoff disease
Sandrock test for thrombosis
sandwich patch closure, anterior
Sanfilippo syndrome
SA (sinoatrial)
SA nodal reentry tachycardia
SA node (also called sinus)
Sansom sign in pericardial effusion
Santiani-Stone classification of pancreatitis
Santorini
  duct of
  papilla of
saphenofemoral junction
saphenous varices
saphenous vein
  greater
  reversed greater
saphenous vein bypass graft
saphenous vein graft (SVG)
saphenous vein incompetence
sarcoid-like reaction
sarcoid of Boeck
sarcoidosis
  hepatic
  spinal cord
sarcoma (see also *carcinoma*, *tumor*)
  Abernethy
  alveolar soft part
  ameloblastic
  angiolithic
  botryoid
  cardiac
  clear cell
  endobronchial Kaposi
  endometrial stromal
  epithelioid
  Ewing

sarcoma *(cont.)*
  gastric Kaposi
  giant cell monstrocellular
  granulocytic
  hemangioendothelial
  high-grade surface osteogenic
  immunoblastic
  intracolonic Kaposi
  intracortical osteogenic
  intrathoracic Kaposi
  Ito cell
  Jensen
  juxtacortical osteogenic
  Kaposi epicardial
  Kupffer cell
  leukocytic
  lipoblastic
  low-grade central osteogenic
  lymphatic
  malignant myeloid
  medullary
  mixed cell
  multicentric osteogenic
  multiple idiopathic hemorrhagic
  myelogenic
  myeloid
  myocardial infiltration by Kaposi
  neurogenic
  osteogenic
  Paget associated osteogenic
  parosteal osteogenic
  periosteal
  postirradiation osteogenic
  primary
  pulmonary Kaposi
  reticulum cell
  right atrial
  small cell osteogenic
  spindle cell
  synovial
  telangiectatic osteogenic
  vasoablative endothelial (VABES)

Sarns wire-reinforced catheter
SAS (supravalvular aortic stenosis)
Sassone score of appearance in transvaginal ultrasound
satellite lesion
satellite nodule
satumomab pentetide (OncoScint CR/OV) imaging agent
saturation
  jugular venous oxygen
  oxygen
  regional cerebral oxygen
saturation inversion projection (SIP)
saturation recovery sequence
saturation recovery technique
saturation stripe
saturation transfer
saucer-shaped excavation
saucerization of vertebra
sausage finger, in syringomyelia
sausaging of vein
sawtooth (also saw-toothed) appearance
sawtooth irregularity of bowel contour
SBDX (scanning-beam digital x-ray)
SBF (systemic blood flow)
SBFT (small bowel follow-through)
SBO (small bowel obstruction)
SBO (spina bifida occulta)
SBP (systolic blood pressure)
SBSP (simultaneous bilateral spontaneous pneumothorax)
SCA (superior cerebellar artery)
SCAD (spontaneous coronary artery dissection)
SCA-EX ShortCutter catheter with rotating blades
scalar quantization, wavelet (WSQ)
scale
  false color
  fish
  gray

scalene fat pad
scalene musculature
scalenus anterior muscle
scalenus anticus muscle hypertrophy
scalenus anticus syndrome
scalenus minimus
scallop of posterior annulus, redundant
scallop, prolapsing
scalloped bowel lumen
scalloped commissure
scalloped luminal configuration
scalloping of margin of vertebral body
scan (scintiscan) (see *imaging; scanner*)
scan decrement
scan defect
Scanditronix PET scanner
Scanmaster DX scanner
Scanmaster DX x-ray film digitizer
scanned-slot detector system
scanner (also digitizer)
  Acoma
  Acuson 128EP
  Acuson ultrasound
  Advanced NMR systems
  Agfa Medical
  All-Tronics
  Aloka ultrasound linear
  Aloka ultrasound sector
  American Shared-CuraCare
  ANMR Insta-scan MR
  Artoscan MRI
  ATL Mark 600 real-time sector
  ATL real-time Neurosector
  Aurora MR breast imaging system
  Biospec MR imaging system
  Bruel-Kjaer ultrasound
  Bruker
  Canon
  Cemax/Icon
  Cencit surface
  charge-coupled device

scanner *(cont.)*
  cine CT (computed tomography)
  Compuscan Hittman computerized electrocardioscanner
  CT Max 640
  CT9000
  CTI 933/04 ECAT
  CTI PET
  Delarnette
  Diasonics ultrasound
  Dornier
  DuPont
  Dynamic Spatial Reconstructor (DSR)
  Eastman Kodak
  electron beam CT
  Elscint CT
  Elscint MR
  Elscint Twin CT
  EMED
  EMI CT
  Fonar
  4096 Plus PET
  Galen Scan
  Gammex RMI
  GE (General Electric)
  GE Advance PET
  GE CT Max
  GE 9800 CT
  GE 8800 CT/T
  GE Genesis CT
  GE GN 500 MHz
  GE HiSpeed Advantage helical CT
  GE Max MR
  GE 9800 high-resolution CT
  GE Omega 500 MHz
  GE 1.5 Tesla Signa
  GE Pace CT
  GE QE 300 MHz
  GE Signa 1.5 Tesla
  GE Signa 4.7 MRI
  GE Signa 5.2 with SR-230 3-axis EPI gradient upgrade

**scanner**

scanner *(cont.)*
   GE single axis SR-230 echo-planar
   GE Vectra MR
   Gyroscan S15
   helical CT
   Hewlett-Packard
   high field open MRI
   high field strength
   Hilight Advantage System
   Hispeed CT
   Hitachi CT
   Hitachi MR
   Hitachi 0.3T unit
   Hitachi Open MRI System
   Hologic 2000
   Howtek Scanmaster DX
   IDSI
   Imatron C-100 ultrafast CT
   Imatron C-100XL CT
   Imatron C-150L EBCT
   Imatron Fastrac C-100 cine x-ray CT
   Imatron Ultrafast CT
   Innervision MR
   InstaScan
   Integris 3000
   intensified radiographic imaging system (IRIS)
   Irex Exemplar ultrasound
   Konica
   large bore 0.6T imaging system
   large bore 1.5T imaging system
   Lumiscan
   Lunar
   LymphoScan nuclear imaging system
   Magna-SL
   Magnetom 1.5 T
   Magnetom SP63
   Magnes 2500 WH (whole blood)
   Magnex MR
   Mallinckrodt

scanner *(cont.)*
   Max Plus MR
   MedImage
   Medison
   Medspec MR imaging system
   midget MRI
   modified electron-beam CT
   MR catheter imaging and spectroscopy system
   multiple jointed digitizer
   multisensor structured light range digitizer
   NeuroSector
   Nishimoto Sangyo
   Norlan pQCT XCT2000
   Olympus endoscopic ultrasound
   Oxford 2T large bore imaging system
   Pace Plus System
   Park Medical Systems
   Perception
   PETite
   Philips CT
   Philips 1.5T NT MR
   Philips 4.7 T small bore system
   Philips Gyroscan ACS
   Philips Gyroscan NT; NT5; NT15
   Philips Gyroscan S5
   Philips Gyroscan T5
   Philips tomoscan 350 CT
   Picker CT
   Picker MR
   Picker PQ 5000 helical CT
   Picker PQ-2000 spiral CT
   Polhemus 3 digitizer
   Posicam HZ PET
   PQCT micro-scanner
   ProSpeed CT
   Quad MRI
   Quick CT9800
   rectilinear
   RT 3200 Advantage ultrasound

scanner *(cont.)*
  RT 6800 ultrasound
  Scanditronix PET
  Scanmaster DX x-ray film digitizer
  scintillation (scintiscanner)
  sector
  Shimadzu CT
  Shimadzu MR
  Siemens CT
  Siemens DRH CT
  Siemens Magnetom GBS II
  Siemens Magnetom Impact
  Siemens Magnetom 1.5 T
  Siemans Magnetom SP 4000
  Siemens Magnetom Vision
  Siemens One Tesla
  Siemens Somaform 512 CT
  Siemens Somatom DR2 whole-body; also DR3
  Siemens Somatom PLUS-S
  Siemens Sonoline Elegra ultrasound
  Siemens SP 4000
  SieScape ultrasound
  Signa 1.5T
  Signa Horizon
  Signa I.S.T. MRI
  single-field hyperthermia combined with radiation therapy and ultrasound
  Smart Prep
  Somatom DR CT
  Somatom Plus-S CT
  spiral CT
  spiral XCT
  Swissray
  TCT900S helical CT
  Tecmag Libra-S16 system
  3D surface digitizer
  3M
  Toshiba CT
  Toshiba helical CT

scanner *(cont.)*
  Toshiba MR
  Toshiba 900S helical CT
  Toshiba 900S/XII
  Toshiba TCT-80 CT
  Toshiba Xpress SX helical CT
  Trionix
  ultrafast computed tomography
  Ultramark
  UM 4 real-time sector
  Vidar
  Vision MRI
  Vision Ten V-scan
  whole-body 1.5T Siemens Vision
  whole-body 3T MRI system
  Xpress/SX helical CT
scanning (see *imaging*)
scanning acoustic microscope (SAM)
scanning-beam digital x-ray (SBDX)
scanning laser ophthalmoscopy
scanning locus
scanogram (see *imaging*)
scanography (see *imaging*)
scan pacing
scan parameters
scan pitch
scan time
scan volume Scan-O-Grams of lower extremities
scan with contrast enhancement
scan without contrast enhancement
scaphocapitate joint
scaphocephalic head shape
scaphocephaly
scaphoid abdomen
scaphoid bone (navicular)
  pole of
  waist of
scapholunate (SL)
scapholunate arthritic collapse (SLAC) wrist
scapholunate dissociation

scapholunate joint
scapholunate ligament (LSS)
scapholunate space
scapholunate widening
scapho-trapezium-trapezoid (STT) joint
scapula
  body of
  high-riding
  inferior tip of
  margin of
  winged
scapular bone
scapular flap
scapular notch
scapular winging
scapuloclavicular
scapulocostal syndrome
scapuloperoneal muscular atrophy
scapulothoracic motion
scapulovertebral border
scar
  dense
  infarcted
  myocardial
  nonviable
  pulmonary
  well-demarcated
  zipper
scar contracture
scar formation
scar tissue
scar tissue reaction
scarification of pleura
scarified duodenum
Scarpa
  canal of
  fascia of
  ganglion of
  ligament of
  method of
  triangle of

scarred duodenum
scarred fibrotic media
scarring
  apical
  basilar pleural
  interstitial
  parenchymal
  pleural
  postnecrotic
  selective
  valve
  valvular
scatoma (stercoroma)
scatter, collimator
scatter compensation
scattered air bronchogram
scattering
  coherent
  Compton
  low angle
  small angle multiple
scattering foil compensator
scattering system
scatter-to-primary ratio
Scerratti goniometer
SCFE (slipped capital femoral epiphysis)
Schatzker fracture classification system
Schatzki ring
Schatzki view
Schaumann body
scheme
  CISS
  computer-aided diagnosis
  encryption
  rule-based
Scheuermann juvenile kyphosis
Schick sign of tuberculosis
Schiefferdecker disk
Schlatter-Osgood disease
Schlesinger, vein of

Schmidt optics system
Schmitt disease
Schmorl disease
Schmorl node
Schneider PTCA instruments
Schneider-Shiley catheter
Schneider Wallstent
Schonander film changer
Schönlein purpura
Schoonmaker multipurpose catheter
Schüller view
Schwann tumor
schwannoma
   facial
   orbital
   vestibular
Schwarten balloon dilatation catheter
Schwartz test for patency of deep saphenous veins
SCI (spinal cord injury)
sciatic artery, persistent
sciatic endometriosis
sciatic foramen
   greater
   lesser
sciatic nerve irritation
sciatic notch
   greater
   lesser
sciatic plexus
sciatica
Sci-Med or SciMed
Sci-Med Express Monorail balloon
Sci-Med SSC "Skinny" catheter
scimitar deformity
scimitar-shaped flap
scimitar-shaped shadow
scimitar sign on chest radiograph
scimitar vein
Scinticore multicrystal scintillation camera
scintigram

scintigraphic imaging
scintigraphic study
scintigraphy
   ACE inhibition
   AMA-Fab (antimyosin monoclonal antibody with Fab fragment)
   antifibrin
   bone
   bone marrow
   brain perfusion
   cortical
   dipyridamole thallium-201
   dual intracoronary
   exercise stress-redistribution
   exercise thallium
   gallium
   gated blood pool
   hepatobiliary
   indium (In)
   $^{111}$In-WBC (indium with white blood cells)
   infarct-avid hot-spot
   iodine (I)
   $^{131}$I-19-iodocholesterol
   $^{131}$I MIBG
   isotope
   labeled FFA (free fatty acid)
   MIBG (metaiodobenzylguanidine)
   microsphere perfusion
   myocardial cold-spot perfusion
   NEFA (non-esterified fatty acid)
   NP-59
   planar thallium
   pulmonary
   pyrophosphate
   quantitative hepatobiliary (QHS)
   radioistope
   resting-redistribution thallium-201
   single photon planar (SPPS)
   SPECT brain perfusion
   SPECT thallium
   technetium $^{99m}$Tc-PYP (pyrophosphate)

scintigraphy (cont.)
   thallium
   thallium perfusion
   thallium-201 myocardial
   three-phase bone (TPBS)
   vesicoureteral
   white blood cell (WBCS) with indium-111 ($^{111}$In)
scintillating scotoma (pl. scotomata)
scintillation camera
scintillation counter
scintillation crystal
scintillation detector
scintillation, migrainous-like
scintillation proximity radioimmunoassay
scintillation scan
scintillation spectrometry
scintillator
   aqueous
   benzene
   CeI
   cyclohexane
   organic liquid
   toluene
scintimammography (SMM)
scintiphotograph
scintirenography
scintiscan (see *imaging*)
scintiscanner (see *scanner*)
scintiscanning
Scintiview nuclear computer system
Scintron IV nuclear computer system
scirrhous carcinoma
scirrhous lesion
scissor gait
scissoring of legs
SCL (sinus cycle length)
SCLC (small-cell lung cancer)
scleroderma of esophagus
sclerosing nonsuppurative osteomyelitis

sclerosis
   Ammon horn (mesial temporal)
   aortic
   arterial
   arteriocapillary
   arteriolar
   Baló
   calcified
   congenital hippocampal
   coronary
   diffuse
   disseminated
   endocardial
   esophageal variceal
   familial amyotrophic lateral
   gastric
   hepatic
   hepatoportal
   hippocampal
   incisural
   Krabbe diffuse
   laser
   lobar
   medial calcific
   mesenteric
   mesial temporal
   Mönckeberg
   multiple (MS)
   pedicle
   posterolateral (of the spinal cord)
   progressive systemic
   pulmonary and cardiac
   renal
   segmental vein
   subchondral
   subendocardial
   tuberous
   valvular
   variceal
   vascular
   venous
sclerotic area

sclerotic coronary arteries
sclerotic degeneration
sclerotic plaque (plaquing)
sclerotic rims in gout
scoliosis
  adolescent idiopathic (AIS)
  Aussies-Isseis unstable
  Cobb measurement of
  dextrorotary
  dextro-
  Dwyer correction of
  Fergusson method for measuring
  fixation of a
  functional
  idiopathic
  King classification of thoracic
  King-Moe
  levorotary
  levo-
  lumbar
  lumbar component of
  Moe and Kettleson distribution of curves in
  rotary
  S-shaped
  thoracic
  thoracolumbar
  uncompensated rotary
  Winter-King-Moe
scoliotic spine
SCOOP 1 transtracheal oxygen catheter
SCOOP 2 catheter with distal and side openings
score
  late effects toxicity
  LENT (late effects of normal tissues)
  mean wall motion
  thallium SPECT
  wall motion
scorings on bone on x-ray

scotoma (pl. scotomata)
  absolute
  bilateral
  cecocentral
  central
  dense
  fortification
  homonymous scintillating
  paracentral
  relative
  scintillating
scotometry
scotomization
scout film
scout image
scout negative film
ScoutView targeting
scrambled image
screen
  guilt
  Lanex Medium
  RF (radiofrequency)
screen craze artifact
screen-film mammogram
screening-detected abnormality
screening mammography
screw
  cancellous
  metallic
  transfixing
screw and plate (screw-plate)
screw fixation
screw-in ceramic acetabular cup
scrotal hernia
SCT (star-cancellation test)
SCTA (spiral CT angiography)
scybalum (pl. scybala)
scyphoid
SDBP (systemic diastolic blood pressure)
SDH (subdural hemorrhage)
S distortion

SDRI (small, deep, recent infarct)
SE (spin-echo) image
SE 1500/40 MR images
SE 300/17 MR images
SEA (spinal epidural abscess)
seal and suction
seat belt fracture
seat belt injury
seat belt sign
sebaceum, adenoma (in tuberous
    sclerosis)
second cranial nerve (optic)
second portion of duodenum
secondary cartilaginous joint
secondary electron production
secondary extravasation of
    intravascular contents
secondary fracture
secondary hypertension
secondary sonographic findings
secondary venous insufficiency
secretin
secretion-filled medium-sized bronchi
secretory capacity of the ACTH
    dependent inner adrenal cortex
section
    axial
    cesarean
    Compton scattering cross-
    coronal
    cross-
    elastic cross-
    flood
    sagittal
    serial
    serpiginous
    step
    transverse
section-select flow compensation
section-select pulse
section-sensitivity profiles

sector
    lower field visual
    Sommer (of the hippocampus)
sector echocardiography
sector probe, biplane
sector scan echocardiography
sector scanning
secundum atrial septal defect (ASD)
Seddon classification of nerve injuries
seeding
    intracranial
    metastatic
    prostate
    radioactive
    TheraSeed (palladium-103) active
        isotope in titanium capsule
    tumor
seed points
seed voxel
segment
    akinetic
    angulated
    anterior
    anterior basal
    anterobasal
    anterolateral
    apex
    apical
    apicoposterior
    arterial
    bronchopulmonary
    cardiac
    coarcted
    contiguous
    diaphragmatic
    distal
    endarterectomized
    expansile aortic
    hypokinetic
    infarcted lung
    inferior

segment *(cont.)*
   inferior basal
   inferoapical
   inferoposterior
   interleaved inversion-readout
   liver
   meatal
   nonfilling venous
   noninfarcted
   posterior
   posterior apical
   posterobasal
   posterolateral
   proximal
   pulmonary
   septal wall
   septum
   superior
   Ta
   vaterian
   venous
segment distraction
segmental atelectasis
segmental bone loss
segmental bowel infarction
segmental branch of artery
segmental bronchus (pl. bronchi)
   cardiac
   lateral
   lateral basal
   medial
   medial basal
   posterior
   posterior basal
   superior
segmental consolidation
segmental defect
segmental distribution of syringomyelia
segmental fracture
segmental ischemia
segmental lesion
segmental limb pressure
segmental lower extremity Doppler pressures
segmental narrowing
segmental orifice
segmental perfusion abnormality
segmental plethysmography
segmental pneumonia
segmental renal artery waveform
segmental sign
segmental symptoms
segmental wall motion abnormality
   akinetic
   dyskinetic
   hyperkinetic
   hypokinetic
segmentation
   automatic lumen edge
   Cannon
   lung
   MR imaging
   rhythmic
   vascular
segmentation method for real-time display
segmented k-space cardiac tagging
segmented k-space time-of-flight MR angiography
segmented k-space turbo gradient echo breath-hold sequence
segmenting dual echo MR head scan
Segond fracture
SEH (spinal epidural hemorrhage)
SeHCAT (selenium-labeled homocholic acid conjugated with taurine) test
SEI (subendocardial infarction)
Seikosha video printer for scans
Seinsheimer classification of femoral fracture

seizure
  generalized
  grand mal
  partial
  petit mal
seizure focus
seizure localization
seizure manifestations
seizure pattern
seizure phenomenon
seizure propagation
seizure threshold
Seldinger catheter
Seldinder technique angiography
selective adenosine A24 antagonist
selective angiography
selective arterial injection
selective arteriogram
selective cannulization
selective catheterization of vessels
selective cerebral arteriography
selective coronary arteriography
selective coronary cineangiography
selective excitation
selective excitation method
selective hole burning
selective injection
selective irradiation
selective osteal salpingography
selective percutaneous transhepatic embolization
selective presaturation MR angiography
selective renal artery embolization
selective saturation method
selective scarring of posterobasal portion of left ventricle
selective separation
selective vascular ligation
selective venography
selective visceral arteriography
selective visualization

selenium (Se)
  Se detector
  $^{77}$Se MRI spectroscopy
  $^{75}$Se selenomethionine radioactive agent
self-aspirating cut-biopsy needle
self-articulating femoral (SAF) hip replacement
self-expanding stent
self-expanding tulip sheath
self-positioning balloon
self-reinforced polyglycolide
sella (pl. sellae)
  atrophy of dorsum
  ballooned
  ballooning of
  decalcified dorsum
  dorsum
  empty
  pressure
  tuberculum
sella-nasion plane
sellar tomography
sella turcica
semiautonomous nodule
semicircular canal
semicoronal plane
semidynamic splint
semilateral position
semilunar aortic valve regurgitation
semilunar bone
semilunar bony formation
semilunar cartilages
semilunar indentations
semilunar pulmonic valve regurgitation
semilunar-shaped fold
semilunar valve cusp
semiquantitative measurement
senescent aortic stenosis
senile ankylosing hyperostosis of spine
senile arteriosclerosis

senile dementia, Alzheimer type (SDAT)
senile emphysema
senile nevus
senile osteoporosis
senile subcapital fracture
Senographe 500 T mammography
sensing coil
sensitive plane projection reconstruction imaging
sensitive point scanning
sensitive volume
sensitivity
   line-shape
   percussion
   uniform
sensitize
sensitization
sentinel fold
sentinel loop
sentinel node
sentinel pile (hemorrhoid)
sentinel transoral hemorrhage
separation
   AC (acromioclavicular)
   aortic cusp
   atlantoaxial
   atlanto-occipital
   carrier-free
   chromatographic
   costochondral junction
   fracture fragment
   leaflet
   selective
   shoulder
sepsis, intra-abdominal (IAS)
septal accessory pathway
septal amplitude
septal arcade
septal area
septal band
septal cardiac defect
septal collateral
septal cusp of valve
septal defect
   atrial
   atrioventricular
   interventricular
septal dip
septal hypertrophy, asymmetric
septal hypokinesis
septal hypoperfusion on thallium scan
septal infarction
septal leaflet
septal necrosis
septal papillary muscle
septal pathway
septal perforation
septal perforator branch
septal perforators
septal region
septal ridge
septal separation
septal thickness
septal wall thickness
septation
septic embolus (pl. emboli)
septic lung syndrome
septic necrosis
septic pleurisy
septic pulmonary emboli
septic pulmonary infarction
septic shock
septic thrombosis
septicemia
septomarginal trabecula
septum (pl. septa)
   alveolar
   anal intermuscular
   anteroapical trabecular
   aortic
   aortopulmonary
   asymmetric hypertrophy of
   atrial

**septum • sequence**      498

septum *(cont.)*
  atrioventricular
  bronchial
  bulbar
  canal
  cartilaginous
  conal
  conus
  crural
  distal bulbar
  dyskinetic
  femoral
  gingival
  infundibular
  intact ventricular
  interatrial (IAS)
  interhaustral
  interlobar
  interlobular
  intermuscular
  internal intermuscular
  interventricular (IVS)
  mediastinal
  membranous
  muscular atrioventricular
  nasal
  perirenal
  posterior median (of cord)
  rectovaginal
  rectovesical
  sinus
  thickened
  ventricular
sequela (pl. sequelae)
  clinical
  late normal tissue
  neuroendocrinological
  significant
sequence (pl. sequences)
  breath-hold GRE
  Carr-Purcell
  Carr-Purcell-Meiboom-Gill

sequence *(cont.)*
  conventional pulse
  CPMG
  DANTE
  diffusion pulse
  diffusion-weighted pulse
  dual echo
  dual GRE pulse
  echo-planar
  echo-planar pulse sequence
  FFE
  FLAIR
  FISP
  FLASH 3D
  flow-compensated gradient-echo
  FMPSRGR
  gradient echo
  gradient-echo imaging
  gradient-echo pulse
  GRASS pulse
  in-phase
  interleaved GRE
  inversion recovery
  Klippel-Feil
  magnetization-prepared rapid
    acqusition gradient-echo
  MP-RAGE (magnetization
    prepared 3D gradient-echo)
  multi-slice spin echo
  multiecho
  opposed-phase
  partial saturation
  PRESS
  pulsed
  saturation recovery
  short T1 inversion recovery (STIR)
  single-shot adiabatic localization
    pulse
  SPAMM
  spin echo
  spin-echo pulse
  spin-echo imaging

sequence *(cont.)*
  spiral pulse
  susceptibility-sensitive
  3DFT-CISS
  3D GRE (gradient-recalled echo)
  3D-PSIF
  3D spoiled GRE
  TONE (tilted optimized nonsaturating excitation)
  Turbo-FLASH
  voiding
  three-dimensional time-of-flight MR angiographic
  turbo SE
sequence processor
sequence time
sequential balloon inflation
sequential bypass graft
sequential dilatations
sequential extraction-radiotracer technique
sequential graft
sequential image acquisition
sequential in situ bypass
sequential monophasic shocks
sequential obstruction
sequential pacing
sequential plane imaging
sequential point imaging
sequential quantitative MR imaging
sequential scalar quantization (SSQ)
sequential compression device, Kendall
sequestered lobe of lung
sequestration
  fluid
  third space
sequestrum (pl. sequestra)
  associated
  bony
  necrotic
  primary

sequestrum *(cont.)*
  secondary
  tertiary
SER-IV (supination, external rotation-type IV) fracture
serendipity view
serial changes
serial contrast MR
serial cut film technique
serial duplex scan
serial images
serial lesions
serialography
serial splinting
serial static image
series
  abdominal
  acute abdominal
  dynamic
  sinus
  small bowel
  upper GI (gastrointestinal)
Series-II humeral head
seriography
seromuscular layer
serosa
serosal surface
serosanguineous fluid
serotonin (5-HIAA)
serotonin (S2) receptors
serous cystadenoma
serous membrane
serous pericardium
serous pleurisy
serpiginous ulceration
serrated catheter
serration, marginal
serratus anterior muscle
Sertoli-Leydig cell tumor
sesamoid bones of foot
  accessory
  bipartite

sesamoid bones of foot *(cont.)*
  entrapped plantar
  fibular
  great toe
  hallux
  Hardy-Clapham classification of
  lateral
  medial
  quadripartite
  symptomatic bipartite
  tibial
  tripartite
sesamoid complex
sesamoid ligament
sesamoid migration
sesamoidometatarsal joint
sesamophalangeal ligament
sessile filling defect
sessile plaque
sessile polyp
sessile tumor
sestamibi polar map (CEQUAL)
sestamibi stress test
sestamibi $^{99m}$Tc SPECT with
  dipyridamole stress test
sestamibi $^{99m}$Tc stress test
set angle of toes
Sethotope radioactive agent
sets, 3D MR imaging data
setting
  quadrature
  wide window
setting-sun phenomenon
7-methoxy $^{11}$C methoxystaurosporine
  imaging agent
seventh cranial nerve (facial nerve)
SFA (superficial femoral artery)
shaded-surface display (SSD)
  algorithm
shaded-surface display CT angiography

shadow (also shadowing)
  acoustic
  band-like
  bat's wing
  breast
  butterfly breast
  cardiac
  centrilobular
  clean
  dirty
  discoid
  effusion
  fusiform
  hilar
  large thymus (obscuring cardiac
    silhouette)
  line
  linear
  paraspinal soft tissue
  Ponfick
  ring
  iliopsoas muscle
  renal
  snowstorm
  spindle-shaped
  toothpaste
  tramlines
  tumorlike
  widened heart
shadowing stone
Shadow over-the-wire balloon catheter
shaft
  bone
  distal third
  femoral
  French
  middle third
  ministem
  proximal third
shaft fracture

shag, aortic
shagging of cardiac borders
shaggy aorta syndrome
shagreen patches in tuberous sclerosis
Shames model
shape (shaped)
    barrel-
    boat
    brachycephalic head
    dumbbell-
    half-moon
    head
    horseshoe
    hourglass
    mesocephalic head
    oval
    ovoid-
    S-
    scaphocephalic head
    scaphoid
    sickle
    spherical
    spheroid-
Shape Maker system
shape recovery
sharp border of lung
sharp carina
sharp dissection
sharp lateral margin
Sharp-Purser test
shaver catheter
shaving
    femoral condylar
    patellar
shavings, residual metal fragment
Shaw catheter
SHC (sclerosing hepatic carcinoma)
shear fracture
shearing forces (on sacroiliac joints in runners)
shearing of white matter (in head injury)
shearing stress
shear rate
shear stress
sheath
    angioplasty
    anterior rectus
    arterial
    carotid
    catheter
    caudal
    check-valve
    common synovial flexor
    Cordis
    crural
    dentinal
    dural
    extensor carpi ulnaris
    fascial
    femoral artery
    fenestrated
    fibrous
    flexor tendon
    ganglionic cyst in synovial tendon
    guiding
    Henle
    intratendon
    introducer
    muscle
    myelin
    nerve
    nerve root
    neural
    peel-away
    periradicular
    pilar
    plicated dural
    posterior rectus
    rectus
    Schwann cell of myelin
    self-expanding tulip
    synovial
    tearaway

sheath *(cont.)*
   tendon
   transseptal
   tulip
   unplicated
   vascular
   venous
sheath and side-arm
Shebele physician reporting workstation
sheetlike
Sheffield modification of Bruce treadmill protocol
Sheffield treadmill exercise protocol
Sheldon catheter
shelf
   Blumer rectal
   buccal
   dental
   lateral
   medial
   mesocolic
   palatine
   patellar
   rectal
shell, acetabular
shelling off of cartilage
Shelton femur fracture classification
shelving edge of Poupart ligament
Shenton line
Shepherd fracture
shepherd's crook deformity
SHG (sonohysterography)
shield
   apron
   Faraday
   lead apron
   lead eye
   RF magnetic
   tungsten eye
shield apron

shift
   anterior capsular
   chemical
   Doppler frequency
   intracranial
   lanthanide-induced
   left-to-right
   mediastinal
   midline
   navigator
   paradigm
   paramagnetic
   phase
   pineal gland
   pivot
   plantar
   reverse pivot (RPS)
   right-to-left
   ST segment
   superior frontal axis
   tracheal
   ventricular
   weight
shift of mediastinal structures
shift of midline structures (of the midbrain)
shift to the left (white blood cells)
shift to the right (white blood cells)
Shiley guiding catheter
Shiley-Ionescu catheter
shill, protrusio
shim coil
shim magnet
shim placement
Shimadzu scanner
Shimazaki area-length method
shimmering, visual
shimming of MRI magnet, poor
shin bone
shin, saber
SHJR4s (side-hole Judkins right, curve 4 French, short)

shock-monitoring method
Shone anomaly
short-arm Grollman catheter
short axis acquisition
short axis images
short axis parasternal view
short axis plane on echocardiography
short axis slice
short bone
short-distance radiotherapy (brachytherapy)
short echo time
short echo time proton spectroscopy
short half-life
short head of biceps
short inversion time inversion recovery (STIR) (MRI)
short pulse
short rib-polydactyly syndrome
short T1 inversion recovery (STIR) sequence
short T1 relaxation time
short TE, long TR
short TR/TE (repetition time/echo time) (T1-weighted image)
shortening
   Achilles tendon
   fractional myocardial
   leg
   mean rate of circumferential
   phalangeal
   skeleton
   suboccipital
   tendon
   T2 (second thoracic vertebra)
shotty lymph node
shoulder
   baseball
   drop
   flail
   frozen
   knocked-down

shoulder *(cont.)*
   Little Leaguer
   loose
   Neviaser classification of frozen
   ring man (in gymnasts)
   sprained
   swimmer's
   tennis
shoulder compression test
shoulder depression test
shoulder-hand-finger syndrome
shoulder immobilizer
shoulder of heart
shoulder pointer
shoulder prosthesis
shoulder rock test
shoulder separation
shoulder-upper extremity-thoracic outlet syndrome
shower of echoes
shrinkage, graft
shrinkage of ganglion cells
shrugging sign
shrunken gallbladder
SHU 454 (Echovist) imaging agent
SHU 508A (Levovist) imaging agent
shudder of carotid arterial pulse
shunt (also shunting)
   aorta to pulmonary artery
   aorticopulmonary
   aortopulmonary
   apicoaortic
   arteriovenous (A-V)
   ascending aorta to pulmonary artery
   atrial right-to-left
   barium-sulfate impregnated
   bidirectional
   biliopancreatic
   Blalock
   Blalock-Taussig
   Buselmeier

**shunt**

shunt *(cont.)*
  cardiac
  cardiovascular
  central aortopulmonary
  Cordis-Hakim
  CSF (cerebrospinal fluid)
  cysto-atrial
  Davidson
  Denver hydrocephalus
  Denver peritoneal venous
  descending aorta-pulmonary artery
  descending thoracic aorta to
    pulmonary artery
  dialysis
  distal splenorenal (DSR)
  DVP flush
  end-to-side portacaval
  esophageal
  extracardiac right-to-left
  gastric venacaval
  Glenn
  Gore-Tex
  Gott
  Hakim-Cortis ventriculoperitoneal
  hermetic external
  Heyer-Schulte neurosurgical
  high-pressure
  Holter
  Hyde
  infant
  intracardiac right-to-left
  intrapericardial aorticopulmonary
  intrapulmonary
  ISCI
  Javid endarterectomy
  left-to-right
  LeVeen peritoneal
  Linton
  low-pressure
  lumbar arachnoid peritoneal
  lumboperitoneal (LP)
  medium-pressure

shunt *(cont.)*
  mesocaval H-graft
  mesocaval interposition
  migration of
  modified Blalock-Taussig
  net
  Ommaya ventriculoperitoneal
  one-piece
  peritoneal-atrial
  peritoneocaval
  peritoneovenous (PVS)
  portacaval
  portopulmonary
  portosystemic vascular
  posterior fossa-atrial
  Potts
  preferential
  proximal splenorenal
  Pruitt-Inahara carotid
  Pudenz
  Quinton-Scribner
  reversed (right-to-left)
  right-to-left (reversed)
  side-to-side portacaval
  small-bowel
  Spetzler lumboperitoneal
  splenorenal
  subclavian artery to pulmonary
    artery
  subclavian-pulmonary
  subdural to peritoneal
  Sundt loop
  supracardiac
  systemic-pulmonary artery
  T-tube
  thecoperitoneal
  transjugular intrahepatic
    portosystemic
  UNI-SHUNT hydrocephalus
  vena cava to pulmonary artery
  venoarterial
  ventriculoatrial (VA)

shunt *(cont.)*
   ventriculojugular (VJ)
   ventriculoperitoneal (VP)
   ventriculopleural
   ventriculovenous
   Wakabaushi
   Warren splenorenal
   Waterston
   Waterston-Cooley
shunted blood
shunted tracer
shunt flow
   anatomic
   physiologic
   relative
shunt function, cerebrospinal fluid
shunting of blood
   left-to-right
   marked
   right-to-left
shuntogram
shunt quantification
shunt reservoir
shunt reversal
shunt syndrome, lumbar thecoperitoneal
shunt valve
shutdown, renal
SI (sacroiliac) joint
   SI joint to sacrum ratio
SI (saturation index) of bile
SI (signal intensity)
SI (sinus irregularity)
SI (stroke index)
Si(Li) x-ray detector
sialography CT
sialography MRI
Sibson fascia
sick sinus node
sick sinus syndrome (SSS)
   extrinsic
   intrinsic

sickle cell disease
sickle-shaped fold
SICOR (computer-assisted cardiac
   catheter recording system)
side branch occlusion
side-by-side transposition of great
   arteries
side-hole catheter
side-to-side anastomosis
siderosis
siderotic splenomegaly
sideswipe elbow fracture
sidewall, pelvic
sidewinder catheter
Siemens AG system
Siemens DRH CT scanners
Siemens gamma camera
Siemens LINAC (linear accelerator)
Siemans Magnetom 1.5 T
Siemans Magnetom SP 4000 scanner
Siemens Mevatron 74 linear
   accelerator
Siemens One Tesla scanner
Siemens Satellite CT Evaluation
   Console
Siemens Somaform 512 CT scanner
Siemens Somatom DR2 whole-body
   scanner (also DR3)
Siemens Somatom PLUS-S imager
   (scanner)
Siemens SP 4000 scanner
sigmoid cavity of radius
sigmoid cavity of ulna
sigmoid colon volvulus
sigmoid curve
sigmoid notch
sigmoid omentum
sigmoid sinus
sigmoid valve
sign
   Aaron
   Abrahams

**sign**

sign *(cont.)*
    ace of spades (on angiogram)
    Achilles bulge
    Adson
    Allen
    Allis
    Amoss
    amputation
    angel wing
    Anghelescu
    antecedent
    anterior tibial
    antler
    anvil
    aortic arch aneurysm
    aortic nipple
    apical cap
    Apley
    applesauce
    Ashhurst
    Auenbrugger
    Babinski
    Baccelli (of pleural effusion)
    bagpipe
    ball-bearing eye
    Ballance
    Bamberger
    banana
    Bancroft
    barber pole
    Barlow
    Battle
    bayonet
    beading
    Becker
    Beevor
    Bethea
    beveled edge
    Biermer
    bilateral pyramidal
    Biot
    Bird

sign *(cont.)*
    Blumberg
    Bouillaud
    bow-tie
    bowler hat
    bowstring
    Boyce
    Bozzolo
    Bragard
    brain stem
    Branham arteriovenous fistula
    Braunwald
    brim
    Broadbent inverted
    Brockenbrough-Braunwald
    Brudzinski
    Bryant
    Burton
    buttock
    camelback
    Cantelli
    Cardarelli
    cardinal
    cardiorespiratory
    Carnett
    carotid string
    Carvallo
    Castellino
    Cegka
    cerebral
    Chaddock
    chain of lakes
    Chilaiditi
    choppy sea
    Christmas tree
    Chvostek-Weiss
    Claybrook
    Cleeman
    clockwise whirlpool
    cobblestoning
    Codman
    Cogan lid twitch

sign *(cont.)*
   cogwheel
   Cole
   Collier
   colon cut-off
   commemorative
   Comolli
   contralateral
   Coopernail
   cord
   Corrigan
   cortical
   corticospinal tract
   coughing
   Courvoisier
   cranial nerve
   crescent
   crescent-in-doughnut (for intussusception)
   cross-chest impingement
   crossed sciatica
   Cruveilhier
   cuff
   Cullen
   D'Amato
   Dance
   Dawbarn
   Dejerine
   de la Camp
   de Musset (aortic aneurysm)
   de Mussey (pleurisy)
   Delbet
   Delmege
   delta
   Demianoff
   dense sigmoid sinus
   dense vein
   Desault
   Deyerle
   displaced fat pad
   doll's eye
   doorbell

sign *(cont.)*
   Dorendorf
   dorsal column
   double bubble
   double-bubble duodenal
   double camelback
   Drummond
   Duchenne
   Dupuytren
   dural trail
   Duroziez
   d'Espine
   E
   Ebstein
   Egawa
   Ellis
   empty delta
   Erb
   Erichsen
   Ewart
   extrapyramidal tract
   Fajersztajn crossed sciatic
   false localizing
   fan
   fat pad
   Federici
   figure 3
   fingertip
   Finkelstein
   Fischer
   fissure
   flapping tremor
   Fleck
   Fleischner
   focal neurologic
   Forestier bowstring
   Frank
   Fränkel
   Franz
   Friedreich
   Froment paper
   frontal lobe

**sign**

sign *(cont.)*
Fürbringer
Gaenslen
Gage
Galant
Galeazzi
Gerhardt
Gilbert
Glasgow
gloved finger
Goldthwait
gooseneck
Gordon
Gowers
Grancher
Green-Joynt
Greene
Grey Turner
Griesinger
Grocco
Grossman
guarding
Guilland
Gunn crossing
Hall
halo
Hamman pneumopericardium
harlequin eye
Hart
Heim-Kreysig
Helbing
Henning
Hill
Hirschberg
Hoffmann
Homans
Honda
Hoover
Hope
Horn
hot-cross-bun skull
hot nose

sign *(cont.)*
Howship-Romberg
Huchard
Hueter fracture
Huntington
hyperdense middle cerebral artery
hyperintensive ring
iliopsoas
inverted V
J
Jaccoud
Jackson
Jenet
jugular
jump
Jürgensen
Kanavel
Kantor
Kaplan
Karplus
Katz-Wachtel
Keen
Kehr
Kellgren
Kellock
Kernig
Kerr
Klemm
knuckle
Kocher-Cushing
Korányi-Grocco
Kussmaul venous
Lachman
Laënnec
Lancisi
Landolfi
Langoria
Lasègue
lateralizing
Laugier
Lazarus
Leichtenstern

sign *(cont.)*
  lemon
  Lennhoff
  Leri
  Leser-Trelat
  Levine
  Lhermitte
  Linder
  linguine (in breast)
  liver flap
  liver-jugular
  Livierato abdominocardiac
  localizing neurological
  lollipop tree
  long-tract
  Lorenz
  Lowenberg
  lower motor neuron
  Ludloff
  Macewen
  Mahler
  Maisonneuve
  Mannkopf
  Marie-Foix
  McBurney
  McCort
  McGinn-White
  McMurray
  Meltzer
  Mendel-Bekhterev
  meningoencephalitic
  meniscus
  Mennell
  Mercedes-Benz
  Minor
  Morquio
  Morton-Horwitz nerve cross-over
  Moschcowitz (of arterial occlusive disease)
  motor
  moulage
  movie

sign *(cont.)*
  Mulder
  Müller (Mueller) aortic regurgitation
  Murphy
  Musset (de Musset)
  mute toe
  Myerson
  Naffziger
  Neer impingement
  negative delta (on CT)
  Negro
  Nelson
  Neri bowing
  neurologic soft
  Nicaladoni-Branham
  nubbin
  obturator
  oculomotor
  Oliver-Cardarelli
  ominous
  Oppenheim
  orbicularis
  organic (of brain damage)
  Ortolani
  Osler
  pad
  panda
  parietal lobe
  Parrot
  patent bronchus
  pathognomonic
  pathologic lid retraction
  Paul
  Payr
  percussion
  Perez
  peripheral washout
  peritoneal
  peroneal
  Pfuhl-Jaffé
  Phalen

**sign**

sign *(cont.)*
   phonatory
   piano key
   pillow
   Pins
   Piotrowski
   piston
   pivot-shift
   plane
   plumb-line
   Plummer
   positive bottle
   postural motor
   Potain
   Pott
   Pottenger
   precursor
   premonitory
   Prevel
   Prévost
   pronation
   pronator
   pruning
   Prussian helmet
   pseudo-Babinski
   pseudobulbar
   pseudo-Foster-Kennedy
   pseudo-Romberg
   psoas
   puddle
   pupillary
   pyloric string
   pyramidal
   Queckenstedt
   Quénu-Muret
   Quincke
   rabbit ear
   raccoon eyes
   rachitic rosary
   radialis
   railroad track
   Raimiste

sign *(cont.)*
   rat-tail
   rebound
   Renee creak
   reversal
   reversed 3
   reversed Mercedes Benz
   Rigler
   rim
   ring of cribriform plate fracture
   Riordan
   Risser
   Rivero-Carvallo
   Riviere
   Robertson
   Romberg
   Rosenbach
   Rotch
   Rothschild
   Rovighi
   Rovsing
   Rust
   Sabathie
   sail
   Sanders
   Sansom
   Sarbo
   sawtooth appearance
   Schepelmann
   Schick
   Schlesinger
   Schoeber
   scimitar
   seat belt
   segmental
   Seguin
   Seitz
   setting-sun
   Shapiro
   Shibley
   shrugging
   Sister Mary Joseph

sign *(cont.)*
Skoda
Smith
soft neurologic
somatic
sonographic Murphy
Soto-Hall
Spalding
Speed
spinal
spread suture
Spurling
square-root
stairs
steeple
Steinberg thumb
Steinmann
Sterles
Sterling-Okuniewski
Sternberg
Stewart-Holmes
Stierlin
Strauss
string
string of pearls
stripe
Strümpell (Struempell)
Strunsky
Sumner
tandem Romberg
target
Terry fingernail
Terry-Thomas
tethered-bowel
theater
Thomas
thorn
thumbprinting
Thurston-Holland
tibialis (of Strümpell)
Tinel percussion
toe spread

sign *(cont.)*
trapezius ridge
Traube aortic regurgitation
Trimadeau
tripod
Troisier
Trömner (Troemner)
Trousseau
Turner
Turyn
Uhthoff
unilateral Babinski
upper motor neuron
VAD (voluntary anterior drawer)
Vanzetti
vein
versive motor
vital
voluntary posterior drawer (VPD)
Voshell
VPD (voluntary posterior drawer)
Waddell
Walter-Murdoch wrist
Wartenberg
Weill
Weiss
Westermark
wet leather
whirlpool
white cerebellum
white matter
Williams
Williamson
Wilson
wind sock (echocardiogram)
windshield wiper
winking owl spinal
Wintrich
Yergason
Signa GEMS MR imaging system
Signa Horizon scanner
Signa I.S.T. MRI scanner

Signa 1.5T scanner
signal
  color Doppler
  D
  differential
  disk water
  Doppler flow
  flow
  hyperintense
  hypointense
  lipid
  magnetic resonance
  mosaic-jet
  NAA metabolite
  stimulus-correlated
  water
signal acquisitions
signal blooming
signal dephasing
signal fallout
signal intensity (SI)
signal intensity curve
signal intensity time curves
signal loss
signal magnification
signal mass
signal time-course
signal-to-clutter ratio
signal-to-noise ratio (SNR or S/N ratio)
signal void
signature, echo
signet ring appearance
signet ring carcinoma
signet ring pattern
significant axis deviation
significant, clinically
significant residual deficit
significant sequelae
Silastic catheter
Silastic stent
silence, electrocerebral (ECS)

silent areas of brain
silent gallstone
silent ischemia
silent mitral stenosis
silent myocardial infarction
silent myocardial ischemia
silent patent ductus arteriosus
silent regurgitation
silhouette
  cardiac (large thymus shadow obscuring)
  cardiovascular
  enlarged cardiac
  luminal
  roentgenographic
  widened cardiac
silhouette image
Silicon Graphics Reality Engine system
silicone implant rupture (seen on MRI)
Silicore catheter
silicosis
silicotic fibrosis of lung
silicotic nodule with central necrosis
silicotic visceral pleura
silicotuberculosis
silver-fork deformity
silver-fork fracture
SIM (small intestine mesentery)
Simmons 1, 2, and 3 catheter
Simmons-type sidewinder catheter
Simon nitinol percutaneous IVC filter
simple dislocation
simple fracture, complex
simple shift
simplex, xanthoma tuberosum
Simplus PE/t dilatation catheter
Simpson atherectomy catheter
Simpson atherectomy device, PET balloon
Simpson Coronary AtheroCath (SCA) system

Simpson-Robert catheter
Simpson rule method for ventricular
　volume
Simpson Ultra-Low Profile II balloon
　catheter
Sims position
simulation-aided field setting
simulated annealing methods
simulated equilibrium factor study
simulation, laboratory
simulation of converging ports
simulation of tangential portals
simulation of treatment area
simulator
　Maxwell 3D Field
　MR
　virtual reality
　Ximatron
simultaneous balloon inflation
simultaneous bilateral spontaneous
　pneumothorax (SBSP)
simultaneous fluoroscopy and
　manometric evaluation of
　pharyngeal swallowing and
　dysphagia
simultaneous pacing and coronary
　blood flow measurement
simultaneous volume imaging
Sincalide (synthetic CCK)
singer's node
Singh index of osteoporosis
single atrium
single-breath hold
single-breath view
single-contrast arthrography
single-dose gadolinium imaging
single extrastimuli
single fill/void technique
single isocenter
single-lumen silicone breast implant
single-lung transplantation
single-outlet heart

single-photon emission CT with MR
single peak
single photon absorptiometry (SPA)
single photon emission computed
　tomography (SPECT)
single photon planar scintigraphy
　(SPPS)
single pleurisy
single port
single-shot adiabatic localization pulse
　sequence
single-shot MR cholangiography
single-slice long-axis tomograms
single-stripe colitis (SSC)
single ventricle with pulmonic stenosis
single-vessel disease
single-vessel runoff
single voxel proton spectroscopy
sink-trap malformation
sinoatrial (SA)
sinoatrial branch
sinoatrial node (SA or S-A node)
　Flack
　Koch
sinoatrial node artery
sinoatrial node dysfunction
sinoatrial node infarction
sinoauricular node
sinodural plate
Sinografin contrast medium
sinogram
sinotubular junction
sintering
sinus
　accessory
　aortic valve
　atlas articular
　barber's pilonidal
　basilar
　Breschet
　carotid
　cavernous

**sinus**

sinus *(cont.)*
  cerebral venous
  cervical
  circular
  coccygeal
  coronary (of Valsalva)
  costomediastinal
  cranial
  distal coronary (DCS)
  draining
  dura mater venous
  dural
  dural venous
  ethmoid
  frontal
  Guérin
  inferior sagittal (ISS)
  lateral
  left coronary
  lumbosacral dermal
  lymph node
  marginal
  mastoid
  maxillary
  medullary
  middle coronary (MCS)
  nasal
  noncoronary
  oblique pericardial
  osteomyelitic
  paranasal
  pericardial
  perineal
  Petit
  petrosal
  pilonidal
  piriform
  precoronal sagittal
  prostatic
  proximal coronary (PCS)
  pulmonary
  pyriform

sinus *(cont.)*
  renal
  Ridley
  Rokitansky-Aschoff
  rudimentary
  sagittal
  sigmoid
  sphenoid
  sphenoparietal
  subeustachian
  superior sagittal (SSS)
  thickened
  transverse pericardial
  Valsalva
  valve of coronary
  venous
  vertebral articular
sinus aneurysm, aortic
sinus irregularity (SI)
sinus lesion, cavernous
sinus mechanism
sinus nodal reentry
sinus node automaticity
sinus node depression
sinus node dysfunction
sinus node recovery time, corrected
sinus node reentry
sinus of Morgagni
sinus of pulmonary trunk
sinus of Valsalva
sinus of venae cavae
sinusoidal vascular spaces
sinusoid reference function
sinusoids, hepatic
sinus pause
sinus retroperfusion, coronary
sinus segment
sinus septum
sinus series
sinus slowing
sinus tarsi syndrome
sinus tract study

sinus venous defect
sinuvertebral nerve (of Luschka)
SIP (saturation inversion projection)
siphon, carotid
SIR angiogram
Sister Mary Joseph node
site
  de-airing
  fracture
  ipsilateral antegrade
  reference
site of arterial puncture
site of maximal intensity
site-specific labeling
sitting-up view
situs ambiguus of atria
situs
  atrial
  D-loop ventricular
  L-loop ventricular situs
situs atrialis solitus
situs concordance
situs inversus
situs inversus totalis
situs inversus viscerum
situs perversus
situs solitus
  atrial
  visceral
situs transversus
situs viscerum inversus
6-[$^{18}$F] fluoro-DOPA
sixth compartment
sixth cranial nerve (abducens nerve)
sixth intercostal space
60° left anterior oblique projection
60 MHz Fourier Transform NMR
  spectrometer
60 MHz Rapid Scan spectrometer
64 x 64 byte mode
size and caliber
size and configuration

size estimation error
size, particle
sizer, prosthetic valve
sizing, balloon
sizing ring
Sjögren syndrome
SJS (Schwartz-Jampel syndrome)
skeletal amyloidosis
skeletal bed
skeletal disruption
skeletal emphysema
skeletal hyperostosis
skeletal hypoplasia
skeletally immature
skeletally mature
skeletal metastases
skeletal radiology
skeletal survey, isotopic
skeletal traction
skeleton
  appendicular
  articulated
  axial
  bony
  cardiac
  fibrous
  gill arch
  spidering
  spiky
  sulcal
  visceral
skeleton shortening
skeletonizing
skier's fracture
skier's thumb
Skillern fracture
skin bridge
skin crease artifact
skin depth
skin fold artifact
skin lesion artifact
skin lines

Skinny over-the-wire balloon catheter
skin-rolling scapular tenderness
skin thickening
Skiodan contrast medium
skip lesions of Crohn disease
Skoda sign
skull
   beaten silver appearance of
   cloverleaf
   foramen magnum of
   hammer-marked, secondary to thinning
   hot-cross-bun
   lytic lesion of the
   molding of
   sonolucent
skull asymmetry
skull base
skullcap
skull defect, postoperative
skull films
skull fracture
   basilar
   compound
   depressed
   depressed and compound
   linear
   simple
   stellate
   undepressed
skull hyperostosis
skull plate
skyline view of patella
SL (scapholunate) joint
slab (pl. slabs)
   coronal
   interleaved axial
SLAC (scapholunate arthritic collapse) wrist
slant hole collimator
SLAP (superior labrum anterior posterior) lesion

slate-gray cyanosis
SLE (systemic lupus erythematosus)
slew rate
slice
   angled
   apical short-axis
   axial
   basal short-axis
   contiguous
   coronal
   digitized CT
   horizontal long-axis
   intermediate CT
   long axis
   mid-ventricular short-axis
   plurality of
   sagittal
   serial CT
   short-axis
   texture
   tissue
   tomographic
   transaxial
   transverse
   vertical long-axis
slice format
slice fracture
slice orientation
slice-overlap artifact
slice sensitivity profile (SSP)
slice thickness
slice volume
slicing planes
sliding-type hiatal hernia
Slinky catheter
slip angle
slip-in connection
slippage, film
slipped capital femoral epiphysis
slipped disk
slipped tendon
slipped upper femoral epiphysis (SUFE)

slipping rib syndrome
slip-ring camera
slip-ring CT
slip-ring technology
SLJD (Sinding-Larsen-Johansson disease)
slope
  closing (on echo)
  D to E (of mitral valve)
  decreased E to F (E-F)
  disappearance
  E to F (of mitral valve)
  flat diastolic
  flattened E to F
  opening (on echo)
  ST/HR (ST segment/heart rate)
  valve opening
slot blot analysis
sloughed mucosa
sloughed papilla
sloughed urethra syndrome
slow-channel blocking drugs
slow filling wave
slow-flow lesions
slow-flow vascular anomaly
slow-flow vascular malformation
slow neutron
sludge
  biliary
  blood
  gallbladder
sluggishly flowing blood
Sm (samarium)
SMA (smooth muscle antibody)
SMA (superior mesenteric artery)
SMALL (same-day microsurgical arthroscopic lateral-approach laser-assisted) fluoroscopic diskectomy
small airway dysfunction
small angle multiple scattering
small aorta syndrome
small bowel contents

small bowel follow-through (SBFT)
small bowel infarct
small bowel series
small bowel transit time
small cardiac vein
small cell carcinoma of the lung
small cell lung cancer (SCLC)
small cuff syndrome
small feminine aorta
small field-of-view (FOV) MR imaging
small-lunged emphysema
small saphenous vein
small vessel stroke
small water-hammer pulse
Smart Prep imaging agent
Smart Prep scanner
SmartSpot high resolution digital imaging system
SMAS (superior mesenteric artery syndrome)
smear fragment
Smec balloon catheter
SMIS console
Smith fracture
SMM (scintimammography)
smokelike echoes
smooth hyperplasia
smooth muscle tumor
SMPTE (Society of Motion Picture and Television Engineers) test pattern (teleradiology)
SMV (superior mesenteric vein)
S/N (signal-to-noise) ratio
snake graft
snapping hip syndrome
snapshot, contrast-enhanced dynamic
Sneppen fracture of talus
snowman appearance of heart
snowman deformity
snowplow occlusion
snowstorm shadow on chest x-ray

SNR (signal-to-noise ratio)
SNRT (sinus node recovery time)
snuffbox, anatomic
snufftaker's pituitary disease
soap bubble appearance of exudate
soap bubble radiolucency
soapsuds enema (SSE)
socket/residuum interface
socket-stump interface
sodium diatrizoate contrast medium
sodium iodide contrast medium
sodium iodide ring
sodium iodipamide contrast medium
sodium iodohippurate contrast medium
sodium iodomethamate contrast medium
sodium iothalamate contrast medium
sodium ipodate contrast medium
sodium methiodal contrast medium
sodium pertechnetate $^{99m}$Tc
sodium thorium tartrate contrast medium
sodium tyropanoate contrast medium
soft-copy computed radiography
soft disk herniation
soft neurologic sign
soft palate
soft photon
softening and swelling of cartilage
softening of brain
Softip diagnostic catheter
soft tissue abnormality
soft tissue calcification
soft tissue contracture
soft tissue contusion
soft tissue defect
soft tissue density structure
soft tissue entrapment
soft tissue interposition
soft tissue mass
soft tissue necrosis
soft tissue ossification
soft tissue osteochondroma
soft tissue radiograph
soft tissue, stippled
soft tissue swelling
soft tissue window
Softouch guiding catheter
Soft-Vu angiographic catheter
Soft-Vu Omni Flush catheter
software (see also *program*)
   DecThreads
   Kodak
   modified vessel image processor
   Neuro Echo
   Neuro Lobe
   Neuro SPGR
   P-LINK
   SPARC
   Starlink
   VERT
   Viewnex
   Voxel-Man
   VoxelView
Solayrès obliquity
soldier's heart syndrome
soldier's patches of pericardium
soldier's spot
soleal line
soleal vein
solenoid surface coil
soleus muscle
solid bolus challenge
solid bone
solid edema of lung
solid lesion, echogenic
solid modeler
solid state manometry catheter
solid state nuclear track detector
solitary cold lesion
solitary lung nodule
solitary mass
solitary pulmonary nodule (SPN)

solitus
  atrial situs
  situs
  visceral situs
Solo catheter with Pro/Pel coating
Solomon syndrome
SoloPass stent and catheter
Solu-Biloptin contrast medium
solution
  Lugol's
  SSKI
SOMA scale
Somatom DR CT scanner
Somatom Plus-S CT Scanner
somatosensory cortex
somatostatin receptor
S1-S5 (five sacral vertebrae)
Sones Cardio-Marker catheter
Sones Hi-Flow catheter
Sones selective coronary arteriography
sonicated albumin microbubbles
sonicated contrast medium
Sonicator portable ultrasound
Sonifer sonicating system
Sonnenberg classification of erosive esophagitis
sonoangiogram
Sonocut ultrasonic aspirator
sonogram (see *ultrasound*)
sonographic feature analysis
sonographic Murphy sign
sonographic parameter
sonography (see *ultrasound*)
sonohysterography (SHG)
Sonoline Elegra ultrasound system
sonologist
sonolucent area or zone
sonolucent cystic lesion or mass
sonolucent fluid-filled area
Sonos 500 2.5 MHz ultrasonographic transducer
Sorbie calcaneal fracture

sorption kinetics
sorption potential
sorption studies
  Joliot
  radiotracer foil method
Soto USCI balloon
sound beam
sound transmission
S/P (status post)
SPA (single photon absorptiometry)
space
  alveolar dead
  anatomical dead
  antecubital
  apical
  apical air
  axillary
  Baros
  Berger
  Bogros
  Bottcher
  Bowman
  Burns
  capsular
  cartilage
  Chassaignac
  Cloquet
  Colles
  Cotunnius
  C-Y color
  dead
  disk
  Disse
  dorsal subaponeurotic
  dorsal subcutaneous
  echo-free
  epicardial
  epidural
  episcleral
  epitympanic
  extradural
  extrapleural

space *(cont.)*
   fifth intercostal
   first intercostal
   foraminal
   fourth intercostal
   free pericardial
   gingival
   Henke
   His perivascular
   Holzknecht
   hyperintense marrow
   increased lateral joint
   intercellular
   intercondylar (ICS) joint
   intercostal
   intermetatarsal
   interpeduncular
   interpleural
   interstitial
   intervertebral disk
   intrathecal
   intravascular
   joint
   K-
   Kiernan
   Kretschmann
   Kuhnt
   lateral joint
   left intercostal (LICS)
   Lesgaft
   Lesshaft
   lung air
   Magendie
   Malacarne
   masticator
   Meckel
   medial joint
   midpalmar
   Mohrenheim
   narrowing of joint
   parapharyngeal
   Parona (subtendinous)

space *(cont.)*
   patellofemoral joint
   peribronchial alveolar
   pericardial
   perineal
   perinephric
   perirenal
   perisinusoidal
   peritoneal
   plane of intercostal
   pleural
   Poirier
   Poiseuille
   popliteal
   posterior septal
   presacral
   Prussak
   pulp
   Q
   Reinke
   retrocardiac
   retromammary
   retro-orbital
   retropancreatic preaortic
   retroparotid
   retroperitoneal
   retrosphenoidal
   Retzius
   scapholunate
   Schwalbe
   subarachnoid
   subdural
   subhepatic
   subperitoneal
   subtendinous
   subumbilical
   suprahepatic
   supralevator
   syndesmotic clear
   Tailarach
   Tarin
   Tenon

space *(cont.)*
  thenar
  tibiocalcaneal
  tissue
  Traube semilunar
  Trautmann triangular
  ventricular
  vesicovaginal
  Virchow-Robin space of the brain
  Waldeyer
  web
  Westberg
  Zang
  zonular
space deficits
Spacemaker balloon dissector
space-occupying lesions
spacing error, raster
spacing, multiple-beam interface
spade-shaped valvotome
Spalding sign
SPAMM sequence
span
  levator
  liver
SPARC software
spare
sparing, arytenoid
sparkling appearance of myocardium
spasm
  artery
  bowel
  bronchial
  catheter-induced coronary artery
  colonic
  coronary artery (CAS)
  coughing
  diffuse arteriolar
  diffuse esophageal (DES)
  hemifacial
  inspiratory
  muscle

spasm *(cont.)*
  muscular
  postbypass
  respiratory
  vascular
  vein
  venous
spastic colon
spastic esophagus
spastic ileus
spatial EPR imaging
spatial mapping
spatial modulation magnetization
spatial peak intensity
spatial presaturation
spatial registration
spatial resolution
spatially selective inversion pulse
specimen, breast core biopsy
speckled pattern
SPECT (single photon emission
    computed tomography)
  acetazolamide-enhanced
  brain perfusion
  dual-head
  dynamic volumetric
  electrocardiogram-gated
  FDG
  ictal
  interictal
  quantitative gated (QGS)
  Tc-99m red blood cell
  Trionix
SPECT brain perfusion scintigraphy
SPECT technetium sestamibi scan
SPECT thallium scintigram
SPECT tomography
SPECT with $^{18}$Fl-2-deoxy-D-glucose
    (FDG)
spectography, nuclear magnetic
    resonance (NMR)
spectra (pl. of spectrum)

spectral analysis
spectral diffusion
spectral Doppler
spectral noise distribution
spectral pattern
spectral US (ultrasound)
Spectranetics excimer laser for
  coronary angioplasty
spectrofluorometry
spectrometer, SISCO (Spectroscopy
  Imaging Systems Corporation)
  4.7T/33 cm diameter imaging
spectrometry
  AMS (accelerator mass)
  Bruker NMR
  Compton suppression
  EDXRF
  4.0T/31cm Surrey Medical
    Imaging Systems (SMIS)
    imaging
  GE NMR
  GN300 7.05T/89 mm bore multi-
    nuclear
  IBM NMR
  liquid scintillation
  Nicolet NMR
  NMR
  PROBE-SV
  pulsed L-band ESR
  scintillation
  60 MHz Fourier Transform NMR
  60 MHz Rapid Scan
  360 MHz VT multinuclear
  270 MHz VT multinuclear
  Varian Associates 11.7T
    (500 MHz)/51 mm bore
  Varian NMR
spectrophotometer
  F-1200 Fluorescence
  F-2000 Fluorescence
  F-4500 Fluorescence
  U-1100 UV-Vis

spectrophotometer *(cont.)*
  U-2001 UV-Vis
  U-2020 UV-Vis
  U-3000 UV-Vis
  U-3010 UV-Vis
  U-3300 UV-Vis
  U-3310 UV-Vis
  UV-Visible
spectrophotometric calculation
spectrophotometric quantity
spectroscopy
  COSY H-1 MR
  CSI
  double-spin echo proton
  fluorescence
  Fourier transform infrared
  Fourier transform Raman
  glutamate
  H-1 MR
  in vivo proton MR
  INVOS 2100 optical
  ISIS
  localized H1
  magnetic resonance (MRS)
  MR H-1 stimulated-echo
    acquisition mode
  NMR (nuclear magnetic resonance)
  nonresonance Raman
  1H magnetic MR
  oxygen-17 NMR
  P-31 MR
  phosphorus nuclear magnetic
    resonance (P-MRS)
  PRESS
  proton magnetic resonance
  Raman
  selenium-77 NMR
  short echo time proton
  single voxel proton
  STEAM
  2D J-resolved 1H MR
spectrum, infinitesimal Z

specular echo
Speedy balloon catheter
Spence, tail of
Spens syndrome
spermatic cord
spermatic vein
SPGR (spoiled gradient-recalled) echo sequences
sphenocephaly
sphenoethmoidal encephalocele
sphenoethmoidal suture
sphenoid bone
sphenoid ridge tumors
sphenoid sinus
sphenoid wing
sphenoidal fissure syndrome
sphenoidal sinusitis
spheno-occipital suture
spheno-occipital synchondrosis
spheno-orbital suture
sphenopalatine ganglion
sphenopalatine neuralgia
sphenoparietal suture
sphenopetrosal suture
sphenopharyngeal meningoencephalocele
sphenosquamous suture
sphenotemporal suture
sphenoturbinal bone
sphenovomerine suture
spherical lesion
spherical map
spherical mass
spherocytosis, hereditary
spheroid-shaped
spheroids, tumor
sphincter
   anal
   antral
   basal
   bicanalicular
   Boyden

sphincter *(cont.)*
   canalicular
   choledochal
   colic
   cricopharyngeal
   duodenal
   duodenojejunal
   external anal
   extrinsic
   first duodenal
   hypertensive lower esophageal
   Hyrtl
   inferior esophageal (IES)
   Lutkens
   Nélaton
   O'Beirne
   Oddi
   pancreatic duct
   pancreaticobiliary
   pharyngoesophageal
   prepyloric
   pyloric
   upper esophageal (UES)
sphingolipidosis
sphingomyelin lipidosis
sphingomyelinase
Sphrintzen velocardiofacial syndrome
sphygmography
sphygmomanometer cuff
spicular density
spicular protrusion
spiculations on colon
spicule of bone
spicules in profile
spider angioma (pl. angiomata)
spidering skeleton
spider-web circulation on angiography of glioblastomas
spider nevus (pl. nevi)
spiderweb appearance
spider x-ray view
spike loading

spiky skeletons
spin (pl. spins)
  flowing
  J-coupled
  stationary
  uncoupled
spina bifida
spina bifida occulta (SBO)
spina bifida posterior
spinal abscess, epidural
spinal accessory nerve (eleventh cranial nerve)
spinal angiogram
spinal angiolipoma
spinal arthritis
spinal axial loading
spinal axis
spinal block by cord compression
spinal canal narrowing
spinal column
spinal cord
  caliber of
  compression of
  decompression of
  hemisection of
  infarction of the
  laceration of the
  multiple focal lesions of (in multiple sclerosis)
  posterolateral sclerosis of
  size of
  tethered
  transection of
spinal cord ependymoma
spinal cord injury (SCI)
spinal cord lesion
spinal cord parenchyma
spinal cord stroke
spinal cord tumor
spinal dural arteriovenous fistula
spinal elements, neoplastic destruction of

spinal ependymoma
spinal epidural abscess
spinal epidural hematoma
spinal fixation
spinal fusion
spinal hemiplegia
spinal hydatid cyst
spinal instability
spinal lordosis
spinal roots
  C1-7 (cervical)
  Co. 1 (coccygeal)
  L1-5 (lumbar)
  S1-5 (sacral)
  T1-12 (thoracic)
spinal subarachnoid hemorrhage
spinal subdural hematoma
spinal tuberculosis
spinal videofluoroscopy
spin coupling
spin density, echo
spindle
  aortic
  His
spindle-shaped shadow
spine
  alar
  angulation of
  anterior column of
  anterior maxillary
  anterior superior iliac
  anteroposterior iliac
  cervical (C)
  Charcot
  coccygeal (coccyx)
  dendritic
  dorsal (D)
  functional units of
  iliac
  ischial
  kinetic cervical
  kissing

spine *(cont.)*
   lateral bending views of the
   lumbar (L)
   lumbarized
   lumbosacral (LS)
   maxillary
   mental
   nasal
   poker
   posterior-inferior
   posterior column of
   posterior-inferior
   rotatory loads on
   rugger jersey
   sacral (S)
   static cervical
   thoracic (T)
   thoracolumbar
   trochanteric
spin echo (SE)
spin-echo imaging sequence
spin-echo pulse sequence
spin-label method
spin-lattice relaxation time
spin-lock and magnetization transfer imaging
spin-lock imaging
spin-lock induced T1rho weighted image
spin-locking, adiabatic off-resonance
spin-lock prepulse
spinocerebellar ataxia
spinocerebellar degeneration
spinoglenoid notch
spinographic angle
spinographic lines
spinography, digitized
spinoreticular tract
spinotectal tract
spinothalamic tract
spinous process
spin-spin relaxation time

spin-warp imaging
SPIO (superparamagnetic iron oxide) oral contrast agent
spiral (also spiraling)
spiral appearance
spiral band of Gosset
spiral computed tomography
spiral CT (computed tomography) angiography (SCTA)
spiral CT pitch
spiral CT scanner
spiral CT with multiplanar reformatting and 3D rendering
spiral dissection
spiral fracture
spiral oblique fracture
spiral pulse sequence
spiral scanning technique
spiral XCT (x-ray computed tomography) scanner
spirometric acquisition
spirometrically controlled CT
splanchnic vascular imaging
splanchnic vasculature
splanchnic vessels
splash, succussion
splashing bruit
splayed
splayfoot deformity
splaying of pedicles
spleen
   accessory
   floating
   inflammatory of
   long axis of
   tip of
spleen-to-liver ratio
splenic artery
splenic flexure
splenic lobule
splenic notch
splenic portography

splenic venography
splenization
splenobronchial fistula
splenography
splenomegaly
  congenital
  congestive
  Egyptian
  fibrocongestive
  Gaucher
  hemolytic
  infectious
  myelophthisic
  Opitz thrombophlebitic
  persistent
  siderotic
splenoportography
splenorenal anastomosis
splenorenal arterial bypass graft
splenorenal recess
splenorenal shunt
splinter hemorrhage
split-brain studies
split-compression fracture
split-course accelerated radiotherapy
split-course hyperfractionated radiation therapy
split hyperfractionated accelerated radiation therapy
split renal function decrease
split sheath catheter
splitting, zero-field
SPN (solitary pulmonary nodule)
SpO$_2$ (oxygen saturation)
spoke bone
spoiled gradient-recalled (SPGR) echo sequences
spoiler, lucite beam
spondylitic change
spondylitis
  ankylosing
  rheumatoid
  tuberculous

spondylitis deformans
spondylolisthesis
  sagittal roll
  slip angle
  traumatic (grades 1-4)
spondylolisthetic pelvis
spondylolysis
spondylomalacia
spondylosis
  cervical
  degenerative
  diffuse
  Nurick classification of
spondylosyndesis
sponge
  Ivalon
  Ray-Tec x-ray detectable surgical sponge
  Vistec x-ray detectable
spongiocytoma
spongiosa of mitral valve
spongy appearance
spongy bone
spongy degeneration leukodystrophy
spontaneous cardioversion
spontaneous closure of defect
spontaneous coronary artery dissection (SCAD)
spontaneous deposition
spontaneous detorsion
spontaneous echo contrast
spontaneous fracture
spontaneous infantile ductal aneurysm
spontaneous involution
spontaneous pneumothorax
spontaneous regression
spontaneous subsidence
spontaneous tension pneumothorax
spontaneous transient vasoconstriction
spoonlike protrusion of leaflets
spot
  capitate soft
  hot

spot compression
spot film
spot-film fluorography
spot images
S-phase fraction
S pouch, ileal
SPP (superparamagnetic particle) contrast medium
SPPS (single photon planar scintigraphy)
SPR (superior peroneal retinaculum)
sprain
  acute
  chronic
  eversion
sprain fracture
sprain-strain
spread, transfascial
Sprengel deformity
Spring catheter with Pro/Pel coating
Springer fracture
spring-loaded vascular stent
sprinter's fracture
sprodiamide imaging agent
SP6 camera
spur (spurring)
  acromial
  anterior
  bone (or bony)
  calcaneal
  calcific
  degenerative
  heel
  hypertrophic marginal
  impingement
  inferior
  marginal
  Morand
  osteoarthritic
  plantar calcaneal
  posterior
  prominent

spur *(cont.)*
  retrocalcaneal
  traction
  uncovertebral
Squibb catheter
Sr (strontium)
SSD (shaded surface display) algorithms
SSFP (steady state free precession)
SSH (spinal subdural hemorrhage)
SSKI (saturated potassium iodide solution)
SSP (slice sensitivity profile)
S-shaped pouch
S-shaped scoliosis
SSQ (sequential scalar quantization)
SSS (subclavian steal syndrome)
stable fracture
stable isotope
stable-state tuberculosis
Stack autoperfusion balloon
stacked foil technique
stacked metaphor workstation
stacked ovoid lesions
stacked scans
stacked tomograms
Stack perfusion coronary dilatation catheter
STAE (subsegmental transcatheter arterial embolization)
staghorn calculus
staging (see also *grading*)
  Berndt-Harty talar lesion
  distraction-flexion (DFS)
  Ficat avascular necrosis
  Gottschalk
  Greulich and Pyle skeletal maturation
  Jackson
  neuroblastoma
  Outerbridge degenerative arthritis
  pre-slip

stagnant loop syndrome
stain, tumor (on cerebral angiography)
stainless steel mesh stent
staircase phenomenon
stairstep air-fluid levels
stairstep artifact
stairstep fracture
stalk
  body
  infundibular
  pituitary
  polyp
  tumor
Stamey-Malecot catheter
standards
  ACR teleradiology standard
  Taveras
  Wilmad reference
standby rate
standing post-void view
standoff
standstill
  atrial
  cardiac
  ventricular
Stand-Up MRI, Fonar
Stanford type B aortic dissection
stannous pyrophosphate
STAR angiography
Starcam camera
star-cancellation test (SCT)
Starling curve
Starlink software
star pattern
STAR registry
STARRT Falloposcopy System
star-shaped vessel lumen
stasis, venous
stasis edema
stasis of blood flow
stasis ulcers
state, chronic constrictive

static 3D FLASH imaging
static image
status post (S/P)
steady state free precession (SSFP)
steal
  arterial
  coronary artery
  subclavian
stealing of cerebral blood by
  subclavian artery
steal phenomenon
STEAM (stimulated echo aquisition
  mode)
STEAM spectroscopy
steep left anterior oblique (LAO) view
steeple sign on chest x-ray
steep Towne projection
steep Trendelenburg position
steerable catheter
steering catheter
steering, electronic independent beam
Steerocath catheter
steganography
stellar nevus
stellate defect
stellate pattern
stellate skull fracture
stellate undepressed fracture
stem
  brain
  bronchus
  reticular formation of the brain
  roundback
  straight
Stener lesion
stenocardia
stenosing ring of left atrium
stenosis
  acquired mitral
  American Heart Association
    classification of
  ampullary

**stenosis** *(cont.)*
- anal
- antral
- aortic (AS)
- aortic valve
- aortoiliac
- aqueductal
- arterial
- atypical aortic valve
- benign papillary
- bicuspid valvular aortic
- bilateral carotid
- bowel
- branch pulmonary
- bronchial
- buttonhole mitral
- calcific aortic
- calcific bicuspid valvular
- calcific senile aortic valvular
- calcific valvular
- cardiac valvular
- carotid artery
- central canal
- central spinal
- cerebral artery
- cervical
- choledochoduodenal junctional
- common pulmonary vein
- concentric hourglass
- coronary artery
- coronary luminal
- coronary ostial
- critical coronary
- critical valvular
- cross-sectional area
- culprit
- diffuse
- discrete subaortic
- discrete subvalvular aortic (DSAS)
- dynamic subaortic
- eccentric
- esophageal

**stenosis** *(cont.)*
- external iliac
- femoropopliteal atheromatous
- fibromuscular subaortic
- fishmouth mitral
- fixed-orifice aortic
- flow-limiting
- focal
- granulation
- hemodynamically significant
- high-grade
- hypercalcemia supravalvular aortic
- hypertrophic infundibular subpulmonic
- hypertrophic pyloric
- hypertrophic subaortic
- idiopathic hypertrophic subaortic (IHSS)
- iliofemoral venous
- infrainguinal bypass
- infrarenal
- infundibular pulmonary
- infundibular subpulmonic
- innominate artery
- interrenal
- linear
- luminal
- membranous subvalvular aortic
- mitral (MS)
- mitral valve
- multifocal short
- muscular subaortic
- napkin-ring
- neoplastic
- noncalcified coronary
- noncritical
- nonrheumatic valvular aortic
- ostial renal artery
- papillary
- peripheral arterial
- peripheral pulmonary artery (PPAS)

stenosis *(cont.)*
  petrous carotid canal
  post-PTCA
  postangioplasty
  preangioplasty
  pulmonary
  pulmonary artery
  pulmonary valve
  pulmonary vein
  pulmonic (PS)
  pyloric
  rectal
  relative mitral
  renal artery
  rheumatic aortic valvular
  rheumatic mitral
  rheumatic tricuspid
  saphenous vein
  segmental
  senescent aortic
  severe
  silent mitral
  spinal
  stomal
  subaortic
  subclavian artery
  subinfundibular pulmonary
  subpulmonic infundibular
  subvalvar aortic
  supra-aortic
  supraclavicular aortic stenosis
  suprarenal
  supravalvular aortic (SAS, SVAS)
  supravalvular pulmonic
  tapering
  tight
  tracheal
  tricuspid (TS)
  true mitral
  truncal renal artery
  tubular
  tunnel subvalvular aortic

stenosis *(cont.)*
  unicuspid aortic valve
  unilateral carotid
  ureteral
  valvar aortic
  valvular pulmonic
  vertebral artery
stenotic but patent tricuspid valve
stenotic isthmus
stenotic lesion
stenotic valve
Stensen duct
stent (stenting)
  ACS Multilink coronary
  activated balloon expandable
    intravascular
  antegrade ureteral
  balloon-expandable flexible coil
  balloon-expandable intravascular
  balloon-expandable metallic
  beStent balloon-expandable
  biliary
  biodegradable
  CardioCoil self-expanding coronary
  coil vascular
  covered Gianturco
  Dacron-covered
  double pigtail
  EndoCoil biliary
  endoluminal
  EsophaCoil biliary stent
  esophageal
  Gianturco-Rösch Z-stent
  heat-expandable
  helical coil
  iliac artery
  indwelling
  interdigitating coil
  intracoronary
  intravascular
  iridium-192 ($^{192}$Ir)-loaded
  Medivent vascular

stent *(cont.)*
   nitinol
   nitinol thermal memory
   Palmaz balloon-expandable iliac
   Palmaz-Schatz coronary
   pancreatic duct
   patent
   percutaneous
   pigtail
   polymer-coated drug-eluting
   polyurethane
   porous metallic
   radioisotope
   Reliance urinary control
   renovascular
   Roubin-Gianturco flexible coil
   Schatz-Palmaz tubular mesh
   self-expanding
   Silastic
   spring-loaded vascular
   stainless steel mesh
   straight
   Strecker balloon-expandable
   Strecker tantalum
   T-tube
   tantalum
   thermal memory
   transhepatic biliary
   U-tube
   Ultraflex self-expanding
   ureteral
   Wallstent spring-loaded
   Wiktor
   wire-mesh self-expandable
   zig-zag
stent deployment
stent embolization
stent expansion
stent-graft
   endovascular
   percutaneous endoluminal
      placement of

stentless porcine aortic valve
stent migration
stent-mounted allograft valve
stent-mounted heterograft valve
stent recanalization
stent thrombosis
stent-vessel wall contact
Stenver view
step-down deformity of shoulder
step-off between bone fracture fragments
step-off, orbital rim
stepped-care antihypertensive regimen
stepup (or step-up)
stepwise regression analysis
stercoral ulcer
stercoroma
stereocinefluorography
stereofluoroscopy
stereographic projections
stereogram
stereolithography
stereologic method of volume estimation
stereoradiography
stereoscopic view
stereoscopic vision
stereotactic (or stereotaxic)
stereotactic ablation
stereotactic add-on device
stereotactically guided
stereotactic biopsy
stereotactic CT scan
stereotactic data
stereotactic localization
stereotactic method for intracranial navigation
stereotactic neurosurgery
stereotactic procedure
stereotactic proton irradiation
stereotactic radiation therapy
stereotactic radiosurgery

stereotactic resection, computer-assisted
stereotactic surface projection (SSP)
stereotaxis
   computer-assisted volumetric
   imaging-based
   volumetric
stereotaxy
sterile
Sterling contrast medium
sternal angle of Louis
sternal border and apex
sternal cartilage
sternal edge
sternal joint
sternal lift
sternal marrow
sternal notch
sternal pleural reflection
sternal splitting
sternal view
Sternberg myocardial insufficiency
sternoclavicular angle
sternoclavicular joint
sternocleidomastoid muscle
sternocostal joint
sternocostal surface of heart
sternohyoid muscle
sternopericardial ligament
sternothyroid muscle
sternum, anterior bowing of
Stertzer brachial guiding catheter
Stieda fracture
Stierlin sign
stiffening
Still disease (juvenile rheumatoid arthritis)
Stiller rib
stimulated echo acquisition mode (STEAM)
stimulated echo artifact
stimulated echo-tagging technique
stimulus-correlated signal

stippled calcification
stippled epiphysis
stippled soft tissue
stippling of lung fields
STIR (short T1 inversion recovery) scan
STIR (Short Tau Inversion Recovery) sequence
stocking-glove distribution
stoma
   abdominal
   bowel
   diverting
   gastrointestinal
   permanent
   prolapsed
   retracted
   Silastic collar-reinforced
stomach
   aberrant umbilical
   antrum of
   bilocular
   canal of
   cardiac
   cascade
   convex border of
   coronary artery of
   cup-and-spill
   distal blind
   distended
   dumping
   greater curvature of
   Holzknecht
   hourglass
   intrathoracic
   leather bottle
   lesser curvature of
   miniature
   Pavlov
   pit of
   riding
   scaphoid

stomach *(cont.)*
  sclerotic
  sour
  thoracic
  trifid
  upset
  upside-down
  water-trap
  waterfall
stomal bag
stone (see also *gallstone*)
  barrel-shaped
  bile duct
  biliary
  biliary tract
  bilirubinate
  black faceted
  bladder
  bosselated
  calcium bilirubinate
  CBD (common bile duct)
  common bile duct
  gall
  gallbladder
  high attenuation
  impacted urethral
  intrahepatic
  intraluminal
  intravesical
  kidney
  lung
  metabolic
  noncalcified
  radiolucent
  renal
  residual
  salivary
  staghorn
  shadowing
  ureteral
  ureteric

stone *(cont.)*
  urinary
  vein
  womb
stone differentiated from tumor
stone formation, vesical
stone manipulation, percutaneous
stop action images
stopcock
stopping power
storage phosphor radiology
storiform pattern
straddle fracture
straight AP pelvic injection
straight chest tube
straight flush percutaneous catheter
straight-line HT (Hough transform) mapping
straight ureter
strain
  ligamentous
  lumbosacral spine
  muscle
strain fracture
strain-rate MR imaging
strain-sprain injury
stranding
  fascial
  mesenteric
  soft tissue
strands of increased density on chest x-ray
strandy pulmonic infiltrate
strangulated bowel
strangulated hernia
stratigraphy
stray neutron field
streaks of atelectasis on chest film
streaks of increased density
Strecker balloon-expandable stent
Strecker tantalum stent

stress
   adduction (to fingers)
   biomechanical
   mediolateral
   shear
   shearing
   torque
   valgus
   varus
stress and rest images
stress cystogram
stress films
stress fracture
stress gated blood pool cardiac examination
stress images (imaging)
stress-induced left ventricular dilatation
stress-injected sestamibi-gated SPECT with echocardiography
stress management
stress perfusion and rest function by sestamibi-gated SPECT
stress radiography
stress-redistribution exam
stress-rest-reinjection examination
stress test
   dipyridamole thallium
   persantine thallium
stress thallium scan
stress thallium-201 myocardial imaging
stress ulcer
stricture
   anal
   anastomotic
   annular esophageal
   antral
   benign biliary
   bile duct
   cicatricial
   contractile

stricture *(cont.)*
   esophageal
   irritable
   longitudinal esophageal
   peptic
   pyloric
   recurrent
   spasmodic
   ureteral
   urethral
string guideline
stringlike bands of fibrous tissue
string of beads appearance
string of pearls nuclear arrangement
string of pearls sign
string sign in terminal ileum
strip, primary motor
stripe
   Baillarger
   central intraluminal saturation
   flank
   Gennari
   paraspinal pleural
   paratracheal
   properitoneal flank
   Retzius
   saturation
   vertebral
   Vicq d'Azyr
stripe sign
striping, horizontal
stroke
   cerebrovascular
   hyperacute
   thromboembolic (TE)
stroke distance, Doppler-derived
stroke ejection rate
stroke force
stroke index (SI)
stroke power
stroke scale score
stroke volume (SV)

stroke volume image
stroke volume index (SVI)
stroke volume ratio
stroma
strontium (Sr)
$^{82}$Sr
$^{89}$Sr bracelet
$^{89}$Sr chloride (Metastron) radioactive drug
$^{90}$Sr-loaded eye applicator
structural epilepsy
structural weakness of bronchial wall supports
structure (pl. structures)
 biliary
 bony
 branching linear
 branching tubular
 calcified density
 central hilar
 cord
 denture-supporting
 elongated
 high-density
 hollow
 intratumoral
 KUB (kidneys, ureters, bladder)
 labyrinthine
 low-contrast
 low-density
 organoid
 osseous
 renal collecting
 ring-like
 satellite
 soft tissue density
 submillimeter
 superior mediastinal
 supraglottic
 tubular
 vascular
structured coil electromagnet

Strümpell-Lorrain disease
Strümpell-Marie disease
strut
 corticocancellous
 optic
 tricuspid valve
 valve outflow
STT (scapho-trapezium-trapezoid) joint
studded fissures
study (see *imaging*)
stump
 appendiceal
 cervical
 duodenal
 gastric
 rectal
Sturge-Weber telangiectasia
S2 (serotonin) receptor
styloid process
subacromial bursitis
subadventitial plane
subadventitial tissue
subannular region
subaortic curtain
subaortic glands
subaortic muscle
subaortic stenosis
subapical
subarachnoid cavity
subarachnoid hemorrhage (SAH)
subarachnoid instillation of contrast material
subarachnoid metastatic disease
subarachnoid phenol block (SAPB) with fluoroscopy
subarachnoid space
subareolar
subarticular cyst
subastragalar dislocation
subatmospheric pressure
sub-band (or subband), wavelet

subcallosal gyrus
subcapital fracture
subcapsular hematoma
subcarina (pl. subcarinae)
subcarinal node
subchondral bone cyst
subchondral bone plate
subchondral microfractures
subchorionic hemorrhage
subclavian aneurysm
subclavian approach for cardiac catheterization
subclavian artery occlusion
subclavian artery steal of cerebral blood
subclavian artery stenosis
subclavian catheter
subclavian loop
subclavian-pulmonary shunt
subclavian steal phenomenon (SSP)
subclavian steal syndrome (SSS)
subclavian vein, blind percutaneous puncture of
subclavian vein catheterization
subclavicular approach
subcollateral gyrus
subcoracoid dislocation of shoulder
subcortical infarct
subcortical ischemic vascular dementia
subcortical intracerebral hemorrhage
subcortical intracranial lesion
subcortical lesion
subcortical tumor
subcostal approach
subcostal artery
subcostal branch
subcostal margin
subcostal nerve
subcostal window
subcu (subcutaneous)
subcutaneous air
subcutaneous array electrode
subcutaneous emphysema
subcutaneous fat line
subcutaneous fracture
subcutaneous hemangioma
subcutaneous injection of contrast artifact
subcutaneous patch
subcutaneous pocket
subcutaneous tissue
subcutaneous tissue gas
subcutaneous tunnel
subcutaneous veins
subcuticular layer
subdeltoid bursal adhesion
subdiaphragmatic abscess
subdural abscess
subdural blood
subdural cavity
subdural clot
subdural effusion
subdural empyema
subdural hematoma
subdural hemorrhage
subdural hygroma
subdural space
subdural window on CT scan
subendocardial infarction (SEI)
subendocardial injury
subendocardial ischemia
subendocardial myocardial infarction
subendocardial necrosis
subendothelial hyalinization
subependymal hemorrhage
subeustachian sinus
subfalcine (subfalcial) herniation
subfascial transposition
subfascially
subfrontal meningioma tumor
subgaleal abscess
subgaleal hematoma
subglenoid dislocation of shoulder
subglottic area

subglottic edema
subhepatic area
subhepatic space
subinfundibular pulmonary stenosis
subintimal cleavage plane
subintimal dissection
sublabral recess
subligamenous disk herniation
sublingual varices
sublux
subluxated
subluxation
    atlanto-axial
    element
    forward
    occult
    patellar
    posterior
    radial head (RHS)
    reduced
    rotary
    tendon
    Volkmann
submandibular ganglion
submandibular triangle
submaxillary
submental vertex view
submillimeter structures
submucosal lesion
submucosal thickening
submucous myoma
suboccipital shortening
suboptimal film due to:
    film quality
    patient cooperation
    positioning
suboptimal results
suboptimal runoff
suboptimal visualization
suboptimally visualized
subpectoral pocket
subperiosteal abscess of frontal sinus

subperiosteal fracture
subperiosteal new bone formation
subperiosteally
subphrenic abscess
subphrenic biloma
subpleural bleb
subpleural curvilinear lines
subpleural dots
subpleural lines
subpubic arch
subpulmonic fluid
subpulmonic infundibular stenosis
subpulmonic obstruction
subrectus placement
subsartorial tunnel
subsegment of lung
subsegmental bibasilar atelectasis
subsegmental bronchus
subsegmental perfusion abnormality
subsegmental transcatheter arterial
    embolization (STAE)
subsegments, right middle lobe
subserosal fibrosis
subserosal layer
subspinous dislocation
substernal angle
substernal goiter
substernal thyroid
substitution bone
substrate, main energy
subtalar articulation
subtalar joint space
subtendinous space
subtentorial lesion
subtotal lesion
subtraction, Epistar
subtraction films
    digital
    manual
    serial
subtraction images
subtraction technique

subtrochanteric fracture
subvalvular aneurysm
subvalvular aortic obstruction
subvalvular aortic stenosis
subxiphoid echocardiography view
subxiphoid implantation
subxiphoid view
sucking pneumothorax
Sucquet-Hoyer anastomosis
Sucquet-Hoyer canal
sucrose dosimeter
sucrose polyester contrast
suction line, aortic vent
Sudbury system
sudden blockage of coronary artery
Sudeck atrophy
SUFE (slipped upper femoral epiphysis)
suite, angiography
sulcal skeleton
sulcation
sulcus (pl. sulci)
  angularis
  basilar
  blunted posterior
  cortical
  costal
  Harrison
  atrioventricular
  calcarine
  callosal
  central
  cingulate
  collateral
  dilatation of the
  effacement of
  frontal
  hypothalmic
  lateral occipital
  lips of lateral
  occipitotemporal
  olfactory

sulcus *(cont.)*
  parieto-occipital
  pontomedullary
  postcentral
  posterior interventricular
  precentral
  pulmonary
  rami of lateral
  rolandic
  superior frontal
  superior temporal
  supracallosal
  temporal
  ulnar
  widened (on scan)
sulfobromophthalein (BSP) imaging agent
sulfur colloid labeled with Tc 99m scan
sulfur colloid, technetium bound to
SULP II catheter
sum-peak method
summation shadow artifact
summing correction
Summit LoDose collimator
summit, ventricular septal
sump catheter
Sun SPARCstation system
Sun workstation
sunburst pattern
sunrise view of patella
sunset view
superabsorbent polymer (SAP) embolic material
super scan appearance
superciliary arch
superconducting magnet
superconductor
superdominant left anterior descending artery
superfical femoral artery
superficial external pudendal artery

superficial femoral arteries (SFAs)
superficial femoral artery occlusion
superficial femoral vein
superficial lesion
superficial palmar arterial arch
superficial posterior compartment
superficial vein
superimposed
superimposition artifact
superimposition of signals
superincumbent spinal curves
superior border of heart
superior border of rib
superior bronchus
superior caval defect
superior caval obstruction
superior colliculus
superior costotransverse ligament
superior epigastric artery
superior facet
superior frontal gyrus
superior frontal sulcus
superior genicular artery
superior intercostal artery
superior intercostal vein
superior lobe of lung
superior margin of inferior rib
superior marginal defect
superior mediastinal structures
superior mediastinum
superior mesenteric artery (SMA)
superior mesenteric vein (SMV)
superior parietal lobule gyrus
superior pubic ramus
superior pulmonary artery
superior pulmonary vein
superior retraction
superior sagittal sinus
superior segment
superior temporal gyrus
superior temporal sulcus
superior thoracic aperture

superior thyroid artery
superior vena cava obstruction
supernormal conduction
supernormal excitation
supernumerary bone
supernumerary sesamoid bones
superoinferior heart
superolaterally
superomedial portal
superparamagnetic contrast agent
superparamagnetic iron oxide-
 enhanced imaging
superparamagnetic iron oxide (SPIO)
 oral contrast agent
superselective (not supraselective)
superselective angio-CT
superselective angiography
superselective catheterization
superselective intra-arterial
 chemotherapy
supination-adduction fracture
supination-eversion fracture
supine film
supine position
supplemental beam filtration
suppression
   Cytomel (thyroid hormone)
   double-echo three-point Dixon
    method
   fat
   paradoxical
suppressor mesh
suppuration
supra-annular constriction
supra-aortic ridge
supra-aortic stenosis
supracallosal sulcus
supracardiac shunt
supracardiac-type total anomalous
 venous return
supraceliac aorta
supraclavicular aortic stenosis

supraclavicular lymph node
supraclavicular node
supraclavicular region
supraclavicular triangle
supraclinoid internal carotid artery
supracolic compartment
supracollicular spike of cortical bone
supracondylar femoral fracture
supracondylar humerus fracture
supracoronary ridge
supracristal ventricular septal defect
supradiaphragmatic aorta
supraduodenal approach
supraepicondylar
supraepitrochlear
supraglottic larynx
supraglottic structures
suprahepatic caval cuff
suprahepatic space
suprahepatic vena cava
suprainterparietal bone
supralevator space
supraligamentous disk herniation
supramalleolar region
supramarginal gyrus
supranuclear lesion
supraoccipital bone
supraorbital fissure
supraorbital ridges
suprapatellar bursa
suprapatellar plica
suprapatellar pouch
suprapharyngeal bone
suprapubic area
suprarenal aneurysm
suprarenal extension of aneurysm
suprarenal gland
suprarenal stenosis
suprascapular nerve entrapment
"supraselective" (see *superselective*)
suprasellar adenoma
suprasellar aneurysm

suprasellar cistern
suprasellar extension of tumor
suprasellar lesion
suprasellar mass
suprasellar region
suprasellar tumor
supraspinatus nerve
supraspinous ligaments
suprasternal bone
suprasternal bulging
suprasternal notch view on
 echocardiogram
suprasternal window
suprasyndesmotic fixation
supratentorial brain tumor
supratentorial cerebral blood flow
supratentorial primitive neuroectodermal tumor (PNET)
suprathreshold
supratip nasal tip deformity
supratrochlear
supravalvular aortic stenosis (SAS,
 SVAS)
supravalvular aortogram
supravalvular mitral stenosis
supravalvular pulmonic stenosis
supravaterian duodenum
supraventricular crest (SVC)
supravesical obstruction
sural nerve
SureStart feature of Aspire continuous
 imaging
surface
 acromial articular
 anterolateral
 anteromedial
 apposing articular
 articular
 articulating
 arytenoidal articular
 auricular
 axial

surface *(cont.)*
  basal
  bone
  bosselated
  buccal
  calcaneal articular
  carpal articular
  cartilaginous joint
  cerebral
  colic
  contiguous articular
  costal
  cuboidal articular
  diaphragmatic
  distal
  endosteal
  endothelial
  fibular
  fibular articular
  gastric
  glenoid
  grooving of articular
  joint articular
  occlusal
  parallelism of articular
  posterior
  radioulnar
  roughened articular
  superomedial
  weightbearing
surface application of radioelement
surface coil localization
surface distance
surface matching technique
surface projection rendering
surface registration
surface tension of lungs
surface variable attenuation correction
surfer's knots
surgery
  salvage
    video-assisted thoracic (VATS)

surgical cardiac tamponade
surgical emphysema
surgical intervention
surgical neck fracture
surgical neck of humerus
surgical revascularization
Surgical Simplex P radiopaque bone cement
surgical simulation CT
surgical staples
surgical venous interruption
Surgilase 150 laser
Surgilase $CO_2$ laser
survey
  bone
  four-view wrist
  joint
  metastatic bone
  osseous
survey-view images
susceptibility artifact
susceptibility, diamagnetic
susceptibility-sensitive sequence
susceptibility-weighted MR
suspended heart syndrome
suspension, barium
suspension characteristics
sustained anterior parasternal motion
sustained apical impulse
sustained left ventricular heave
sutural bone
sutural diastasis
suture
  apical
  basilar
  biparietal
  bregmatomastoid
  coronal
  cranial
  delayed closure of
  dentate
  diastasis of the

suture *(cont.)*
  ethmoidolacrimal
  ethmoidomaxillary
  frontal
  frontoethmoidal
  frontolacrimal
  frontomaxillary
  frontonasal
  frontoparietal
  frontosphenoid
  frontozygomatic
  Gillies
  Gruber
  interparietal
  jugal
  lambdoidal cranial
  mamillary
  metopic
  nonfusion of cranial
  occipital
  occipitomastoid
  occipitoparietal
  occipitosphenoid
  overlapping
  parietal
  parietomastoid
  parieto-occipital
  petrobasilar
  petrosphenobasilar
  petrospheno-occipital
  petrosquamous
  prematurely closed
  radiopaque
  rhabdoid
  sagittal
  sagittal cranial
  sphenoethmoidal
  spheno-occipital
  spheno-orbital
  sphenoparietal
  sphenopetrosal
  sphenosquamous

suture *(cont.)*
  sphenotemporal
  sphenovomerine
  splayed cranial
  spread (cranial sign)
  squamosomastoid
  squamosoparietal
  squamososphenoid
  squamous
  temporal
Sv (sievert) radiation absorbed dose
SV (stroke volume)
SVAS (supravalvular aortic stenosis)
SVC (superior vena cava)
SVC (supraventricular crest)
SVI (stroke volume index)
SvO$_2$ (venous oxygen saturation)
SVR (systemic vascular resistance)
SVRI (systemic vascular resistance index)
swallow
  barium
  dry
  Gastrografin
  ice-water
  water-soluble contrast esophageal
  wet
swallowing artifact
swallowing center
swallowing dysfunction
swallowing function
swallowing mechanism, video fluoroscopy of
swallow syncope
swamp-static artifact
Swan-Ganz balloon-flotation catheter
Swan-Ganz thermodilution catheter
swan-neck catheter
swan-neck deformity
swan neck shape of ventricular outflow
Swediaur disease

sweep, duodenal
sweeper
Sweet sternal punch
swelling, soft tissue
SWI (stroke work index)
swimmer's view
swinging flashlight test
swirling smokelike echoes
Swiss cheese appearance
Swiss cheese ventricular septal defect
Swissray scanner
swiss roll technique
swivel dislocation (of midfoot)
swollen tissues
Swyer-James unilateral hyperlucency of lung
SXA (single-energy x-ray) absorptiometer
SXCT (spiral x-ray computed tomography )
Sydenham chorea
Syed-Neblett brachytherapy method
sylvian aqueduct syndrome
sylvian candelabra
sylvian fissure
sylvian operculum
sylvian/rolandic junction
Sylvius
   aqueduct of
   cistern of
   fossa of
Syme amputation
symmetrical chest
symmetrical narrowing
symmetrical phased array
symmetric distribution
symmetric pulmonary congestion
symmetry
sympathetic chain
sympathetic denervation
sympathetic ganglia
sympathetic innervation
sympathetic nervous tissue
sympathetic vascular instability
symphysis, pubic
symphysis pubis
symptomatic metastatic spinal cord compression
symptomatology
symptom complex
synaptic cleft
synaptic dopamine concentration
synaptic pathways
synchronicity
synchronization device
synchronous carotid arterial pulse
synchrotron, monochromatic
synchrotron radiation
syndactylization of digits
syndactyly
syndrome
Synergy ultrasound system
synkinesis (pl. synkineses)
synostosis
   cervical
   congenital radioulnar
   coronal
   lambdoid
   multiple-suture
   nonsyndromic bicoronal
   nonsyndromic unicoronal
   premature suture
   radiographically firm
   sagittal
   single suture
   terminal
   tibiofibular
synovial cavity
synovial membrane
synovial plica
synovial proliferation
synovial sarcoma of heart
synovial surface
synovial thickening

synoviogram
synovium
  boggy
  exuberant
  hyperplastic
  opaque
synpneumonic empyema
synthesis
  automated
  facile
synthetase, nitrous oxide
syringe, Ultraject pre-filled contrast media
syringobulbia
syringocele
syringocoele
syringoencephalia
syringoencephalomyelia
syringomeningocele
syringomyelia
syringopontia
syrinx cavity
syrinx, traumatic
system (see also *scanner*; *ultrasound*)
  Acuson 128XP ultrasound
  Agfa CR
  Agfa PACS
  AI 5200 diagnostic ultrasound
  ALT Ultrasound
  Angiomat 6000 contrast delivery
  AngioVista angiographic
  AquaSens FMS 1000 fluid monitoring
  Arcitumomab diagnostic imaging
  Artoscan MRI
  Aspen digital ultrasound
  Aspire continuous imaging (CI)
  Aurora dedicated breast MRI
  Aurora MR breast imaging
  automated angle encoder
  BAK-1 interbody fusion
  Bard percutaneous cardiopulmonary support (CPS)

system *(cont.)*
  Biad SPECT imaging
  biliary
  Biosound AU
  Biospec MR imaging
  biphasic
  Bracco
  Bristol-Myers
  Bruker CSI MR
  caliceal
  Cartesian reference coordinate
  CathTrack catheter locator
  central nervous (CNS)
  CGR biplane angiographic
  Chemo-Port perivena catheter
  circumflex coronary
  collateral
  collecting
  Compass stereotactic frame
  Compton-suppression
  continuous-wave high frequency Doppler ultrasound
  continuous-wave laser
  contoured tilting compression mammography
  Contour mammography
  Cordis endovascular
  COROSKOP C cardiac imaging
  CT-MRI-compatible stereotactic headframe
  Curix Capacity Plus film processing
  Cyberware
  dedicated breast biopsy
  DELTAmanager MedImage
  Desilets introducer
  Diasonics
  DICOM
  Dictaphone Digital Express clinical reporting
  Digital Equipment
  digital mammographic
  DIMAQ integrated ultrasound

system *(cont.)*
  directly coupled sample changer
  dominant left coronary artery
  dominant right coronary
  dual-head gamma camera
  Dynarad portable imaging
  Echovar Doppler
  Elscint
  endocavitary applicator
  engorged collecting
  external jugular
  extracranial carotid
  FlimFax teleradiology
  FluoroPlus angiography
  Fonar
  foreign body retrieval
  full-field digital mammography
  Galen teleradiology
  GE (General Electric)
  greater saphenous
  Greenfield vena cava filter
  HDI (high-definition imaging) 3000 ultrasound
  hepatic ductal
  Hewlett Packard
  high-field
  Hi-Star midfield MRI
  homonuclear spin
  House grading
  HyperPACS
  IBM Speech Server clinical reporting
  IMAC
  image analysis
  Imatron
  immunomedics
  Impax PACS
  Instrumentation Laboratory
  internal carotid
  intrahepatic
  Isocam scintillation imaging
  Jackson staging

system *(cont.)*
  Lanier clinical reporting
  lesser saphenous
  Liebel-Flarsheim CT 9000 contrast delivery
  lipophilic sequestration
  LymphoScan nuclear imaging
  Magnes biomagnetometer
  Magnetom Open
  Magnetom Vision MR
  Magnex Alpha MR
  Marex MRI
  MEDDARS cardiac catheterization analysis
  Medspec MR imaging
  Medweb clinical reporting
  multidetector
  Novacore left ventricular assist (LVAS)
  Octreoscan
  OEC Series 9600 cardiac
  1.5T Signa Advantage
  open architecture
  open-configuration MR
  OpenPACS
  OSCAR ultrasonic bone cement removal
  OsteoView x-ray
  Ovation Falloposcopy
  Paris
  PenRad mammography clinical reporting
  PF-PACS
  Philips
  Picker
  Pinnacle 3 radiation therapy planning
  PMT robotic fulcrumless tomographic
  polar coordinate
  PortalVision radiation oncology
  PowerVision Ultrasound

system *(cont.)*
   Probe balloon-on-a-wire dilatation
   Profile Mammography
   ProstaScint
   pulmonary venous
   PulseSpray pulsed infusion
   Q-cath catheterization recording
   quadrature surface coil MRI
   radiation therapy planning (RTP)
   radionuclide carrier
   RadNet radiology information
   Redi-Vu teleradiology
   reference coordinate
   renal collecting
   reticuloendothelial
   Retzius
   ring-type imaging
   Rogan teleradiology
   RTP (radiation therapy planning)
   saphenous
   Scanmaster DX
   scanned-slot detector
   scanning beam digital
   scattering
   Schmidt optics
   Scintiview nuclear computer
   Scintron IV (four) nuclear computer
   sequestration
   Shape Maker
   Shimadzu
   SICOR (computer-assisted cardiac catheter recording)
   Siemens AG
   Signa GEMS MR imaging
   Signal
   Silicon Graphics Reality Engine
   SmartSpot high resolution digital imaging
   Sonoline Elegra ultrasound
   Squibb
   STARRT Falloposcopy

system *(cont.)*
   Sudbury
   Summit LoDose collimator
   Sun SPARCstation
   SureStart imaging
   Synergy ultrasound
   thermal dosimetry
   TMS 3-dimensional radiation therapy planning
   transluminal lysing
   Triad SPECT imaging
   TRON 3 VACI cardiac imaging
   UltraPACS diagnostic imaging
   UltraSTAR computer-based ultra sound reporting
   uPACS picture archiving system
   upper collecting
   USCI Probe balloon-on-a-wire dilatation
   Varian brachytherapy
   VARIS radiation oncology
   VasoView balloon dissection
   VAX 4100
   ventricular
   VentTrak monitoring system
   vertebral artery
   Vingmed Sound CFM ultrasound
   Vitrea 3-D
   VoiceRAD clinical reporting
   VoxelView
   Xillix LIFE-GI fluorescence endoscopy
   XKnife stereotactic radiosurgery
   x-ray shadow projection microtomographic
systematic ultrasound-guided biopsies
systemic anticoagulation with heparin
systemic arterial circulation
systemic arterial oxygen desaturation
systemic arterial vasoconstriction
systemic AV $O_2$ difference
systemic blood

systemic carnitine deficiency
systemic circulation
systemic diastolic blood pressure (SDBP)
systemic disorder affecting heart function
systemic heparinization
systemic hypoperfusion
systemic inflammatory response syndrome
systemic lupus erythematosus (SLE)
systemic mean arterial pressure (SMAP)
systemic mercury intoxication
systemic oxygen saturation measured after balloon-occluding each collateral
systemic perfusion, diminished
systemic pressure
systemic-pulmonary artery shunt
systemic vascular resistance (SVR)
systemic vascular resistance index (SVRI)
systemic venous hypertension
systemic venous return

systolic acceleration time
systolic and diagnostic gating
systolic anterior motion (SAM) on 2D echocardiogram
systolic blood pressure (SBP)
systolic-diastolic blood pressure
systolic ejection period (SEP)
systolic fractional shortening
systolic gradient
systolic heart failure
systolic hypertension
systolic impulse
systolic mammary souffle
systolic pressure
systolic pressure determination (SLP)
systolic pressure-time index
systolic prolapse of mitral valve leaflet
systolic reserve
systolic retraction of apex
systolic S waves
systolic time interval (STI)
systolic upstroke time
systolic velocity-time integral

# T, t

T (temporal)
T (tesla)
T (thoracic)
Ta (tantalum)
table
    dual lookup
    Hydradjust IV
    pivoting
    tilt
TAE (transcatheter arterial embolization)
tag image file format (TIFF)
tag of cartilage
tag plane
Tagarno 3SD cine projector for angiography
tagged antibody, fluorescently
tagged atom
tagged, radioactively
tagging cine magnetic resonance
tail-like segment
tail of breast in mammography
tail of pancreas
tail of Spence in mammography
Tailarach space
takeoff of vessel
takeup of radioactive material

talar dome
talar impingement
talar osteochondral fracture
talar tilt angle
talc plaque
talipes arcuatus
talocalcaneal angle
talocalcaneal articulation
talocalcaneal index
talocalcaneal joint
talocalcaneal ligament
talocrural angle
talocrural fusion
talocrural joint
talofibular joint
talofibular ligament
talometatarsal angle
talonavicular angle
talonavicular beaking
talonavicular capsule
talonavicular joint
talonavicular ligament
talus (ankle)
    congenital vertical
    flat top
    neck of
        Sneppen fracture of the

talus *(cont.)*
  sulcus
  vertical
tamponade
  balloon
  cardiac
  chronic
  esophagogastric
  ferromagnetic
  florid cardiac
  full-blown cardiac
  heart
  low-pressure cardiac
  pericardial chyle with
  subacute cardiac
  surgical cardiac
tandem and ovoids
tandem, external beam with
tandem lesion
tangential
tangentially
tangential breast fields
tangential constriction
tangential cut
tangential layer of hand
tangential ports
tangential scapular view
tangential view
tantalum bronchogram
tantalum (Ta) (see *imaging agent*)
tantalum stent
tapering occlusion
tapering off
tapering stenosis
tapers, fiberoptic
TAPVR (total anomalous pulmonary venous return)
Tar symptoms
target (targeting)
  angiographic
  gas
  internal cyclotron

target *(cont.)*
  metal technetium
  three-dimensional reconstructed
  tungsten
target appearance
target calcification
target lesion
target MIPcor
target organ
target sign
target tissues
target-to-background ratio
tarsal-metatarsal (or tarsometatarsal) joint space
tarsal arch
tarsal bone
tarsal canal
tarsal coalition
tarsal navicular
tarsal tunnel syndrome
tarsometatarsal (or tarsal-metatarsal) joint space
T artifact
task-activated brain regions
task-rest pattern
Taussig-Bing congenital malformation of heart
Taussig-Snellen-Alberts syndrome
taut pericardial effusion
TAV (transcutaneous aortovelography)
Taveras, standards of
Tawara atrioventricular node
TB (tuberculosis)
TBNA (transbronchial needle aspiration)
TBT (transcervical balloon tuboplasty)
Tc HIDA (technetium hepatoiminodi-acetic acid) ("tek-high-dah") scan
TCA (transcondylar axis)
TCBF (total cerebral blood flow)
TCD (transcranial Doppler) ultrasonography

Tc99m or $^{99m}$Tc (see *imaging agent, technetium*)
T condylar fracture
TCP/IP (transmission control protcol/Internet protocol)
TCS (tethered cord syndrome)
TCT900S helical CT scanner
T/D (thickness-to-diameter of ventricle) ratio
TE (echo delay time)
TE (echo time)
TE (tracheoesophageal) fistula
tear (rupture)
  attritional
  bowstring
  bucket-handle
  cleavage
  dural
  entry
  fishtail
  flap
  full-thickness
  ligament
  Mallory-Weiss
  micro
  parrot-beak
  partial-thickness
  radial
  rotator cuff
  serosal
  tendon (types I-IV)
tearaway sheath
teardrop-shaped flexion-compression fracture
teboroxime cardiac scan for myocardial infarction
teboroxime resting washout (TRW)
TEC (transluminal endarterectomy catheter)
TEC (transluminal extraction catheter)
TECA (technetium albumin) study
Technegas
TechneScan MAG3 (99mTc mertiatide) renal diagnostic imaging
technetium (Tc99m or $^{99m}$Tc) (see *imaging agent*)
Technicare camera
technique (see also *method*)
  acquisition
  Amplatz
  background subtraction
  bayesian
  blended
  brain surface matching
  bread-loaf
  Brown-Roberts-Wells
  bull's-eye
  coronal oblique
  cross-correlation
  cuboid squeeze
  cuboid whip
  cut-film
  deblurring
  deconvolution
  double contrast
  double umbrella
  echo-tagging
  Egan
  EPISTAR perfusion
  equilibrium radionuclide angiocardiography
  esophageal balloon
  exclusion-HPLC
  fast-FLAIR
  field-fitting
  first-pass
  flow mapping
  full bladder
  gated
  gradient echo cine
  Gruentzig PTCA
  half-wedged field
  HARC-C wavelet compression

technique *(cont.)*
  in vivo
  inhalation
  intercomparison measurement
  inverse radiotherapy
  inversion-recovery
  isolation-perfusion
  Judkins
  kissing atherectomy
  kissing balloon
  Leksell
  loading
  low-angle shot (flash)
  low-dose film mammographic
  Markov chain Monte Carlo
  MIDCAB (minimally invasive direct coronary artery bypass)
  ML/EM reconstruction
  multimodal image fusion
  multiphasic multislice MRI
  multiplanar
  multislice multiphase spin-echo imaging
  multislice spin-echo
  navigator echo motion correction
  NEUGAT (neutron/gamma transmission)
  neutron/gamma transmission (NEUGAT)
  no-gap
  noncoplanar arc
  noninvasive
  packing, extraction, and calculation
  papillon
  partial saturation
  PASTA (polarity-altered spectral-selective acquisition)
  PCICO (pressure-controlled intermittent coronary occlusion)
  percutaneous transfemoral
  pharmokinetic
  pressure half-time

technique *(cont.)*
  radiotracer
  region-of-interest imaging
  Riechert-Mundinger
  road-mapping
  robus registration
  scintillation counting
  Seldinger percutaneous
  sequential extraction-radiotracer
  serial cut film
  silhouette
  single-field hyperthermia combined with radiation therapy and ultrasound
  single fill/void
  sliding thin-slab, minimum intensity projection
  Sones cineangiography
  spin echo
  spin-label
  stacked-foil
  stereotactic or stereotaxic
  stimulated echo-tagging
  subclavian turndown
  subtraction
  tetrahedral interpolation
  three-dimensional (3D)
  tissue characterization
  Todd-Wells
  transcatheter
  transgluteal CT-guided
  trephine
  two-dimensional (2D)
  upgated
  ureteral compression
  volumetric mapping
technology, slip-ring
Tecmag Libra-S16 system
tectal lesion
tectoral ligament
tectospinal tract
TED (thromboembolic disease)

Tedlar bags
TEE (transesophageal echocardiography) imaging with DTI
teeth
  Hutchinson
  incisor
  milk
  molar
  premolar
  primary
  secondary
  wisdom
TEF (tracheoesophageal fistula)
Teflon ERCP catheter
tegmental tract
tegmentum
  medullary
  midbrain
  pontine
tegmentum of pons
Teichholz ejection fraction in echocardiogram
Teichholz equation for left ventricular volume
"tek-high-dah" (Tc HIDA) scan
telangiectatic osteosarcoma
telangiectatic vessel
telecobalt
telecom integration
telecurietherapy (radiotherapy)
Telepaque contrast medium
teleradiology videoconferencing
teletherapy, C-60
telos radiographic stress device
temperature, firing
temperature sensors
template irradiation
temporal aliasing
temporal artery
temporal bone fracture
temporal horn
temporal instability artifact

temporal lobe lesion
temporal lobe tumor
temporal-occipital junction
temporal phase delay
temporally
temporo-occipital region
temporomandibular joint (TMJ)
temporoparietal region
temporopontine tract
temporozygomatic region
tendinosis, patellar
tendo (pl. tendines)
tendo Achillis (Achilles tendon)
tendo calcaneus (Achilles tendon)
tendon
  Achilles
  calcaneal
  central (of diaphragm)
  central perineal
  collagen fibrils within
  common
  conjoined
  conjoint
  coronary
  cricoesophageal
  hamstring
  heel (tendo calcaneus)
  membranaceous
  patellar
  peroneal
  rider's
  slipped
  Todaro
  Zinn (common tendinous ring)
tendon rupture
tendon-sheath space infection
tendon sling
tendon tear (types I-IV)
tennis elbow
tennis leg (plantaris rupture)
tennis shoulder
tennis toe

Tennis Racquet angiography catheter
tension pneumothorax
tension-time index (TTI)
tentative diagnosis
tented up
tenth cranial nerve (vagus nerve)
tenting of diaphragm
tentorial edge
tentorial herniation
tentorial meningioma
tentorial notch herniation
TER (therapeutic external radiation)
teratoma
  cystic
  ovarian
  pineal
  sacrococcygeal
  solid
  suprasellar atypical
  testis
terminal
  character cell
  dumb
  X-
terminal air sac
terminal air space
terminal bronchiole
terminal crest
terminal ileum
terminal inversion
terminal reservoir syndrome
terminal thrombosis
termination
  early-phase
  late-phase
Terry-Thomas sign
tertiary collimation
tertiary contraction
tesla (T)
tesla field
test (see *imaging*)

test meal
test-retest precision
testicle
testicular adrenal rest tissue
testicular artery
testicular infarction
testicular torsion
testis (pl. testes)
  appendix
  descended
  ectopic
  efferent ductules of
  infarcted
  rete
  torsion of
  undescended
"tet" (tetralogy) of Fallot
tethered bowel sign
tethered cord
tethered spinal cord
tetrad, Fallot
tetrahedral interpolation technique
tetralogy of Fallot (TOF)
tetrapolar esophageal catheter
texture, echo
texture mapping
texture slice
TFA (thigh-foot angle)
TFA (tibiofemoral angle)
TFC (triangular fibrocartilage)
TFCC (triangular fibrocartilaginous
  complex)
T fracture
TGA (transposition of great arteries)
thalamic fracture of the calcaneus
thalamic infarct
thalamic lesion
thalamocaudate artery
thalamoperforate artery
thalamostriate vein
thalamotegmental involvement

thalamus
thallium (Tl) (see *imaging agent*)
   $^{201}$Tl imaging agent
   $^{201}$Tl myocardial scintigraphy
   $^{201}$Tl stress imaging
thallium SPECT score
thallium-to-scalp ratio
thatched-roof worker's lung
THC (transhepatic cholangiography)
THE (transhepatic embolization)
thebesian circulation
thebesian foramen
thebesian valve
thebesian vein
theca (pl. thecae)
theca externa
theca interna
theca lutein ovarian cyst
thecal sac
thecoperitoneal shunt
thenar eminence
thenar muscle
thenar space abscess
theophylline attenuation
theory
   Beer-Bouguer
   density matrix
   fuzzy set
   Kubelka-Munk
   quantum
therapeutic application of radioactive
   source
therapeutic embolization
therapeutic external radiation (TER)
therapeutic pneumothorax
therapeutic radiation
therapeutic radiology
therapy (see also *radiation therapy*
   adjunctive
   adjuvant radiation
   antineoplastic
   antitubercular

therapy *(cont.)*
   arc
   brachytherapy
   Bragg-peak photon-beam
   brisement
   chemo-
   chemoradiation
   combined-modality radiation
   conformal radiation (CRT)
   conventionally fractionated
      stereotactic radiation
   craniospinal axis radiation
   electron arc
   electron beam
   endoscopic sclerosing
   endovascular
   ethanol
   eye-view 3D-CRT radiation
   fast-neutron
   fibrinolytic
   fluoroscopy-guided subarachnoid
      phenol block (SAPB)
   four-fiber
   fractionated radiation
   fragmentation
   grid
   hyperfractionated radiation
   hypertonic glucose
   hypofractionated
   $^{192}$I high-dose rate single catheter
   immunosuppressive
   indicator dilution
   indomethacin
   interstitial radioactive colloid
   intra-articular radiopharmaceutical
   intracavitary radioactive colloid
   intracoronary thrombolytic
   intraoperative radiation (IORT)
   intravascular radiopharmaceutical
   IORT (intraoperative radiation)
   laser
   megavoltage grid

therapy *(cont.)*
  megavoltage radiation
  megavoltage x-ray
  neoadjuvant hormonal
  neutron
  neutron capture
  neutron/gamma transmission
  orthovoltage radiation
  palliative
  partial-brain radiation
  radiation
  radio-
  radiofrequency ablation
  radiopharmaceutical
  rotation
  salvage
  split hyperfractionated accelerated radiation
  split-course hyperfractionated
  stereotactic radiation
  supportive
  three-dimensional conformal radiation (3D-CRT)
  thrombolytic
  tiered
  total androgen suppression
  transcatheter
  ultraearly thrombolytic
  updraft
  whole-brain radiation
therapy tomographs
therapy zones
TheraSeed (palladium-103) active isotope in titanium capsule
thermal ablation
thermal convection patterns
thermal diffusion
thermal dosimetry system
thermal equilibrium
thermal memory stent
thermal neutron
thermal treatment parameters
therminoluminescent dosimetry
thermistor catheter
thermistor plethysmography
thermoacoustics
thermochemotherapy
thermodilution balloon catheter
thermodilution cardiac output
thermodilution catheter
thermodilution ejection fraction
thermodilution method of cardiac output measurement
thermodilution Swan-Ganz catheter
thermogram, liquid crystal
thermography
  blood vessel
  laser-induced (LITT)
  liquid crystal contact (LCT)
thermoluminescence
thermoluminescent dosimeter
thermoradiotherapy, interstitial
thermotherapy
  laser-induced (LITT)
  MR imaging-guided laser-induced interstitial
thickening
  diffuse
  focal intimal
  intimal
  mottled
  partial
  wall
thickness, full
thick-slice image
thick-walled
Thiemann disease
thigh-foot angle
thin border
thin cylindrical uniform field volumes
thin film analysis
thin fibrous cap
thin-collimation images
thin-plate spline

thin-section (or slice) CT
thin-slice (or section) CT
thin-slice image
thin-walled
third cranial nerve (oculomotor nerve)
third intercondylar tubercle of Parsons
third intercostal space
third left interspace
third order chordae
third portion of duodenum
third space sequestration
third ventricle tumors
30° position
30° right anterior oblique projection
Thixokon contrast medium
thoracentesis, ultrasonic guidance for
thoraces (see *thorax*)
thoracic aortic aneurysm
thoracic aortography
thoracic asymmetry
thoracic cage configuration
thoracic catheter
thoracic cavity
thoracic component of scoliosis
thoracic deformity
thoracic duct
thoracic empyema
thoracic esophagus
thoracic fistula
thoracic gas volumes
thoracic inlet
thoracic inlet (Pancoast) syndrome
thoracic kyphosis, loss of
thoracic outlet syndrome (TOS)
thoracic scoliosis
thoracic spine (T spine)
thoracic stomach
thoracic vertebrae (T1-T12)
thoracic wall
thoracoabdominal aorta
thoracoabdominal aortic aneurysm
thoracoabdominal wall

thoracoepigastric vein
thoracofemoral conversion
thoracolumbar scoliosis
thoracolumbar spine
thoracoport
thorax (pl. thoraces, thoraxes)
    asymmetrical
    bony
    cylindrical
    squared off
    symmetrical
thorax view
Thorel bundle of muscle fibers in heart
Thorel pathway
thorium dioxide granuloma
thorium dioxide imaging agent
Thorotrast contrast medium
threatened vessel closure post-PTCA
30 sec./frame time
3:2 block ("three-to-two")
three-axis gradient coil
three-compartment wrist angiography
three-dimensional (3D or 3-D)
    3D anthropometry
    3D connect operation
    3D CRT (conformal radiation therapy)
    3D dose profile
    3D echocardiography
    3D freehand ultrasound
    3DFT (three-dimensional Fourier transform)
    3DFT GRASS MR imaging
    3DFT magnetic resonance angiography
    3DFT-CISS sequence
    3DFT SPGR MR imaging
    3D gadolinium-enhanced magnetic resonance angiography for aortoiliac inflow
    3D GRE (gradient-recalled-echo) MRI

**three-dimensional • thymus**

three-dimensional *(cont.)*
  3D H-1 magnetic resonance spectroscopic imaging
  3D helical computerized tomographic angiography (3D helical CTA)
  3D holography
  3D image reconstruction
  3D inflow MR angiography
  3D MRI data sets
  3D magnetic resonance microscopy
  3D magnetic source imaging (MSI)
  3D modeling
  3D MSI (magnetic source imaging)
  3D phase-contrast magnetic resonance angiography
  3D processed ultrafast computerized imaging
  3D-PSIF sequence
  3D spoiled gradient-recalled sequences
  3D stereotaxic surface projections
  3D surface anthropometry
  3D surface digitizer
  3D technique
  3D time-of-flight magnetic resonance (3D TOF MR) angiographic sequences
  3D transesophageal echocardiography
  3D Turbo-FLAIR (fluid-attenuated inversion recovery)
  3D turbo SE imaging
  3D ultrasound
three-head camera
three-head scan
3M scanner
three-part fracture
three-phase bone scintigraphy (TPBS)
three-vessel coronary disease
three-vessel runoff
three-way stopcock

thresher's lung
threshold, malignancy
thresholding method
thrombi (pl. of thrombus)
thromboatherosclerotic process
thromboembolus
thromboembolism
thromboembolization
  catheter-induced
  deep venous
  pulmonary
  venous
thrombolysis
  mechanical
  pharmacomechanical
  pulse-spray
thrombolytic therapy
thrombo-obliterative process
thromboresistance
ThromboScan MRU (molecular recognition units)
thrombosed
thrombosis
  intentional reversible
  syndrome of impending
  therapeutic
thrombostasis
thrombosuction catheter
thrombus
  calcified
  intramural
  mural
thrombus formation
through-and-through fracture
Thruflex PTCA balloon catheter
thumb, gamekeeper's
thumbprints (or thumbprinting) on surface of colon in barium enema
Thurston Holland sign
thymic cyst
thymoma of heart
thymus gland

thyrocardiac disease
thyrocervical trunk of subclavian artery
thyroglossal duct cyst
thyroid
  lingual
  multinodular
  substernal
thyroid artery
thyroid cartilage
thyroid dysgenesis
thyroid gland
  accessory
  enlarged
thyroid isthmus
thyroid lobe
thyroid nodule
thyroid radioiodine uptake
thyroid scan
thyroid stunning
thyroid suppression test
thyroid uptake
thyroiditis
thyroxine radioisotope assay ($T_4RIA$)
TI (inversion time)
TIA (transient ischemic attack)
TIB (tree-in-bud) pattern
"tib-fib" (tibia-fibula)
tibial artery disease
tibial crest
tibial flare
tibial obliterative thrombi
tibial outflow tracts, blind
tibial plafond fracture
tibial plateau fracture
tibial sesamoid ligament
tibial tendon
tibial torsion
tibial tuberosity
tibial-peroneal trunk
tibioastragalocalcaneal canal of Richet
tibiocalcaneal fusion
tibiocalcaneal joint complex

tibiocalcaneal ligament
tibiocalcaneal space
tibiofibular diastasis
tibiofibular fracture
tibionavicular ligament
tibioperoneal occlusive disease
tibiotalar angle
tibiotalocalcaneal fusion
tibiotarsal dislocation
TICA (traumatic intracranial aneurysm)
tidal wave of carotid arterial pulse
Tietze syndrome
TIFF (tag image file format)
tight lesion
Tillaux-Kleiger fracture
tilted optimized nonsaturating
  excitation (TONE)
time
  acceleration
  acquisition
  asymmetric appearance
  atrial activation
  atrioventricular
  data acquisition
  deceleration
  diastolic perfusion
  dwell
  echo (TE)
  echo delay
  ejection (ET)
  emptying
  esophageal transit
  gastric transit
  image acquisition
  interpulse
  inversion (TI)
  isovolumic contraction
  isovolumic relaxation (IVRT)
  left ventricular ejection (LVET)
  maximum inflation
  maximum walking (MWT)
  mean

time *(cont.)*
   myocardial contrast appearance (MCAT)
   perfusion
   pulmonary transit (PTT)
   pulse reappearance
   pyelographic appearance
   radionuclide esophageal dead
   reaction recovery
   real-
   recovery
   relaxation
   repetition (TR)
   resolving
   right ventricle-to-ear
   scan
   short echo
   sinoatrial conduction (SACT)
   sinus node recovery (SNRT)
   small-bowel transit
   spin-lattice proton relaxation
   systolic acceleration
   systolic upstroke
   T1 relaxation
   T2 relaxation
   transit
   venous filling (VFT)
   venous return (VRT)
   ventricular activation (VAT)
   ventricular isovolumic relaxation
time activity curve of contrast agent
time-attenuation curve
time-averaged flow
timed bolus delivery
time-density curve
timed imaging
time-insensitive
time-intensity curve
time-lapse quantitative computed tomography lymphography
time-of-flight (TOF)
time-of-flight angiography
time-of-flight echoplanar imaging
time-of-flight (TOF) magnetic resonance angiography
time-of-flight measurement
time-of-flight (TOF) PET imaging systems
time-out, ventriculoatrial
time-resolved imaging by automatic data segmentation (TRIADS)
time-sensitive
time to peak activity
time to peak contrast (TPC)
time to peak filling rate (TPFR)
TIMI (thrombolysis in myocardial infarction) classification
TIPS (transjugular intrahepatic portosystemic shunt)
tissue
   aberrant
   abnormal
   adventitial
   aerated
   areolar
   bony
   cartilaginous
   cavernous
   chondroid
   chorionic
   collagenous
   connective
   cortical
   crushed
   damaged
   dartoic
   dead
   degenerated
   dense
   destruction of
   ectopic
   exuberant
   fatty
   fibroadipose

tissue *(cont.)*
  fibroareolar
  fibrocartilaginous
  fibrofatty
  fibroglandular
  fibromuscular
  fibrosing
  fibrotic
  fibrous
  fibrous scar
  fibrovascular
  gangrenous
  gelatinous
  glandular
  granulation
  grumous
  hyperplastic
  hypertrophic
  interlobular
  isointense soft
  joint
  lipomatous-like
  lymph node
  lymphatic
  lymphoid
  lymphoreticular
  mesenchymal
  mesenteric
  muscle
  muscular
  necrotic
  neoplastic
  nodal
  noncritical soft
  nonviable
  osseous
  ossification of soft
  parenchymal
  periarticular
  proliferation of fibrous
  regeneration of
  scar

tissue *(cont.)*
  soft
  subadventitial
  subcutaneous
  synovial
  taenia
  tendon
  tuberculosis granulation
  underlying
tissue-based T2 relaxation
tissue-borne
tissue characterization technique
tissue contrast
tissue deficit compensator
tissue density
tissue Doppler imaging
tissue inhomogeneity factors
tissue mass
tissue migration
tissue outflow valve
tissue perfusion
tissue sequelae
tissue slice
tissue veil
tissue viability
titanium capsule
titanium plate
Tl (thallium)
TLC (triple-lumen catheter)
TLD (thermoluminescent dosimeter)
  rod
TLI (total lymphoid irradiation)
T loop (vectorcardiography)
TMA (true metatarsus adductus)
TME (trapezium-metacarpal
  eburnation)
TMJ (temporomandibular joint)
  syndrome
TMS three-dimensional radiation
  therapy planning system
TMST (treadmill stress test)
TNM classification of carcinoma

Todaro, triangle of
Todd cirrhosis
TOF (tetralogy of Fallot)
TOF (time-of-flight) magnetic resonance angiography
TOF PET (time-of-flight positron emission tomography)
Tolosa-Hunt syndrome
toluene scintillator
Tomocat contrast medium
tomogram (see *imaging*)
tomographic cut
tomographic section
tomographic slice
tomography (see *imaging*)
tomomyelography
tomoscanner, Philips T-60
tomoscintigraphy
T1 (longitudinal or spin-lattice relaxation time) constant
   T1 pulse sequence
   T1 relaxation time
   T1 weighted coronal image
   T1-weighted fat-suppressed images (T1FS)
   T1-weighted image (short TR/TE)
   T1-weighted sagittal image
T (thoracic)
T1-T12 (twelve thoracic vertebrae)
TONE (tilted optimized nonsaturating excitation)
tongue and trough bone
tongue of tissue
tongue-type fracture
tonsil, herniated cerebellar
tonus
toothpaste shadow
top normal limits in size
tophaceous gout
tophus (pl. tophi) formation
topical water-soluble contrast media
topodermatography

topogram (see *topography*)
topograph
topographic identification
topographic measurement
topography
   balloon
   scintigraphic balloon
   vessel
   x-ray
Torcon NB selective angiographic catheter
Tornwaldt cyst in nasopharynx
torr pressure
torsed appendage
torsion fracture
torsion of fracture fragment
torsional abnormalities
torsional alignment
torsional impaction force
torsional stress
torso phased-array coil (TPAC)
tortuosity and elongation
tortuosity precluding catheter passage
tortuous emptying
torus fracture
TOS (thoracic outlet syndrome)
Toshiba Aspire CI (continuous imaging)
Toshiba CT scanner
Toshiba echocardiograph machine
Toshiba helical CT scanner
Toshiba MR scanner
Toshiba 900S helical CT scanner
Toshiba 900S/XII scanner
Toshiba TCT-80 CT scanner
Toshiba Xpress scanner
Toshiba Xpress SX helical CT scanner
Toshiba Xvision scanner
total anomalous pulmonary venous drainage (TAPVD)
total atrial refractory period (TARP)

total body irradiation
total body scanning
Total-Cross PTA catheter
total fracture
total lymphoid irradiation (TLI)
Towne projection in skull x-rays
Towne view
toxic adenoma
toxic nodular goiter
toxicity, flutamide-associated liver
TPAC (torso phased-array coil)
TPBS (three-phase bone scintigraphy)
TPC (time to peak contrast)
TPFR (time to peak filling rate)
Tpot, flow cytometry
TPR (total peripheral resistance)
TPR (total pulmonary resistance)
TR (repetition time)
TR (tricuspid regurgitation)
TR/TE (repetition time/echo time),
    long (T2-weighted image)
    short (T1-weighted image)
trabecula (pl. trabeculae)
trabecular bone
trabecular pattern
trabeculated atrium
trabeculated outline
trabeculation, endocardial
trace (see *imaging agent*)
trace amount of radiopharmaceutical
trace element distribution
tracer accumulation
tracer activity
tracer bolus
tracer dose
tracer, neutron-rich biomedical
tracer uptake
trachea
    annular ligament of
    carina of
    scabbard
tracheal anastomosis

tracheal bifurcation
tracheal deviation
tracheal displacement
tracheal ring
tracheal shift
tracheal stenosis
tracheobronchial fistula
tracheobronchial foreign body
tracheobronchial tree
tracheoesophageal fistula (TEF)
tracheomalacia
tracing, vessel-
track cone length
Tracker catheter
track etching
tracking
    bolus
    magnetic resonance needle
    real-time biplanar needle
    real-time magnetic resonance
        imaging
tracking limit
tract
    alimentary
    ascending
    atriohisian
    Bekhterev
    biliary
    Bruce and Muir
    bulbar
    Burdach
    central tegmental
    cerebellorubral
    cerebellorubrospinal
    cerebellospinal
    cerebellotegmental
    cerebellothalamic
    comma tract of Schultze
    conariohypophyseal
    corticobulbar
    corticopontine
    corticorubral

**tract**

tract *(cont.)*
  corticospinal
  corticotectal
  crossed pyramidal
  cuneocerebellar
  Deiters
  dentatothalamic
  descending
  digestive
  direct pyramidal
  dorsolateral
  extracorticospinal
  extrapyramidal
  fastigiobulbar
  fistulous
  Flechsig
  flow
  frontopontine
  frontotemporal
  gastrointestinal (GI)
  geniculocalcarine
  geniculostriate
  genital
  genitourinary
  GI (gastrointestinal)
  Goll
  Gombault-Philippe
  Gowers
  habenulopeduncular
  Helweg
  hepatic outflow
  hypothalamicohypophysial
  ileal inflow
  intermediolateral
  internodal
  intersegmental
  interstitiospinal
  intestinal
  intrahepatic biliary
  Lissauer
  long
  Lowenthal

tract *(cont.)*
  lower
  Maissiat
  mammilopeduncular
  mammilotegmental
  mammilothalamic
  Marchi
  mesencephalic
  Meynert
  Monakow
  motor
  Muir and Bruce
  nigrostriate
  occipitopontine
  pancreaticobiliary
  paraventriculohypophysial
  parietopontine
  patent needle
  peduncular
  Philippe-Gombault
  pilonidal
  posterior spinocerebellar
  pulmonary conduit outflow
  pulmonary outflow
  pyramidal
  respiratory
  reticulospinal
  rubrobulbar
  rubroreticular
  Schultze comma
  Schutz
  semilunar
  sensory
  septomarginal
  sinus
  spinal
  spinocerebellar
  spinocervical
  spinocervicothalamic
  spinothalamic
  Spitzka-Lissauer
  strionigral

tract *(cont.)*
  sulcomarginal
  tectobulbar
  tectocerebellar
  tegmental
  tegmentospinal
  temporopontine
  testobulbar
  thalamo-olivary
  transverse
  triangular
  trigeminal nerve
  trigeminothalamic
  tuberohypophysial
  upper
  upper gastrointestinal (UGI)
  urinary
  uveal
  ventral amygdalofugal
  vestibulocerebellar
  Vicq d'Azyr
tract embolization
traction diverticulum
tragus
train, fast SE
tram track pattern on x-ray in Sturge-Weber syndrome
tramline cortical calcification
tramlines shadow
transabdominal scanning
transaortic radiofrequency ablation
transapical endocardial ablation
transarterial embolization
transaxial CT scan
transaxial images
transaxial maximum-intensity projection (MIP)
transaxial slice
transaxillary lateral view
transbronchial lung biopsy
transbronchial needle aspiration (TBNA)

transcapitate fracture
transcatheter ablation
transcatheter arterial chemo-embolization
transcatheter arterial embolization (TAE)
transcatheter filter placement
transcatheter introduction of intravascular stent
transcatheter oily chemoembolization
transcatheter therapy
  embolization
  infusion
transcatheter variceal embolization
transcervical balloon tuboplasty (TBT)
transcervical catheterization of fallopian tube
transcervical fracture
transchondral talar fracture
transchoroidal approach
transclival approach
transcondylar axis (TCA)
transcondylar fracture
transcranial color-coded duplex sonography
transcranial color-coded real-time sonography
transcranial Doppler (TCD) ultrasound (sonography)
transcutaneous extraction catheter atherectomy
transducer, sector
  Acuson linear array
  broadband
  catheter-borne
  epicardial Doppler flow
  linear
  M-mode
  magnetic resonance imaging-guided focused ultrasound
transect, transected
transection

transependymal uptake of tracer
transepiphyseal fracture
transesophageal Doppler color flow
   imaging
transesophageal echocardiography
   (TEE)
transesophageal imaging
transesophageal transducer
transfemoral arteriogram
transfer
   energy
   magnetization
   rapid image
   saturation
   ultrafast video
transfer mode, asynchronous (ATM)
transferrin receptor
transform
   cosine
   fast Fourier
   Fourier
   K-L
transformation matrix
transgluteal CT-guided technique
transhamate fracture
transhepatic cholangiography
transhepatic embolization (THE)
transient ischemic attack (TIA)
transient shunt obstruction
transillumination
transit, bolus
transit time
transition zone
transitional rhythm
transitional vertebra
transjugular cholangiogram
transjugular intrahepatic portosystemic
   shunt (TIPS)
translation-invariant filter
translocation of coronary arteries
translucency, first-trimester nuchal

translucent depression in interatrial
   septum
translumbar aortogram
translumbar aortography
transluminal angioplasty, percutaneous
   (PTA)
transluminal atherectomy
transluminal balloon angioplasty
transluminal coronary angioplasty
transluminal coronary artery
   angioplasty complex
transluminal dilatation
transluminal endatherectomy catheter
   (TEC)
transluminal extraction catheter (TEC)
transluminal lysing system
transluminally placed stented graft
transmalleolar axis (TMA)-thigh angle
transmedial plane
transmesenteric plication
transmetatarsal amputation (TMA)
transmission block
transmission control protocol/Internet
   protocol (TCP/IP)
transmission CT
transmission data
transmission dosimetry
transmission scan
transmitral flow
transmitral gradient
transmitted carotid artery pulsations
transmural cryoablation
transmural fibrosis
transmural match
transmural myocardial infarction
transmural steal
transmutation
transmyocardial perfusion pressure
transnasal endoluminal ultrasonography
   of GI tract
transnasally

transoral
transorally
transparent rendering
transpedicular decompression
transphyseal
transplant (or transplantation)
transport
  forward
  reverse
transporter, dopamine
transposed aorta
transposition
  atrial
  carotid-subclavian
  congenitally corrected
  corrected great arteries
  gastric
  great vessel
  Jatene
transposition cipher
transposition of great arteries (TGA)
  (great vessels)
  complete
  corrected (CTGA)
  partial (of great vessels)
transpulmonary echo ultrasound
  reflectors
transpulmonary pressure (PTP)
transpulmonic gradient
transradial styloid perilunate
  dislocation
transradiancy
transradiant air
transradiant zone
transrectal echography
transrectal ultrasound (TRUS)
transscaphoid perilunate dislocation
transsection, spinal cord
transseptal angiocardiography
transseptal left heart catheterization
transseptal perforation
transseptal puncture

transseptal radiofrequency ablation
transsyndesmotic screw fixation
transtentorial herniation
transtentorial
transtentorially
transthoracic echocardiography (TTE)
transthoracic imaging
transthoracic needle aspiration,
  ultrasound-guided
transthoracic needle biopsy (TNB)
transthoracic three-dimensional
  echocardiography
transtriquetral fracture-dislocation
transudate
transudation
transudation of fluid
transudative pericardial fluid
transurethral ultrasound-guided laser-
  induced prostatectomy (TULIP)
transurethral
transurethrally
transvaginal echography
transvaginal oocyte retrieval
transvaginal sonography
transvaginal ultrasound (TVS)
transvaginal uterine cervical dilation
  with fluoroscopic guidance
transvalvar (or transvalvular) gradient
transvenous implantation
transverse arch
transverse colon
transverse cord lesion
transverse diameter
transverse fracture
transverse heart
transverse hypoplasia
transverse ligaments of atlas
transverse magnetization
transverse orientation
transverse pelvic diameter
transverse plane
transverse plane forces

transverse presentation
transverse process
transverse relaxation rate
transverse section
transverse slice
transverse sinus
transverse ultrasound
trapeziometacarpal joint
trapezioscaphoid joint
trapeziotrapezoid joint
trapezium (greater multangular) bone
trapezius muscle
trapezoid (lesser multangular) bone
trapezoid bone of Henle
trapezoid bone of Lyser
trapezoid ligament
Trapper catheter exchange
trapping, air
trapping of radioisotope
Traube aortic regurgitation sign
Traube semilunar space
trauma
  acoustic
  birth
  blunt
  multiple
  penetrating
  physical
traumatic aneurysm
traumatic avulsion
traumatic brain injury (TBI)
traumatic dislocation
traumatic disruption
traumatic emphysema
traumatic infarct
traumatic intracranial aneurysm
traumatic meningeal hemorrhage
traumatic pneumothorax
traumatic pseudoaneurysm
traumatic rupture
traumatic spondylolisthesis (grades 1-4)
traumatic spondylolysis

traumatic thrombus
traumatogenic occlusion
traversing the fracture
Treacher Collins syndrome
treadmill exercise stress test
treadmill exercise test (TET)
treadmill inclination, incremental
  increases in
treadmill slope
treadmill speed, incremental
  increases in
treadmill stress test (TMST)
treatment energy
treatment port
tree
  arterial
  biliary
  bronchial
  coronary artery
  hepatobiliary
  iliocaval
  intrahepatic biliary
  lower extremity arterial
  tracheobronchial
tree artifact
tree-in-bud (TIB) pattern
tree-in-winter appearance
tree-like airway structure
tree-shaped spot on radiograph
trefoil balloon catheter
Treitz hernia
Treitz ligament
trend-correction
Trendelenburg position
Trevor disease
TRH (thyrotropin releasing hormone)
  stimulation test
$T_4$RIA (thyroxine radioisotope assay)
triad
  acute compression
  Charcot
  Dieulafoy

triad *(cont.)*
  hepatic
  portal
  Saint
  Whipple
TRIADS (time-resolved imaging by automatic data segmentation)
Triad SPECT imaging system
triangle
  anal
  aponeurotic
  auricular
  axillary
  Burger scalene
  Calot
  cardiohepatic
  carotid
  cephalic
  cervical
  clavipectoral
  Codman
  crural
  cystohepatic
  deltoideopectoral
  digastric
  Einthoven
  facial
  femoral
  Garland
  Gerhardt
  Grynfeltt
  Henke
  Hesselbach
  iliofemoral
  inguinal
  insular
  internal jugular
  Koch
  Korányi-Grocco
  Labbé
  Langenbeck
  Lesgaft

triangle *(cont.)*
  Livingston
  lumbocostoabdominal
  mesenteric
  paramedian
  Pawlik
  posterior
  scalene
  Scarpa
  submandibular
  supraclavicular
  Todaro
  urogenital
  vertebrocostal
  Ward
triangular area of dullness
triangular bone
triangular defect
triangular external ankle fixation
triangular fibrocartilage (TFC)
triangular fibrocartilage complex (TFCC)
triangular ligament
triangulation of Carrel
tributary (pl. tributaries)
trichinous embolism
tricuspid aortic valve
trifid stomach
triflanged nail
trifoil balloon
trifurcation of artery
trigeminal cavernous fistula
trigeminal cavity
trigeminal hemangioma
trigeminal nerve (fifth cranial nerve)
trigeminal pattern
trigeminy
triggering ventricular contraction
trigonal hypertrophy
trigone
  angles of
  collateral

trigone *(cont.)*
   deltoideopectoral
   fibrous
   Henke
   hypertrophied
   hypoglossal
   inguinal
   lateral ventricle
   Lieutaud
   Müller
   Pawlik
   vertebrocostal
Triguide guide catheter
triisocyanide $^{99m}$Tc imaging agent
trilaminar appearance
trilayer appearance
trileaflet
trilinear interpolation
trimalleolar fracture
Trionix camera
Trionix scanner
Trionix SPECT
triphasic spiral CT
triplane fracture
triple-dose gadolinium imaging
triple-head SPECT with FDG
triple-lumen central venous catheter
triple label
triple match
triple resonance NMR probe circuit
triple ripple
triplet beat
tripod position
tripolar electrode catheter
triquetral bone
triquetral fracture
triquetrohamate joint
triquetrohamate ligament
triquetrolunate dislocation
triradiate cartilage
trisacryl gelatin microspheres
tristimulus values

trochanter
   greater
   lesser
trochlear nerve (fourth cranial nerve)
trochlear notch
trochlear process
Troisier node
TRON 3 VACI cardiac imaging
   system
trophedema
trophic fracture
trophoblastic material
true channel
true conjugate
true lumen
truncal artery
truncal renal artery stenosis
truncal valve
truncated NMR probe
truncation band artifact
truncus arteriosus
   embryonic
   persistent
trunk
   articulations of
   atrioventricular (AV)
   bifurcation of
   brachiocephalic
   bronchomediastinal
   bronchomediastinal lymph
   celiac
   cordlike
   costocervical
   joints of
   lumbosacral
   lymph
   nerve
   posterior vagal
   thyrocervical
   vagal
Trunkey fracture classification system
TRUS (transrectal ultrasound)

Tru-Scint AD imaging agent
Tru-Trac high-pressure PTA balloon
TRW (teboroxime) resting washout
TS (tricuspid stenosis)
T-shaped fracture
TSH (thyroid-stimulating hormone)
  TSH-dependent functioning nodule
  TSH stimulation test
T spine (thoracic spine)
TSPP (technetium stannous pyrophos-
  phate) rectilinear bone scan
TTC (T-tube cholangiogram)
TTE (transthoracic echocardiography)
T3 resin uptake test
TTS (tarsal tunnel syndrome)
T-tube cholangiogram
T tubogram
T2 (transverse or spin-spin relaxation
    time) constant
  T2 pulse sequence
  T2 QMRI (T2 quantitative MRI)
  T2 relaxation time
  T2 shortening
  T2 star relaxation
  T2 time constant
  T2 weighted image (long TR/TE)
  T2 weighted spin-echo image
tubal insufflation
tubal pregnancy
tubal ring
tube
  anode
  auditory
  bilateral pleural
  blocked shunt
  bronchial
  calices (calyces)
  capillary
  cathode-ray
  Chaoul voltage x-ray
  chest
  collecting

tube *(cont.)*
  corneal
  cuffed endotracheal
  digestive
  double-lumen endobronchial
  endobronchial
  endotracheal (ET)
  enterolysis
  Eppendorf
  ET (endotracheal)
  eustachian
  fallopian
  feeding
  fenestrated
  J-shaped
  large-caliber
  muscular
  nasogastric (NG)
  nasotracheal
  neural
  NG (nasogastric)
  obstructed shunt
  oroendotracheal
  orogastric
  pharyngotympanic
  pickup
  pleural
  polyethylene
  right-angle chest
  separator
  Shiner radiopaque
  shunt
  solid-phase extraction
  stomach
  straight chest
  suction
  T-
  T self-retaining drainage
  tracheal
  uterine
  water-seal chest
  x-ray

tube current
tube drainage
tube geometry module of VIDA
tube position rotation
tuber cinereum
tubercle
  accessory
  acoustic
  adductor
  amygdaloid
  articular
  auricular
  calcaneal
  carotid
  Chaput
  conoid
  corniculate
  costal
  crown
  cuneiform
  darwinian
  dental
  dissection
  epiglottic
  fibrous
  genial
  genital
  Gerdy
  Ghon
  greater
  iliac
  intercondylar
  lesser
  Lister
  Parsons
  prominent
  pubic
  rib
  scalene
  sella turcica
  tibial

tubercle bacillus
tubercular empyema
tuberculoma
tuberculosis (TB)
  bone
  disseminated
  exudative
  fulminant
  genitourinary
  hematogenous
  inhalation
  meningeal
  miliary
  postprimary
  primary
  pulmonary
  renal
tuberosity (pl. tuberosities)
  bicipital
  calcaneal
  coracoid
  costal
  deltoid
  femoral
  greater
  iliac
  infraglenoid
  ischial
  lesser
  navicular
  omental
  radial
  tibial
  ulnar
tuberous sclerosis
tubogram
tuboplasty, balloon
tubular bone
tubular lesion
tubular magnet
tubular stenosis

tubular structure
tubule
  collecting
  connecting
  convoluted
  dental
  dentinal
  discharging
  distal convoluted
  proximal convoluted
  renal
  seminiferous
  straight
  tortuous
tuft fracture
tulip sheath
TULIP (transurethral ultrasound-guided laser-induced prostatectomy)
tumor
  apple core
  Askin
  benign
  Brenner
  carcinoid
  cavernous
  chondrogenic
  chordoma
  chromophobe adenoma
  clivus meningioma
  CNS (central nervous system)
  colloid cyst
  craniopharyngioma
  cutaneous
  cystic
  deep-seated
  discrete
  dumbbell
  echogenic
  embryonal
  ependymoma
  epidermoid
  Ewing

tumor *(cont.)*
  extension of
  extracompartmental
  extramedullary
  fatty
  fibroadenoma
  fibroid
  finger of
  focal
  ganglion
  globular
  gross
  highly vascular
  hourglass
  hypoechogenic
  intra-axial brain
  intracompartmental
  intracranial
  intradural
  intramedullary
  invasive
  Krukenberg
  lobulated
  locally invasive
  lymphoid
  main
  malignant
  metastatic
  microadenoma
  napkin ring
  nonechogenic
  non-neoplastic
  Pancoast
  papilloma
  pedunculated
  phyllodes
  pilocytic
  pinealoma
  pontine glioma
  poorly circumscribed
  poorly differentiated
  Pott puffy

tumor *(cont.)*
  primary
  prolactin-secreting adenoma
  pseudo-
  pseudomalignant
  radiosensitive
  RIF-1
  scirrhous
  secondary
  seeding of
  sessile
  smooth muscle
  solid
  spread of
  subcortical
  submucosal
  subserosal
  vascular
  Warthin (adenolymphoma)
  well-circumscribed
  Wharton (cystadenoma)
  Wilms
tumor-bearing bone
tumor bed
tumor blush on cerebral angiography
tumor boundary
tumor capillary permeability
tumor cleavage plane
tumor embolism
tumor embolization
tumor extirpation
tumorlike shadow
tumor marker
tumor mass
tumor matrix
tumor osteoid
tumor recurrence
tumor staining on cerebral angiography
tumor-to-normal brain ratio
tumor vascularity
tumor volume
tumor volumetry
tungsten eye shield
tungsten target
tunica adventitia
tunica intima
tunica media
tunica propria
tuning unit, reflectometer
tunnel
  carpal
  cubital
  retropancreatic
  tarsal
tunnel view
turbid effusion
turbinate bone
Turbo-FLAIR imaging
Turbo-FLASH sequence
turbo SE sequences
turbulence
turbulent flow
turbulent signal
turcica, sella
turf-toe
Turkish sabre syndrome
Turner marginal gyrus
turning-point morphology (TPM)
turricephaly
TV (tricuspid valve)
TV-interlaced (TVI)
T vector
TVS (transvaginal ultrasound)
twelfth cranial nerve (hypoglossal nerve)
twig
  cutaneous
  muscular
twinkling artifact
twin-to-twin transfusion syndrome (TTTS)
twin trunk
2-nitroimidazole nucleoside analog

24-bit image
270 MHz VT multinuclear spectrometer
two-channel phased array RF receiver coil system
2D (see *two-dimensional*)
two-dimensional (2D or 2-D)
    2D B-mode ultrasound machine
    2D color-coded imaging of blood flow
    2D echocardiography (sector scan)
    2D format
    2D Fourier imaging
    2D Fourier transform (2DFT)
    2DFT (two-dimensional Fourier transform)
    2D GRE dynamic protocol
    2D J-resolved 1H MR spectroscopy

two-dimensional *(cont.)*
    2D portal image registration
    2D pulsatility index mapping
    2D resistance index mapping
    2D sector scan
    2D spatially selective radiofrequency (RF) pulses
two-frame gated imaging
two-part fracture
two-phase computed tomographic imaging
two-phase helical computed tomography
two-vessel runoff
two-view chest x-ray
Tygon catheter
tympanic bone
type I, II, and III dens fracture
tyropanoate sodium contrast medium

# U, u

U (uranium)
UBM (ultrasound backscatter microscopy)
UC (ulcerative colitis)
UCG (ultrasonic cardiography)
UCL (ulnar collateral ligament)
UCLA imaging protocol
UEs (upper extremities)
UES (upper esophageal sphincter)
UFCT (ultrafast computed tomography)
UGI (upper gastrointestinal) series
UGI SBF (upper GI series with small-bowel follow-through)
Uhl syndrome
UHMM (ultra-high magnification mammography)
UJ (uncovertebral joint)
ulcer (ulceration)
   acid peptic
   active duodenal
   acute peptic
   amebic
   anastomotic
   anterior wall antral
   antral
   aortic

ulcer *(cont.)*
   arteriolar ischemic
   atheromatous
   atherosclerotic aortic
   Barrett
   bear claw
   benign
   bleeding
   bulbar peptic
   chronic
   chronic peptic
   collar button
   colonic mucosal
   craterlike
   Cruveilhier
   Curling
   Cushing
   Cushing-Rokitansky
   duodenal
   esophageal
   flask-shaped
   focal
   gastric
   gastrointestinal
   giant peptic
   greater curvature
   healing

ulcer *(cont.)*
    Hunner
    indolent
    intestinal
    intractable
    ischemic
    jejunal
    juxtapyloric
    kissing
    Kocher dilatation
    lesser curvature
    linear
    malignant
    marginal
    minute bleeding
    necrotic
    patchy colonic
    penetrating
    peptic
    perforated
    perforating
    postbulbar duodenal
    postsurgical recurrent
    prepyloric gastric
    punched-out
    punctate
    puncture
    pyloric channel
    radiation-induced
    rake
    recurrent
    Rokitansky-Cushing
    thorn
    round
    sea anemone
    secondary
    serpiginous
    stercoral
    stomach
    stomal
    stress
    trophic

ulcer *(cont.)*
    urinary
    V-shaped
ulcer base
ulcer bed
ulcer crater
ulcer osteoma
ulcer with heaped-up edges
ulcerated atheromatous plaque
ulcerated plaque
ulcerative colitis (UC)
ulna
ulnar abutment syndrome
ulnar bone
ulnar bursa
ulnar collateral ligament
ulnar deviation
ulnar extensor
ulnar facing of metacarpal heads
ulnar hand
ulnar nerve entrapment
ulnar nerve lesion
ulnar notch
ulnar pulse
ulnar sesamoid bone
ulnar styloid process
ulnar tubercle
ulnarward
ulnocarpal ligament
ulnolunate ligament
ulnotriquetral ligament
ULP (ultra low-profile) catheter
ultraearly thrombolytic therapy
ultrafast computed tomography
    (UFCT) scanner
ultrafast CT electron beam
    tomography
ultrafast video transfer
ultra-high magnification
    mammography (UHMM)
Ultraject pre-filled contrast media
    syringe

UltraLite flow-directed microcatheter
ultra-low profile fixed-wire balloon
    dilatation catheter
Ultramark 4 ultrasound
Ultramark 8 transducer
Ultramark 9 scanner
UltraPACS diagnostic imaging system
ultrasmall superparamagnetic iron
    oxide (USPIO) imaging agent
ultrasonically activated scalpel
ultrasonic aortography
ultrasonic aspiration
ultrasonic assessment
ultrasonic cardiogram
ultrasonic cardiography (UCG)
ultrasonic guidance for interstitial
    radioelement application
ultrasonic guidance for intrauterine
    fetal transfusion
ultrasonic guidance for placement of
    radiation therapy fields
ultrasonic knife, UltraCision
ultrasonic lithotripsy
ultrasonic nebulizer (USN)
ultrasonic scalpel
ultrasonic tomographic image
ultrasonographic catheter
ultrasonographic images,
    cross-sectional
ultrasonography
ultrasound (US)
    abdominal
    ACM (automated cardiac flow
        measurement)
    Acuson
    ADR
    AI 5200 diagnostic
    Aloka linear
    Aloke sector
    A-mode
    Aspen digital
    ATL real-time
ultrasound *(cont.)*
    BladderManager
    BladderScan
    B-mode
    breast
    Bruel-Kjaer
    color-coded duplex
    color-coded real-time
    color Doppler
    color duplex
    color power transcranial Doppler
    compression
    contact B-scan
    continuous wave
    contrast-enhanced
    cranial
    CUSALap
    diagnostic
    diagnostic range
    Diasonics
    diathermy
    DIMAQ integrated
    Doppler
    duplex
    duplex B-mode
    duplex carotid
    duplex Dopper
    duplex pulsed-Doppler
    DUST (dynamic ultrasound of
        shoulder)
    Echo-Gen enhanced
    endoanal
    endorectal
    endoscopic (EUS)
    endovaginal
    endovascular
    EUS (endoscopic ultrasonography)
    fatty meal (FMS)
    fetal
    5 MHz
    freehand interventional
    frequency domain imaging (FDI)

ultrasound *(cont.)*
  full-bladder
  gallbladder
  gastrointestinal endoscopic
  GI (gastrointestinal) endoscopic
  graded compression
  gray-scale
  Hewlett-Packard
  high-frequency therapeutic
  high-intensity focused (HIFU)
  high-resolution
  Hitachi
  immersion B-scan
  intracaval endovascular (ICEUS)
  intracavitary prostate
  intracoronary
  intraoperative
  intraportal endovascular
  intrarectal
  intravascular (IVUS)
  Irex Exemplar
  laparoscopic (LUS)
  laparoscopic contact (LCU)
  laparoscopic intracorporeal (LICU)
  low-intensity pulsed
  M-mode
  MUSTPAC (medical ultrasound 3D portable, with advanced communications)
  neonatal adrenal
  NeuroSector
  noninvasive
  obstetric
  Olympus endoscopic
  pancreaticobiliary (or pancreatic-biliary)
  pelvic
  Pentax EUP-EC124 ultrasound gastroscope
  Pentax-Hitachi FG32UA endosonographic system
  photoacoustic

ultrasound *(cont.)*
  power Doppler
  PowerVision
  pulsed
  pulsed Doppler
  real-time
  rectal endoscopic
  renal
  RT 3200 Advantage
  RT 6800
  sagitta
  Siemens Sonoline Elegral
  SieScape
  single-field hyperthermia combined with radiation therapy and
  Sonicator portable
  Synergy
  three-dimensional (3D) freehand
  two-dimensional (2D) B-mode
  transcranial color-coded duplex
  transcranial Doppler (TCD)
  transnasal endoluminal
  transrectal (TRUS)
  transthoracic
  transvaginal (TVS)
  transverse
  TRUS (transrectal ultrasound)
  Ultramark 4
  VingMed
ultrasound backscatter microscopy (UBM)
ultrasound diffraction tomography
ultrasound echocardiography
ultrasound-enhanced stylet, INRAD HiLiter
ultrasound for foreign body detection
ultrasound gel
ultrasound-guided percutaneous interstitial laser ablation
ultrasound-guided stereotactic biopsy
ultrasound-guided transthoracic needle aspiration

ultrasound-guided TULIP (transurethral laser-induced prostatectomy)
ultrasound hyperthermia treatment
ultrasound imaging technology
ultrasound monitoring
ultrasound pad
ultrasound probe, Olympus UM-1W transendoscopic
ultrasound scanning, high-resolution
ultrasound system (see *ultrasound*)
ultrasound venography
UltraSTAR computer-based ultrasound reporting system
ultrastructural abnormality
Ultravist (iopromide) imaging agent
UM 4 real-time sector scanner
umbilical artery
umbilical catheter
umbilical cord
 three-vessel
 two-vessel
umbilical hernia
UMI catheter
unattached fractions
unbuttoning of device
uncalcified pleural plaque
uncal gyrus
uncal herniation syndrome
uncertainty principle
unciform bone
uncinate aura
uncinate gyrus
uncinate process of pancreas
uncinate region of temporal lobe
uncommitted metaphyseal lesion
uncommon pneumoconioses
uncomplicated myocardial infarction
uncontrolled bronchospasm
uncoupled spins
uncovertebral joint (UJ)
uncovertebral spurring

uncus, arachnoid of
uncus corporis
undercorrection
underdetection
underdrive termination
under fluoroscopic guidance
underinflation of lung
underloading, ventricular
underperfused
underperfusion
under-scan method/projection
undersurface
underventilation
undifferentiated nasopharyngeal carcinoma (UCNT)
undisplaced fracture
undulant impulse
undulating contour
undulating course
unenhanced magnetic resonance imaging scan
unfused physis
unguicular tuberosity
unicameral bone cyst
unicameral brain
unicommissural aortic valve
unicommissural valve
unicompartmental knee prosthesis
unicorn
unicornuate uterus
unicoronal synostosis
unicortical screw
unicusp with central raphe
unicuspid aortic valve
unidirectional lead configuration
unifascicular block
unifocal
unifocalization
uniform attenuation coefficient
uniform loading
uniform resource locator (URL)
uniform sensitivity

uniform TR (repetition time)
   excitation
uniformly progressive deterioration
unigravida
unilateral fragmentation
union
   bony
   delayed fracture
   faulty
   fibrous
   osseous
   secondary
   vicious
union of fracture fragments
unipara
uniphasic contrast medium
unit
   BICAP
   EMI
   gamma
   Hounsfield (HU)
   HU (Hounsfield)
   Leksell gamma
   linear accelerator
   musculotendinous
   reflectometer tuning
   rutherford (rd)
   Sheffield gamma
   stepdown
   Wood (of pulmonary vascular resistance)
unit of measure
   becquerel (Bq)
   centigray (cGy)
   centimeter (cm)
   cubic centimeter (cc)
   deciliter (dl)
   femtoliter (fL)
   gauss (G)
   gram (g)
   gray (Gy)
   international unit (IU)

unit of measure *(cont.)*
   joule (J)
   kelvin (K)
   kiloelectron volt (keV or kev)
   kilogram (kg)
   kilohertz (kHz)
   kilometer (km)
   liter (L)
   megacurie (MCi)
   megahertz (MHz)
   meter (m)
   microcurie
   milliampere (mA)
   millicurie (mCi)
   milliequivalent (mEq)
   milligram (mg)
   milliliter (ml)
   millimeter (mm)
   millimeter of mercury (mm Hg)
   millimole (mmol)
   milliroentgen (mR)
   milliunit (mU)
   rad (radiation absorbed dose)
   roentgen (R)
   tesla (T)
univentricular heart
University of Florida LINAC (linear accelerator)
Unix/X11 workstation
unleveling, pelvic
unmitigated (unrelieved)
unmodulated radiofrequency current
unmyelinated nerve fibers
unopacified
unopacification
unopposed images
unreliable marker
unresectable
unresolved pneumonia
unresponsive programming
unroofed coronary sinus syndrome
unroofing of nerve

unshunted hydrocephalus
unstable angina
unstable fracture
unsuppressed exam
untether
untethered
ununited (nonunited) fracture
U-1100 UV-Vis spectrophotometer
   (also U-2001, U-2010, U-3000,
   U-3010, U-3300, U-3310)
U1-NA cephalometric measurement
up-regulation, radiation-induced
uPACS picture archiving system
updraft therapy
UPJ (ureteropelvic junction)
upper airway obstruction, foreign
   body
upper collecting system
upper gastrointestinal series
upper GI (gastrointestinal) series
upper GI with small bowel follow-
   through
upper-limb cardiovascular syndrome
upper limits of normal
upper lobe vein prominence
upper lung field
upper mantle radiotherapy
upper pole collecting system
upper pole moiety
upper pole ureter
upper rate interval
upper respiratory tract disease
upright chest film
upright PA (posteroanterior) film
upright post-void view
upright view
UP7 film
Upshaw-Schulman syndrome
upstairs-downstairs heart
upstream blood
upstroke, carotid pulse
upstroke phase of cardiac action
   potentials

uptake (of organ)
   contrast
   diffuse
   dye
   fluorescein
   focal
   heterogeneous
   localized
   observed maximal
   predicted maximal
   radioiodine
   radioisotope
   radiotracer
   tracer
   uniform
uptake and excretion
uptake and retention
uptake in radionuclide scan
upward and backward dislocation
upward retraction
uranium (U)
   $^{235}$U (uranium-235)
uremia
uremic pneumonitis
ureter
   atonic
   circumcaval
   dilatation of
   dilated
   ectopic
   intravesical
   kinked
   moderately dilated
   orthotopic
   postcaval
   retrocaval
   retroiliac
   rigid
   straight
   tortuosity of
ureteral achalasia
ureteral bud, accessory

ureteral calculus
ureteral catheter
ureteral compression technique
ureteral dilatation
ureteral distention
ureteral division
ureteral filling defect
ureteral fistula
ureteral notching
ureteral occlusion
ureteral reflux study
ureteral stasis
ureteral stenosis
ureteral stent
ureteral stricture
ureterectasis
ureterocele
ureterocutaneous fistula
ureterogram, retrograde
ureterography
ureterohydronephrosis
ureteropelvic junction (UPJ) obstruction
ureteropyelogram, retrograde
ureteropyelography
ureterovaginal fistula
ureterovesical junction, competence of
urethra
   angle of inclination of
   anterior
   bulbous
   membranous
   pendulous
   penile
   posterior
   prostatic
urethral atresia
urethral induration
urethral stricture
urethral trauma
urethral valve
urethrocystogram

urethrocystography
   retrograde
   voiding (VCU)
urethrogram, retrograde
urethrovesical angle (UVA)
urinary extravasation
urinary fistula
urinary tract
urine
   postvoid residual
   radiopaque
   residual
   retained
URL (uniform resource locator)
urogenital diaphragm
Urografin 290 imaging agent
urogram
urography
   antegrade
   excretory
   intravenous
   retrograde
urokinase protocol
UroLume flow-directed microcatheter
urothelial striations
Urovist Cysto imaging agent
Urovist Meglumine imaging agent
Urovist Sodium imaging agent
US (ultrasound, ultrasonography)
US (under-scan) method/projection
USCI Mini-Profile balloon dilatation catheter
uterine adenomyosis
uterine cirsoid aneurysm
uterine didelphia
uterine fibroid, pedunculated
uterine myoma (pl. myomata)
uterine neck
uterocervical
uterogram
uterography
uteropelvic

uterosalpingography
uterotubography
uterovesical
uterus
   anteflexed
   anteverted
   aplastic
   bicameral
   bicornis
   bicornuate
   biforate
   bilocular
   bipartite
   cervix of
   cochleate
   cornu of
   Couvelaire
   didelphic
   double
   double-mouthed
   duplex
   fetal
   fibroid
   gravid

uterus *(cont.)*
   heart-shaped
   horn of
   infantile
   isthmus of
   pear-shaped
   pregnant
   pubescent
   retroflexed
   retroverted
   ribbon
   round ligament of
   saddle-shaped
   septate
   unicornuate
   prostatic
   urethral
utricle
utricular
utriculus (utricle)
UV (ultraviolet)
UVA (urethrovesical angle)
uvula, cerebellar
uvula palatina

# V, v

V (lung volume)
V (ventricular)
VA (ventriculoatrial)
    VA conduction
    VA interval
V-angle, femoral torsion
VABES (vasoablative endothelial sarcoma)
vacuum cleft
vacuum disk
vacuum, facet joint
vacuum joint phenomenon
vagina
    anterior fornix of
    azygos artery of
    double
    fornix of
    vestibule of
vaginal cone irradiation
vaginal ligament of hand
vaginogram
vagus (tenth cranial) nerve
vagus trunk
valgus
    adolescent hallux
    hallux (HV)

valgus *(cont.)*
    hindfoot
    metatarsus
    pes
    talipes
valgus carrying angle
valgus deformity
valgus foot
valgus fracture, impacted
valgus heel
valgus tilt
vallecula cerebelli
valley-to-peak dose rate
Valsalva maneuver
value
    attenuation
    bright pixel
    comparative
    CT attenuation
    dark pixel
value flips
    negative predictive
    P
    positive predictive
    predictive
    tristimulus

valvar aortic stenosis
valve
  absent
  aortic (AV)
  Bauhin
  bicuspid
  bileaflet
  billowing mitral
  blunting of
  calcified
  capillary
  cardiac
  caval
  cleft
  competent
  conduit
  congenital absence of
  coronary
  coronary sinus
  disc-type
  doming of
  dysplastic
  early opening of
  echo-dense
  eustachian
  extirpation of
  failed
  fibrotic
  flail
  flexible
  floppy
  foramen ovale
  frenulum of
  globular
  hammocking of
  Heimlich
  Heister
  Houston
  hypoplastic
  ileocecal
  Kerckring
  leaky

valve *(cont.)*
  mitral (MV)
  monocusp
  narrowed
  native
  notching of
  parachute mitral
  premature closure of
  prosthetic heart
  pulmonic
  pulmonary (PV)
  pyloric
  quadricuspid pulmonary
  rectal
  regurgitation of
  rheumatic heart
  semilunar (aortic and pulmonary)
  sigmoid
  spiral
  stenotic
  synthetic
  thebesian
  tilting-disk valve
  track
  tricuspid (TV)
  tricuspid aortic
  trileaflet aortic
  truncal
  unicommissural
  urethral
  vegetation of
  venous
  Vieussens
  xenograft
valve attenuation
valve calcification
valve cusps
valved conduit
valve dehiscence
valve incompetence
valve leaflets
valve outflow strut

valve plane
valve pockets
valve replacement
valve scarring
valve strut
valve thickening and scarring
valve tip
valviform
valvular aortic insufficiency
valvular aortic stenosis
valvular apparatus
valvular atresia
valvular cardiac defect
valvular damage
valvular disease
valvular dysfunction
valvular heart disease
valvular incompetence
valvular opening
valvular orifice
valvular pneumothorax
valvular pulmonic stenosis
valvular regurgitant lesion
valvular regurgitation
valvular stenosis
VAN (vein, artery, nerve)
vanishing lung syndrome (on x-ray)
Vaquez disease
variability
   anatomic
   beat-to-beat
   interpretive
   peak flow
variable-angle uniform signal excitation (VUSE)
variable energy
variable flip angle excitation
variable murmur
variable response rate
Varian Associates 11.7T (500 MHz)/51 mm bore spectrometer
Varian brachytherapy system

Varian LINAC (linear accelerator)
Varian NMR spectrometer
variance images
variant
   anatomic
   labral
   ossification
variant angina pectoris
variation
   area/hemidiameter
   BO field
   exposure
   normal anatomic
   positional
variation in density
variceal column
variceal hemorrhage
variceal sclerotherapy
varices (pl. of varix)
varicocele, idiopathic
varicography
varicose aneurysm
varicose bronchiectasis
varicose vein
varicosity (pl. varicosities)
Variflex catheter
VARIS radiation oncology system
varix (pl. varices)
varum, genu
varus
   metatarsus
   rearfoot
   subtalar
   talipes
   tibial
varus angle
varus deformity
varus heel
varus metatarsophalangeal (MTP) angle
varus tilt
VAS (vestibular aqueduct syndrome)

Vas-Cath catheter for percutaneous thromboarterectomy
Vas-Cath PTA balloon catheter
Vascoray imaging agent
vascular access
vascular accident
vascular anastomosis
vascular anomaly
vascular atrophy
vascular attachments
vascular bed, pulmonary
vascular blush (on carotid angiography)
vascular bud
vascular bundle
vascular catastrophe
vascular channels, aberrant
vascular cirrhosis
vascular compromise
vascular congestion
vascular cord damage
vascular disease, peripheral
vascular ectasia
vascular encasement
vascular engorgement
vascular enhancement
vascular flasks
vascular flow imaging
vascular graft
vascular hamartoma
vascular hemangioma
vascular heterograft
vascular hydraulic conductivity
vascular impedance
vascular insult
vascular invasion
vascular lumen
vascular malformation
vascular markings
vascular network
vascular obstruction
vascular occlusive disease
vascular patency
vascular pedicle
vascular phase
vascular plexus
vascular protrusion
vascular redistribution
vascular reserve
vascular resistance
vascular ring
vascular segmentation and extraction
vascular sling
vascular spasm
vascular supply
vascular syndrome
vascular systemic resistance
vascular tone
vascular tuft
vascular wall
vascular xenograft
vascularity
vasculature
vasculitic lesion
vasoconstriction
vasodepressive
vasodepressor reaction (VDR)
vasodilate
vasodilation
vasodilatation
vasography
vasopressor
vasoreactivity, pulmonary
vasospasm
vasospastic vessel
vasovagal phenomenon
VasoView balloon dissection system
vastus lateralis muscle
vastus medialis advancement (VMA)
vastus medialis muscle
vastus medialis obliquus (VMO)
VAT (vaso-occlusive angiotherapy)

VAT (ventricular activation time)
Vater
　ampulla of
　papilla of
VATER (acronym for vertebral or vascular defects, anorectal malformation, tracheoesophageal fistula, and radial, ray, or renal anomaly)
Vater diverticulum
vaterian segment
VATS (video-assisted thoracic surgery)
vault
　cranial
　plantar
　rectal
VAX 4100 system
VBI (vertebrobasilar insufficiency)
VC (vital capacity)
VCB (ventricular capture beat)
VCF (ventricular contractility function)
VCG (vectorcardiogram)
$VCO_2$ (venous $CO_2$ production)
VCUG (vesicoureterogram)
VCUG (voiding cystourethrogram)
VD (valvular disease)
VDI (venous distensibility index)
VDR (vasodepressor reaction)
VDS (ventral derotating spinal)
VEA (ventricular ectopic activity)
VEB (ventricular ectopic beat)
vector
　expression
　mean cardiac
vectocardiogram
vectorcardiography
　Frank
　frontal plane
　sagittal plane
　spatial
　transverse plane
vector loop

vegetation of valve
vein (pl. veins)
　accessory cephalic
　accessory hemiazygos
　accessory saphenous
　accessory vertebral
　accompanying
　anal
　anastomosing
　anastomotic
　aneurysmal
　angular
　anonymous
　antebrachial
　antecubital
　anterior cardiac
　anterior jugular
　anterior terminal (ATV)
　appendicular
　aqueous
　arciform
　arcuate
　arterial
　ascending lumbar
　auditory
　auricular
　autogenous
　axillary
　azygos
　basal
　basal vein of Rosenthal (BVR)
　basilic
　basivertebral
　Boyd perforating
　brachial
　brachiocephalic
　bronchial
　bulb of
　cannulated central
　capacious
　capillary
　cardiac

**vein**

vein *(cont.)*
    cardinal
    cavernous
    central
    cephalic
    cerebral
    cervical
    choroid
    ciliary
    circumflex
    colic
    common basal
    common cardinal
    common facial
    communicating
    companion
    condylar emissary
    congenital stenosis of
    conjunctival
    coronary
    costoaxillary
    cutaneous
    cystic
    deep
    digital
    dilated
    diploic
    distended
    Dodd perforating group of
    dorsispinal
    duodenal
    embryonic umbilical
    emissary
    engorged
    epigastric
    episcleral
    esophageal
    ethmoidal
    external jugular
    external pudendal
    facial
    familial varicose

vein *(cont.)*
    feeder
    femoral
    fibular
    flat neck
    frontal
    gastric
    gastroepiploic
    great cardiac
    great cerebral vein of Galen
    great saphenous
    harvested
    hemiazygos
    hepatic
    ileocolic
    iliofemoral
    inferior pulmonary
    inferior rectal
    inferior thyroid
    infradiaphragmatic
    innominate
    intercostal
    internal cerebral (ICV)
    internal jugular
    internal thoracic
    intussusception of
    jugular
    Labbé
    labial
    leaking
    left hepatic
    lesser saphenous
    lobe of azygos
    marginal
    Marshall
    median antebrachial
    medullary
    meningeal
    mesenteric
    middle cardiac
    middle rectal
    nodularity

vein *(cont.)*
  oblique
  palmar cutaneous
  pancreatic
  paraumbilical
  parent
  pericardial
  peroneal
  portal
  posterior auricular
  posterior interventricular
  posterior terminal (PTV)
  prepyloric
  pudendal
  pulmonary
  pulsating
  renal
  Retzius
  reversed
  Rosenthal basal
  saphenous
  sausaging of
  Schlesinger
  scimitar
  scrotal
  septal
  small cardiac
  small saphenous
  soleal
  spermatic
  splenic
  subclavian
  subcutaneous
  superficial
  superficial femoral
  superior intercostal
  superior mesenteric (SMV)
  superior pulmonary
  superior rectal
  systemic
  testicular

vein *(cont.)*
  thalamostriate
  thebesian
  thoracoepigastric
  tortuous
  varicose
  vermian
  vertebral
vein graft
  blood flow patterns in
  color-flow duplex imaging of
  patency of
vein graft occlusion
vein graft stenosis
vein graft thrombosis
vein of Retzius
vein patch angioplasty
vein patency
vein sign
velocimetry, laser Doppler
velocity
  blood flow
  closing
  coronary blood flow (CBFV)
  decreased closing
  diastolic regurgitant
  fiber-shortening
  forward
  maximal transaortic jet
  mean aortic flow
  mean posterior wall
  mean pulmonary flow
  meter per second (m/sec)
  muzzle velocity in handgun injury
  peak aortic flow
  peak flow
  peak pulmonary flow
  peak systolic
  peak transmitted
  regurgitant
velocity-encoded magnetic resonance imaging

velocity encoding on brain magnetic
   resonance angiography
velocity mapping, phase
velocity-time integral of early diastole
velocity-time integral of late diastole
velocity waveforms (VWFs)
velopharyngeal closure
velum
vena cava (pl. venae cavae)
   inferior (IVC)
   infrahepatic
   superior (SVC)
   suprahepatic
vena cava (or caval) filter
vena cava syndrome
vena comitans (pl. venae comitantes)
venacavography
venetian blind artifact
venoarterial shunting
venodilators
venofibrosis
venogram
venography
   adrenal
   cerebral CT
   contrast
   conventional
   epidural
   free hepatic
   hepatic
   iliac
   intraosseous
   isotope
   lower limb
   MR
   portal
   radionuclear
   radionuclide
   selective
   splenic
   technetium Tc99m

venography *(cont.)*
   vertebral
   wedged hepatic
veno-occlusive disease (VOD)
venostasis
venous access
venous angioma
venous anomaly
venous backflow
venous blood, arterialization of
venous blood gas values
venous cannula
venous capillaries
venous catheter
venous channel, deep
venous circulation
venous congestion
venous decompensation
venous defects
venous distention
venous Doppler exam
venous embolus
venous engorgement
venous excursion
venous filling
   early
   late
venous gangrene
venous hyperemia
venous hypertension
venous injection
venous insufficiency
venous junction
venous lake
venous malformation (VM)
venous motion
venous obstruction
venous oxygen content
venous plexus
venous pooling
venous pressure

venous pulse, trough of
venous refill time (VRT)
venous reflux
venous reservoir
venous return
   anomalous pulmonary
   total anomalous
venous scan
venous segment, nonfilling
venous sinus
venous spasm
venous stasis
venous thromboembolic disease (VTED)
venous thromboembolism
venous thrombosis
venous ulcer
venous valve
venous vascular malformation
venous wave form
ventilation
   airway pressure release
   alveolar (VA)
   high minute
   maximal voluntary (MVV)
   mechanical
   minute
   partial liquid
   reduced alveolar
   uneven
   volume-controlled inverse ratio
   volume-cycled
ventilation defect
ventilation image
ventilation lung scan
ventilation-perfusion defect
ventilation-perfusion ratio
ventilation-perfusion (V/Q) lung scan
ventilation phase
ventilation scan
ventilatory capacity-demand imbalance
ventilatory defect, restrictive

ventilatory dysfunction
ventilatory effort
ventilatory failure
Ventra PTA catheter
ventral aorta
ventral branch
ventral cochlear nucleus
ventral hernia
ventral spinocerebellar tracts
ventral spinothalamic tracts
ventral surface
ventricle (of brain, heart, larynx)
   absent
   akinetic left
   apex of left
   Arantius
   atrialized
   atrium of
   augmented filling of
   auxiliary
   ballooned floor of
   cephalic
   cerebral
   common
   compensatory enlargement of
   dilatation of
   dilated
   double-inlet
   dual
   Duncan (fifth)
   dysfunctional
   effacement of
   elongation of
   enlargement of
   fifth
   floor of
   fourth
   frontal horn of lateral
   Galen
   hypokinetic
   hypoplastic
   laryngeal

ventricle *(cont.)*
   lateral
   left (LV)
   loculate
   Mary Allen Engle
   Morgagni
   outflow of
   papilloma of the fourth
   parchment right
   pineal
   primitive
   right (RV)
   roof of
   rudimentary
   shift of
   single
   sixth (Verga)
   slit
   Sylvius
   temporal horn of lateral
   terminal
   thick-walled
   third
   thrusting
   tiny
   trigone of
   tubular
   Verga
ventricles of brain
ventricular aberration
ventricular activation time (VAT)
ventricular actuation, direct mechanical (DMVA)
ventricular afterload
ventricular aneurysm
ventricular apex
ventricular assist device (VAD)
ventricular capture beat
ventricular catheter blockage
ventricular cavity
ventricular cineangiogram
ventricular contraction pattern

ventricular couplets
ventricular D-loop
ventricular decompensation
ventricular depolarization
ventricular depression
ventricular dilatation
ventricular disproportion
ventricular drainage
ventricular dysfunction
ventricular dysrhythmia
ventricular ectopy
ventricular effective refractory period (VERP)
ventricular ejection fraction
ventricular elastance, maximum (EMAX)
ventricular electrical instability
ventricular enlargement
ventricular escape mechanism
ventricular extrastimulation
ventricular failure
ventricular filling
ventricular free wall thickness
ventricular function, compromised
ventricular function curve
ventricular function parameters
ventricular gallop
ventricular gradient
ventricular hypertrophy
ventricular intracerebral hemorrhage
ventricular inversion
ventricular irritability
ventricular left-handedness
ventricular myocardium
ventricular myxoma
ventricular obstruction
ventricular overdrive pacing
ventricular paroxysmal tachycardia
ventricular perforation
ventricular pre-excitation
ventricular premature contraction couplets

ventricular pressure, right
ventricular pseudoperfusion beats
ventricular puncture
ventricular rate
ventricular reflux
ventricular refractoriness
ventricular refractory period
ventricular repolarization
ventricular reservoir
ventricular response
ventricular right-handedness
ventricular segmental contraction
ventricular sensed (VS) event
ventricular septal (VS)
ventricular septal aneurysm
ventricular septal defect (VSD), Swiss cheese
ventricular septal summit
ventricular shift
ventricular single and double extrastimulation
ventricular size
ventricular space
ventricular span
ventricular standstill
ventricular status
ventricular stiffness
ventricular synchrony
ventricular system
ventricular systole
ventricular tachycardia (VT, V tach)
ventricular transposition
ventricular wall motion
ventricularization of pressure
ventriculoarterial conduit
ventriculoarterial connections
ventriculoarterial discordance
ventriculoatrial (VA) conduction
ventriculoatrial effective refractory period
ventriculoatrial time-out

ventriculogram
  axial left anterior oblique
  bicycle exercise radionuclide
  biplane
  bubble
  digital subtraction
  dipyridamole thallium
  exercise radionuclide
  first-pass radionuclide
  gated blood pool
  gated nuclear
  gated radionuclide
  intraoperative
  LAO (left anterior oblique) projection
  left (LVG)
  metrizamide
  radionuclide (RNV)
  RAO (right anterior oblique) projection
  retrograde left
  single plane left ventriculography
  xenon 133 ($^{133}$Xe)
ventriculogram
ventriculography
ventriculoinfundibular fold
ventriculomegaly
ventriculoperitoneal (VP)
ventriculoradial dysplasia
ventriculovenous shunt
ventriculus cordis
ventriculus terminalis
Venturi effect
venule (pl. venules)
Verbatim balloon catheter
verge, anal
vergence, downward
vermian medulloblastoma
vermian veins
vermicular appendage

vermicular appendix
vermiform process
vermis
  cerebellar
  folium
vernix membrane
VERP (ventricular effective refractory period)
vertebra (pl. vertebrae)
  arch of
  articular process of
  basilar
  caudal
  cervical (C1 through C7)
  coccygeal
  codfish
  cranial
  displaced
  dorsal (D)
  facet surface of
  false
  fractured
  fused
  last normal (LNV)
  lumbar (L1 through L5)
  midbody of
  olisthetic
  pear-shaped
  sacral (S1 through S5)
  scalloping of
  subluxed
  thoracic (T1 through T12)
  transitional
  transverse process of
  true
  wedging of olisthetic
vertebral ankylosis
vertebral arterial dissection
vertebral artery occlusion
vertebral artery syndrome
vertebral artery system
vertebral-basilar artery syndrome
vertebral-basilar ischemia
vertebral basilar insufficiency
vertebral body collapse
vertebral body endplate
vertebral collapse
vertebral column
vertebral endplate
vertebral pleural reflection
vertebral scalloping
vertebral segmentation anomaly
vertebral steal phenomenon
vertebral stripe
vertebral vein
vertebral venous plexus
vertebra plana fracture
vertebrobasilar circulation
vertebrobasilar disease
vertebrobasilar distribution stroke
vertebrobasilar insufficiency (VBI)
vertebrobasilar ischemia
vertebrobasilar occlusion
vertebrobasilar system
vertebrocostal rib
vertebrophrenic angle
vertebrosternal rib
vertex, cube
vertex presentation
Vertex camera
vertex (pl. vertices)
vertical fracture
vertical heart
vertical-long axial (VLA) images
vertical long-axis slice
vertical plane
vertical shear fracture
vertical talus
VERT software
vesalianum of vertebral body
vesical (adj.)
vesical calculus, radiopaque
vesical distention
vesical injury

vesical neck
vesical outlet obstruction
vesical stone
vesicle
  acoustic
  acrosomal
  air
  allantoic
  auditory
  cerebral
  cervical
  encephalic
  graafian
  malpighian
  pulmonary
  seminal
vesicoureteral reflux
vesicoureteral scintigram
vesicoureterogram
vesicoureterography (VCUG)
vesicourethral angle
vesicovaginal fistula
vesicula (pl. vesiculae)
vesicular emphysema
vesiculography
vessel (pl. vessels)
  afferent
  afferent lymph
  angiographically occult
  anomalous
  arcuate
  atherectomized
  blood
  brachiocephalic
  caliber of
  capillary
  chyle
  circumflex
  codominant
  collateral
  collecting
  commencement of

vessel *(cont.)*
  contralateral
  cranial
  cross-pelvic collateral
  culprit
  curved
  deep lymph
  diminutive
  disease-free
  distal runoff
  dominant
  eccentric
  efferent
  efferent lymph
  end-on
  extracranial
  feeding
  gastroepiploic
  great
  heart and great
  in-plane
  infrapopliteal
  intercostal
  interlobular
  internal pudendal
  intracranial
  intradural
  kidney
  lymph
  lymphatic
  musculophrenic
  nondominant
  occipital
  origin of a
  patent
  perforator
  peripelvic collateral
  peripheral
  peroneal
  pial
  plump
  pole of

vessel *(cont.)*
　posterior lumbar
　renal
　runoff
　splanchnic
　splenic
　superficial lymph
　superior gluteal
　takeoff of a
　tortuous
　transposition of
　vasospastic
　vessels
　wraparound
vessel caliber
vessel closure, abrupt
vessel cutoff of contrast material
vessel loop
vessel rupture
vessel test-occluded
vessel topography
vessel tracing
vest, halo
vestibular apparatus
vestibular aqueduct syndrome (VAS)
vestibular canal
vestibular division of the eighth
　cranial nerve
vestibular schwannoma
vestibule
vestibulocochlear nerve
vestigial commissure
vestigial left sinoatrial node
VF, V fib (ventricular fibrillation)
V5 area
V5M Multiplane transducer
VFT (venous filling time)
VHL (von Hippel-Lindau) syndrome
VHP (Visible Human Project)
viable
viability
vibration frequency

vibratory motion
Vicq d'Azyr, band of (in brain)
VIDA 29 (Volumetric Image Display
　and Analysis)
Vidar scanner
videoangiography, digital
videoconferencing, teleradiology
videodensitometry
videodensity curves
videoendoscopic surgical equipment
videofluoroscopy
videoradiogram
videoradiography
videothoracoscopy
Vieussens
　annulus of
　ansa of
　circle of
　isthmus of
　limbus of
　loop of
　ring of
　valve of
view (see also *position, projection*)
　abdominal
　afferent
　anterior
　AP (anteroposterior)
　AP inversion stress vagina
　AP supine
　apical
　apical and subcostal
　　four-chambered
　apical four-chamber
　　(echocardiogram)
　apical lordotic
　apical two-chamber
　Arcelin
　axial sesamoid
　axillary
　baseline
　beam's eye

view *(cont.)*
  Beath
  biplane orthogonal
  bird-eye
  Boehler (Böhler) calcaneal
  Boehler lumbosacral
  Breuerton
  Brodan
  brow-down skull
  brow-up skull
  Bucky
  Caldwell
  cardiac long axis
  cardiac short axis
  carpal tunnel
  Carter-Rowe
  caudal
  Chamberlain-Towne
  Chausse
  chest (CXR)
  cine
  cineradiographic
  clenched fist
  close-up
  coalition
  comparison
  cone
  coned
  coned-down
  coronal
  coronal bending
  couch
  cranial angled
  craniocaudad, craniocaudal
  cross-table lateral
  cross-table
  CTLV (cross-table lateral view)
  decubitus
  dens
  dorsiflexion
  dorsoplantar
  Dunlop-Shands

view *(cont.)*
  efferent
  en face
  equilibrium
  erect
  expiration
  FCS (full cervical spine)
  Ferguson
  first-pass
  five-
  flexion
  fluoroscopic
  follow-through
  four-chamber apical
  frogleg
  frontal
  full length
  gated
  Granger
  Harris
  Harris-Beath axial hindfoot
  heavily penetrated
  hemiaxial
  hepatoclavicular
  hip-to-ankle
  Hobb
  Hughston
  ice-pick M-mode echocardiogram
  infrapatellar
  inspiration
  intraoperative
  inversion ankle stress
  Jones
  Jude pelvic
  kidneys, ureters, bladder (KUB)
  Knuttsen bending
  KUB (kidney, ureters, blader)
  LAO (left anterior oblique)
  lateral
  lateral anterior drawer stress
  lateral bending view of spine
  lateral decubitus

view *(cont.)*
- lateral oblique
- lateral tilt stress ankle
- Laurin x-ray
- Law
- left anterior oblique (LAO)
- limited
- long axial oblique
- long axis
- long-axis parasternal
- lordotic
- Low-Beers
- Mayer
- mediolateral
- mediolateral oblique
- Merchant
- mortise
- multiplanar reformatting (MPR)
- navicular
- Neer lateral
- Neer transscapular
- nonstanding lateral oblique
- nonweightbearing
- notch
- oblique
- occipital
- odontoid
- open-mouth
- optimally positioned
- orthogonal
- outlet
- over couch
- overhead
- overhead oblique
- Owen
- PA (posteroanterior)
- parasternal long-axis
- parasternal short-axis
- patellar skyline
- Pillar
- plain
- planar

view *(cont.)*
- plantar axial
- plantarflexion
- plantarflexion stress
- portable
- postvoid
- postevacuation
- postoperative
- preliminary
- preoperative
- prereduction
- prone
- prone lateral
- push-pull ankle stress
- push-pull hip
- RAO (right anterior oblique)
- ray-sum
- recumbent
- retromammary space
- Rhees
- right anterior oblique (RAO)
- right lateral decubitus
- right ventricular inflow
- routine magnification
- Schatzki
- Schüller
- scout
- selective coronary arteriography
- serendipity
- short-axis
- short-axis parasternal
- single breath
- sitting-up
- skijump
- skyline
- spider
- spot
- standing
- standing dorsoplantar
- standing lateral
- standing post-void

view *(cont.)*
   standing weightbearing
   static
   steep LAO oblique
   steep left anterior oblique
   Stenver
   stereoscopic
   stress
   stress Broden
   stress eversion
   stress inversion
   subcostal four-chamber
   subcostal long-axis
   subcostal short-axis
   submental vertex
   submentovertex
   subxiphoid
   sunrise
   sunset
   supine
   supine full
   suprasternal notch
   swimmer's
   tangential
   tangential scapular
   tomographic
   Towne
   transaxillary lateral
   transcranial lateral
   transscapular
   true lateral
   tunnel
   two-plane
   upright
   upright post-void
   von Rosen
   washout
   Waters
   weeping willow
   weightbearing
   weightbearing dorsoplantar
   White leg-length

view *(cont.)*
   x-ray
   Y
viewbox, virtual reality
viewing, cine-based
viewing, film-based
viewing, group
viewing, PVR fly-through
view microtomography
view shadow projection microtomographic system
view sharing
view tray, Bucky
Viewnex software
Villaret-Mackenzie syndrome
villoglandular polyp
villous adenoma
villous atrophy
villous fronds
villous proliferation
villus (pl. villi)
   anchoring
   arachnoidal
   chorionic
   duodenal
   fingerlike
   floating
   gallbladder
   intestinal
   leaflike
   placental
   ridged-convoluted
   tongue-shaped
vinculum breve
vinculum longum
VingMed ultrasound system
VIPER PTA catheter
vipoma (or VIPoma)
VIPoma (vasoactive intestinal polypeptide)
viral pneumonia
Virchow law of skull growth

Virchow perivascular space
Virchow psammoma
Virchow-Robin space
Virchow sentinel node
Virchow thrombosis triad
Virchow triad
Virchow-Troisier node
virtual angioscopy
virtual bronchoscopy
virtual colonsocopy
virtual endoscopy
virtual reality imaging
virtual reality simulator
virtual reality viewbox
virus
viscera (pl. of viscus)
   abdominal
   abdominopelvic
   hollow
   intra-abdominal
   intraperitoneal
   pelvic
visceral angiogram
visceral cholesterol embolization
   syndrome
visceral embolus
visceral layer
visceral pericardium
visceral peritoneum
visceral pleura
visceral pleurisy
visceral situs solitus
visceromegaly
visceroptosis
viscid
viscous (adj.)
viscus (pl. viscera)
   hollow
   perforated
   strangulated
VISI (volarflexed intercalated segment
   instability) deformity

visible anterior motion
Visible Human Project (VHP)
Vision camera
Vision MRI scanner
Vision Ten V-scan scanner
Vistec x-ray detectable sponge
visual cortex
visual
visualization
   delayed
   inadequate
   optimal
   poor
   suboptimal
visualization and quantification
vital capacity (VC)
Vitalcor venous catheter
vitelline duct
Viterbi decoding
Vitrea 3-D system
VJ (ventriculojugular) shunt
VLA (vertical-long axial) images
VMO (vastus medialis obliquus)
vocal cords
   true
   false
VOD (veno-occlusive disease)
Voda catheter
VoiceRAD clinical reporting system
void (verb)
void
   flow
   signal
void determination
voiding cystogram
voiding cystourethrogram (VCUG)
voiding sequence
voiding study
volar angulation
volar capsule
volar carpal ligament
volarly

volar wrist
volarward
Volkmann deformity
volume
   adequate stroke
   alveolar
   articular cartilage
   atrial emptying
   augmented stroke
   blood
   cavity
   central blood
   chamber
   circulating blood
   circulation
   closing
   decreased stroke
   decreased tidal
   determination of lung
   diastolic atrial
   diminished lung
   Dodge area-length method for ventricular
   EDV
   end-diastolic (EDV)
   end-expiratory lung
   end-systolic (ESV)
   end-systolic residual
   endocardial
   epicardial
   ESV
   expiratory reserve (ERV)
   extracellular fluid
   flow
   forward stroke (FSV)
   fractional moving blood
   gland
   hippocampal
   image
   increased extracellular fluid
   inspiratory reserve (IRV)
   left ventricular chamber

volume *(cont.)*
   left ventricular end-diastolic
   left ventricular inflow (LVIV)
   left ventricular outflow (LVOV)
   left ventricular stroke
   LV (left ventricular) cavity
   minute
   pericardial reserve
   plasma
   prism method for ventricular
   pulmonary blood
   pyramid method for ventricular
   radionuclide stroke
   reduced plasma
   reduced stroke
   regurgitant
   regurgitant stroke (RSV)
   residual (RV)
   respiratory
   right ventricular
   right ventricular end-diastolic
   right ventricular end-systolic
   scan
   Simpson rule method for ventricular
   slice
   stroke (SV)
   SV (stroke)
   systolic atrial
   Teichholz equation for left ventricular
   thermodilution stroke
   thin cylindrical uniform field
   total stroke (TSV)
   TSV (total stroke)
   ventricular end-diastolic
volume acquisition
volume averaging
volume depletion, intravascular
volume element (voxel)
volume estimation
volume in abstract stereotactic space

volume loss
volume overload
volume regulation
volume replacement
volume-rendered image
volumetric analysis
volumetric computed tomography
volumetric data
volumetric dataset
volumetric image (imaging)
volumetric image data
volumetric mapping technique
volumetric minimally invasive stereotaxis
volumetric multiplexed transmission holography
volumetric resampling
volumetric scan
volumetric stereotaxis
volumetry
  hippocampal magnetic resonance
  tumor
voluming artifact
volvulus
  cecal
  colonic
  midgut
  sigmoid
vomer bone
von Gierke disease
von Hippel tumor
von Hippel-Lindau (VHL) syndrome
von Meyenburg complex
von Recklinghausen syndrome
von Rosen view

Von Rokitansky syndrome
Vostal classification of radial fracture
voxel (volume element) (pl. voxels)
  cubic
  isotropic
  seed
voxel array
voxel gradient rendering
Voxel-Man software
VoxelView software
Voxgram multiple exposure hologram
VP (ventriculoperitoneal) shunt
VPB (ventricular premature beat)
VPC (ventricular premature complex)
VPC (ventricular premature contraction)
VPD (ventricular premature depolarization)
V peak of jugular venous pulse
VQ or V/Q (ventilation-perfusion) scan
V/Q mismatch
VRT (venous refill time)
VRT (venous return time)
VS (ventricular septal)
VSD (ventricular septal defect)
VSD and absent pulmonary valve syndrome
V-shaped fracture
VTED (venous thromboembolic disease)
VUSE, variable-angle uniform signal excitation
v wave (on cardiac catheterization)
VWFs (velocity waveforms), Doppler

# W, w

wafer of endocardium
wagon wheel fracture
Wagstaffe fracture
waist (of anatomical structure)
Walcher position
Waldenström disease
Waldeyer fascia
wall
  abdominal
  aneurysmal
  anterior abdominal
  anterolateral
  apical
  axial
  bladder
  body
  bowel
  carotid
  cavity
  chest
  cyst
  cystic
  gallbladder
  inferior
  inferoapical
  intestinal
  left anterior chest wall

wall *(cont.)*
  luminal
  midabdominal
  nasal cavity
  posterior
  posterior abdominal
  posterolateral
  septal
  stomach
  thickened gallbladder
  thoracic
  vaginal
  variceal
  ventricular
wall akinesis
Wallenberg lateral medullary
  syndrome
wall filter
wall hypokinesis
wall motion study
wall motion abnormalities (WMA)
wall shear stress
wall thickening
wall thickness
wallerian degeneration
Wallstent
wand, programmer

Wanderer microcatheter
Ward triangle
warm nodule
washboard effect on myelography in cervical spondylosis
wash-in phase
washout
  delayed
  lung
  nitrogen
  teboroxime resting (TRW)
washout curve
washout gradient
washout kinetics
washout phase
washout view
Wassel classification of thumb polydactyly
wasting
  muscle
  muscle fiber
wasting syndrome
Watanabe classification of discoid meniscus
water
  doped
  purified (contrast)
water bath
water bolus
water-contrast computed tomography
water density
waterfall stomach
Waterhouse-Friderichsen syndrome
water path
water perfusable tissue index
water range
water retention
water selective SE imaging sequence
water signal on magnetic resonance imaging scan
watershed infarct (infarction)
water-soluble contrast media

Waters projection
Waterston groove
Waters view
Watson-Jones classification of spinal fractures
wave
  abdominal fluid
  fluid
  peristaltic
  primary peristaltic
  secondary
  secondary peristaltic
  tertiary
waveform, segmental renal artery
waveforms, gradient
wavelength
  de Broglie
  readout
wavelet compression
wavelet-encoded
wavelet scalar quantization (WSQ)
wavelet sub-band (or subband)
WBCS (white blood cell scintigraphy) with indium-111 ($^{111}$In)
weak carotid upstroke
weak signal
weaver's bottom
web
  duodenal
  esophageal
  fibrous
  finger
  hepatic
  intestinal
  laryngeal
  postcricoid
  terminal
  thumb
  venous
Web browser (World Wide Web in teleradiology)
Weber C fracture

Weber, circle of
Weber-Osler-Rendu syndrome
web space
wedge
    dynamic
    match-line
    mediastinal
wedge bonds
wedge compression fracture
wedged beam
wedged hepatic venography
wedge factors
wedge flexion-compression fracture
wedge fracture
wedge isodose angle
wedge-shaped mass
wedge position, pulmonary capillary
wedge pressure
wedge-shaped vertebra
wedge-pair beam
wedge-shaped density
wedge-shaped lobe
wedge-shaped zone
wedging deformity
wedging of olisthetic vertebra
wedging of vertebral interspace
weeping willow appearance on venogram
weeping willow view
Wegener granulomatosis
weight, estimated fetal
weight loading, axial
weightbearing (also weight-bearing)
weightbearing dome of acetabulum
weightbearing rotational injury
weightbearing films
weighted spin-echo column (MRI)
weighting, human visual sensitivity
Weil disease or syndrome (Adolf Weil)
Weill sign of pneumonia in infant (Edmond Weill)

Weinberg-Himelfarb syndrome
Weingarten syndrome
Weisenburg syndrome
Weiss-Baker syndrome
Weitbrecht ligament
welder's lung
well-inflated lung
well-preserved ejection fraction
well-type ionization chamber
Wenckebach AV (atrioventricular) block
Wenckebach phenomenon
Werner syndrome
Wernicke-Korsakoff syndrome
Wernicke region
Westermark sign
Westphal-Strumpell disease
wet lung syndrome
wet pleurisy
wet reading of x-ray film
wet swallow (on esophageal manometry)
Wexler catheter
wheelchair artifact
whettle bone
whiplash injury
Whipple disease
whirlpool sign
Whitacre spinal needle
Whitaker test
white-appearing blood pool
white blood cell scintigraphy (WBCS) with indium-111
white cerebellum sign
white clot syndrome
white commissure of spinal cord
white echo writing
Whitehead deformity
White leg-length view
white light pattern projector
white lung syndrome
white matter infarct

white matter signal hyperintensity
white metastasis
white noise
white-out of lungs
white point
white noise artifact
whitlow, melanotic
whole blood monoclonal antibody
whole body 29FDG scanning
whole body imaging with magnified views
whole brain mean CBF
whole-body imaging
whole-body 1.5T Siemens Vision MRI scanner
whole-body PET scan
whole-body 3T MRI system scanner
whole-brain radiation therapy
whorl, coccygeal
whorled appearance
WHVP (wedged hepatic venous pressure)
Wiberg, CE angle of
Wiberg classification of patellar types
wide-beam scanning
wide-mouth sac
wide pulse
wide window setting
widened heart shadow
widened mediastinum
widened sulci
widened teardrop distance
widened thoracic outlet
widening
   ankle mortise
   crural cistern
   growth plate
   interpedicular distance
   interspinous
   joint
   mediastinal
widespread metastases

width
   collimation
   isodose
   pulse
   window
Wiener MRI filter
Wiktor stent
Wilcoxon signed-rank test
Wilkins classification of radial fracture
Williams-Beuren syndrome
Williams-Campbell syndrome
Williamson sign
Willis
   antrum of
   arterial circle of
   artery of
   circle of
Willis pancreas
Willis pouch
willow fracture
Wilmad reference standards
Wilms tumor
Wilson cloud chamber
Wilson disease
Wilson-Mikity syndrome
winding, zero-pitch solenoidal
window
   acquisition
   acoustic
   aorticopulmonary
   apical
   bone
   brain
   cortical
   esophageal
   gastric
   parasternal
   pericardial
   pulmonary parenchymal
   soft tissue
   subcostal

window *(cont.)*
  subdural
  suprasternal
window width
window ductus
window/level settings
window settings
windowing, intensity
windsock aneurysm
windup injury
wing
  iliac
  sphenoidal
winged scapula
Winiwarter-Buerger disease
Winiwarter-Manteuffel-Buerger disease
Winprint imaging laser printer
Winquist-Hansen classification of femoral fracture
Winslow, foramen of
Winslow pancreas
Winston-Lutz for LINAC-based radiosurgery
Winter-King-Moe scoliosis
Wintrich sign
wire
  calibrated guide
  encircling
  figure-of-8
  guide
  Ilizarov
  interfragment
  intravascular guide
  lead
  monitoring
wire fixation
wire localization
wire-related defect
Wirsung duct
Wishard catheter
Wiskott-Aldrich syndrome

wispy connection
Wits cephalometric measurement
WMA (wall motion abnormalities)
Wolf-Hirschhorn syndrome
Wolfe mammographic parenchymal patterns
Wolff law (bone structure)
Wolff-Chaikoff effect
Wolff-Parkinson-White (WPW) syndrome
Wolin meniscoid lesion
Wolman xanthomatosis
womb
woody mass
woolsorter's inhalation disease
word segmentation algorithm
workstation
  imaging
  ISG medical imaging
  MacSpect real-time NMR
  Radstation radiology
  Shebele physician reporting
  stacked-metaphor
  Sun
  Unix/X11
workup (n.), work up (v.)
wormian bone
wound
  exit
  gunshot (GSW)
  missile
  penetrating
  perforating
  puncture
  stab
WPW (Wolff-Parkinson-White) syndrome
wrap-around ghosting artifact
wrestler's elbow
wrinkle artifact
wrinkled pleura
Wrisberg cardiac ganglion

Wrisberg, intermediate nerve of
Wrisberg ligament
wrist
  gymnast's
  palmar
  SLAC (scapholunate arthritic
    collapse)
  volar
  Volz
wrist capsule
wristdrop
wryneck (torticollis)
W-shaped ileal pouch
WSQ (wavelet scalar quantization)
Wyburn-Mason arteriovenous
  malformation

# X, x

x ("by" or "times")
xanthelasma
xanthoastrocytoma, pleomorphic
xanthogranulomatous cholecystitis
xanthoma
   gastric
   malignant fibrous
xanthomatosis, cerebrotendinous
xanthomatosis of long bones with
   spontaneous fracture
xanthomatosis, Wolman
XCT (x-ray computed tomography)
Xe (xenon)
XeCT (xenon computed tomography)
xenograft valve
xenon (Xe)
   $^{127}$Xe imaging agent
   $^{133}$Xe imaging agent
xenon chloride (XeCl) excimer
xenon computed tomography (XeCT)
xenon energy window
xenon trap system
xenon washout studies
xenotransplantation
xerography
xeromammogram
xeromammography

xeroradiogram
xeroradiographic selenium plate
xeroradiography
x-height
Xillix LIFE-GI fluorescence
   endoscopy system
Ximatron simulator
XIP (x-ray in plaster)
xiphisternal joint
xiphoid angle
xiphoid bone
xiphoid cartilage
xiphoid process syndrome
xiphopubic area
x-irradiation
XKnife stereotactic radiosurgery
   system
XMG (x-ray mammogram)
XOP (x-ray out of plaster)
X-Prep bowel prep
Xpress/SX helical CT scanner
XRA (x-ray arteriography)
x-ray (pl. x-rays) (see *imaging*;
   *projection*; *view*)
   baseline
   portable
x-ray C-arm

**x-ray • Xylocaine** 614

x-ray detector, Si (Li)
x-ray film jacket
x-ray in plaster (XIP)
x-ray out of plaster (XOP)
x-ray sensitive vidicon
x-ray topography

X-terminal
X trough
X, Y, and Z coordinates for target lesion
xylenol orange
Xylocaine

# Y, y

Y (yttrium)
YAG (yttrium, aluminum, garnet) laser
Yb (ytterbium)
Y bone plate
Y configuration, inverted
Yergason test of shoulder subluxation
Y fracture
yield comparison
yoke
yokelike
yolk sac (YS) diameter
Y plate
YS (yolk sac)
Y-shaped distortion
Y-T fracture
Y trough
ytterbium (Yb)
    $^{169}$Yb (Yb-169) brachytherapy
yttrium radioactive source
yttrium-90 microspheres
Y view

# Z, z

Zahn
   lines of
   pockets of
Zang space
Z axis
Z-dependent computed tomography
Z disk
zebra artifact
Zeek syndrome
Zellweger syndrome
Zener diode
Zenker diverticulum
Zenker pouch
zero-field splitting
zero-fill artifact
zero-pitch solenoidal winding
zeugmatography, Fourier transformation
Z interpolation algorithms
Zickel fracture classification system
Ziegler syndrome
Zielke derotation level
zinc, irradiated
Zinn, tendon of
zipper artifact
ZK44012 contrast medium

Z-line of esophagus
Zlotsky-Ballard classification of acromioclavicular injury
Z-Med balloon catheter
Zollinger-Ellison syndrome (ZES)
zonal gastritis
zone
   fracture
   Rolando
   slow conduction (ZSC)
   sonolucent
   Westphal
z point pressure
ZSC (zone of slow conduction)
Zucker catheter
Zuckerkandl bodies
Zuckerkandl convolution
ZY plane
zygapophyseal articulation
zygapophyseal joint
zygoma
zygomatic arch
zygomatic bone
zygomatic process
zygomaticomalar area
zygomaticomaxillary fracture